Anatomy

An easy-to-read book written by students for students, edited by senior clinicians and anatomy academics, with contributions from leading anatomists and clinicians. Anatomical facts are correlated with clinical settings, especially medical emergencies, and important points are highlighted with clear learning points. The text is supplemented by diagrams and images, which form an essential part of this book. It covers the students' learning objectives in undergraduate anatomy curricula and helps in preparing them for practical and written exams. It forms a solid foundation for future clinical exams based on the knowledge of anatomical facts in a clinical setting.

Key Features

- Presents a concise, accessible guide to regional and clinically applied anatomy, which clearly demonstrates to students the level of knowledge required for medical and healthcare-related curricula
- Uses high-quality clinical and intraoperative images integrated into the text to emphasize important topics through bullet points
- Features seven logically arranged sections, each devoted to a body region or system, which includes a self-test quiz, with the single best answer and spotter-style questions

Anatomy
Regional, Surgical, & Applied

Edited by

Qassim F. Baker, MBChB FRCS (Eng.)
Royal College of Surgeons of England
United Kingdom

Philip J. Adds, BSc MSc FAS FIBMS SFHEA
St. George's
University of London
London, United Kingdom

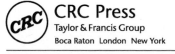

CRC Press
Taylor & Francis Group
Boca Raton London New York

CRC Press is an imprint of the
Taylor & Francis Group, an **informa** business

Cover art: Skeleton drawing by Nigel Rose

First edition published 2023
by CRC Press
6000 Broken Sound Parkway NW, Suite 300, Boca Raton, FL 33487-2742

and by CRC Press
4 Park Square, Milton Park, Abingdon, Oxon, OX14 4RN

CRC Press is an imprint of Taylor & Francis Group, LLC

Library of Congress Cataloging-in-Publication Data

Names: Baker, Qassim F., editor. | Adds, Philip James, editor.
Title: Anatomy : regional, surgical, and applied / edited by Qassim F.
Baker, Philip J. Adds.
Other titles: Anatomy (Baker)
Description: First edition. | Boca Raton, FL : CRC Press, 2023. | Includes
bibliographical references and index. | Summary: "An easy-to-read book
written by students for students, edited by senior clinicians and
anatomy academics, with contributions from leading anatomists and
clinicians. Anatomical facts are correlated with clinical settings,
especially medical emergencies, and important points are highlighted
with clear learning points"-- Provided by publisher.
Identifiers: LCCN 2022027069 (print) | LCCN 2022027070 (ebook) | ISBN
9781032321165 (hardback) | ISBN 9781032321141 (paperback) | ISBN
9781003312895 (ebook)
Subjects: MESH: Anatomy, Regional | Handbook
Classification: LCC QM25 (print) | LCC QM25 (ebook) | NLM QS 39 | DDC
611/.9--dc23/eng/20220830
LC record available at https://lccn.loc.gov/2022027069
LC ebook record available at https://lccn.loc.gov/2022027070

ISBN: 9781032321165 (hbk)
ISBN: 9781032321141 (pbk)
ISBN: 9781003312895 (ebk)

DOI: 10.1201/9781003312895

DEDICATIONS

*To my mother, my first teacher, whom I lost during the preparation of
this book, and to my wife, who has supported me all the way.*

-Qassim F. Baker

To the students who have inspired me, and to my wife for supporting me.

-Philip J. Adds

CONTENTS

Foreword...vii

Preface..viii

Editors..ix

Contributors...x

Artists and Technical Support...xii

Acknowledgements (Clinicians Who Contributed Images)...xiii

List of Abbreviations..xiv

1A   Neuroanatomy: Anatomy of the Brain...1
     Reviewed by Richard Dyball

1B   Neuroanatomy: Anatomy of the Spinal Cord...15
     Reviewed by Valentina Gnoni

2   Anatomy of the Head and Neck..33
     Reviewed by Qassim F. Baker, David Sunnucks, and Georga Longhurst

3   Anatomy of the Upper Limb...80
     Reviewed by Philip J. Adds and Joanna Tomlinson

4   Anatomy of the Thorax..109
     Reviewed by Qassim F. Baker and Mohammed Al Janabi

5   Anatomy of the Abdomen...149
     Reviewed by Qassim F. Baker and David Sunnucks

6   Anatomy of the Pelvis and Perineum...197
     Reviewed by Paul Carter, Qassim F. Baker, and Philip J. Adds

7   Anatomy of the Lower Limb..234
     Reviewed by Philip J. Adds and Joanna Tomlinson

Index..271

FOREWORD

"Anatomy ... teaches us a rational Method of curing Diseases ..." with these words, John Hunter, widely regarded as the "father of the scientific basis of surgery", began his anatomy lectures in the late eighteenth century. Those sentiments have not changed significantly in the intervening years, although a modern surgeon's clinical repertoire includes procedures that Hunter, who worked long before the introduction of anaesthesia, antisepsis, and technological advances such as functional MRI and robotic surgery, could not have anticipated.

Learning anatomy for the first time has always been a daunting task, possibly even more so in today's overcrowded timetables: without appropriate guidance, undergraduate medical and dental students often struggle in a minefield of details while missing clinically relevant points. This user-friendly book, based on the undergraduate anatomy course taught at St. George's, University of London, inhabits the middle ground between textbooks that are too basic and those that contain detail that is not required until the postgraduate level, and then only for specific groups of trainees.

The text is heavily informed by medical students at the sharp end of their anatomical learning, some of whom have taken an intercalated BSc in anatomy, and all of whom have been involved in near-peer anatomy teaching, demonstrating to students of medicine and related healthcare professions. Their experience is therefore very close to that of the intended audience; the tips that helped them grapple with anatomical "tiger territories" will be welcomed by their readers. The line drawings are by medical students, underlining the authors' intention that this should be a book "BY students FOR students", filled with tips, revision and spotter questions, clinical images, and labelled photos of cadaveric specimens. It deserves to be popular with all students learning clinically relevant anatomy.

Susan Standring
Emeritus Professor of Anatomy
King's College, London

PREFACE

It all began with a meeting of a small group of students and anatomy staff on 31 May 2017, in Room 1, Jenner Wing, St. George's, University of London (SGUL). The idea was simple: to put together an anatomy handbook containing all the anatomy that was taught to medical and other healthcare science students at SGUL, together with relevant clinical details. If the idea was simple, the challenge was anything but: to change the concept of anatomy from a massive and rather intimidating obstacle to a lively, energetic, engaging subject that constitutes a vital part of the medical curriculum and is practically applied within the surgical theatres and clinical setting. Who better to advise on this aspect but the students themselves, who are at the sharp end of anatomy curriculum, not only learning the subject but also helping as anatomy demonstrators in the DR, teaching junior students of medicine, biomedical science, physiotherapy, and paramedic science, among others. Our student collaborators, then, played a pivotal role in writing this book and became involved in putting the sections together, digging into references and further reading, to enable them to give their best input. As the book progressed, the number of student contributors grew, involving writers and artists from SGUL and other universities. Truly, we could not have done it without them.

We were also fortunate to have had the input of clinical colleagues from the UK and around the world, who supplied many of the images and gave helpful feedback on the text. Special thanks must go to Prof Stephen Carmichael and Associate Prof Stephanie Woodley for taking the time to review the book and giving valuable feedback, and to Prof Susan Standring for kindly agreeing to write the Foreword.

Many years ago, while a student myself, I remember being told "there is no such thing as the perfect anatomy book, so you will have to write your own". It has taken 40 years, but we got there in the end.

So, is this the perfect anatomy book? Perhaps not, but we believe that it will fill a gap in the literature, and we hope that future generations of students will find it lively, interesting, and not too daunting!

Note: In each section, we have provided some exam-style revision questions and some self-test quiz questions – some without answers – to encourage readers to dig deeper and consolidate their understanding.

Qassim F. Baker and Philip J. Adds

EDITORS

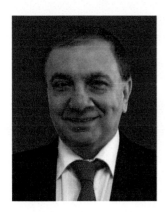

Qassim F. Baker, MBChB FRCS (Eng.), has been an international and UK examiner for the Royal College of Surgeons England since 2015, and before that was an examiner and tutor for the Iraqi Medical Specialisation Board (1996–2004). He was previously a Professor of Surgery at two universities in Malaysia (2013–2016); Assistant Professor at the Department of Surgery, Medical College, University of Baghdad; and the Head of the Department of Surgery at two teaching hospitals in Iraq between 1990 and 2004. Mr. Baker has dedicated his career to teaching and mentoring medical, biomedical, and postgraduate students and edited two books in clinical surgery. His second book, *Clinical Surgery: A Practical Guide,* for candidates sitting their FRCS/MRCS exams (London: Hodder/Arnold, 2009), received a 4-star review from the Annals of Royal College of Surgeons England and Yearbook of ASiT (Association of Surgeons in Training). He frequently talks at grand rounds, seminars, and conferences in the Middle East on breast cancer, thyroid surgery, and medical education. He was awarded the "Best Lecturer" at the Educational and Qualifying Course for Teaching and University Staff Training, March 2000, University of Baghdad, Iraq.

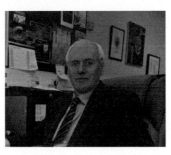

Philip J. Adds, BSc MSC FAS FIBMS SFHEA, retired in 2021 as Reader in Anatomical Sciences and Head of Anatomy at St. George's, University of London. He has had over 20 years of experience teaching anatomy to medical and other students of healthcare sciences and has published widely, with over 50 peer-reviewed papers, specialising in musculoskeletal anatomy and the detailed anatomy of the orbit. Before starting his teaching career, he worked for the Tissue Services arm of the National Blood Service, retrieving tissues including bone, skin, and tendons from donors post-mortem. While at Tissue Services, he established the first national Amniotic Membrane Bank for ocular surface reconstruction surgery. He is a Fellow of the Anatomical Society, Fellow of the Institute of Biomedical Science, and Senior Fellow of the Higher Education Academy. Although retired from full-time teaching, his interests include anatomy and anatomical education. He is the UK Editor for the journal *Clinical Anatomy* and the Editor-in-Chief of the *Journal of Plastination*. His previous books are Adds & Shahsavari *The Musculoskeletal System* (London: Informa Healthcare, 2011) and Degueurce *Fragonard Museum: The Ecorchés* (New York: Blast Books, 2011) (as translator).

CONTRIBUTORS

Ahmad Abdallah
St. George's
University of London
London, United Kingdom

Philip J. Adds
St. George's
University of London
London, United Kingdom

Tara Al-Hamami
St. George's
University of London
London, United Kingdom

Asha Isse Ali
St. George's University Hospital
London, United Kingdom

Mohammed G. Al Janabi
SHARP Health & Eisenhower
    Health
San Diego, United States

Hafssa Anfishi
St. George's
University of London
London, United Kingdom

Qassim F. Baker
Royal College of Surgeons
England, United Kingdom

Naomi Bartholomew
GKT Medical School
King's College London
London, United Kingdom

Jordan Bethel
Kings College Hospital
London, United Kingdom

Jared Bhaskar
St. George's
University of London
London, United Kingdom

Michael Burrows
St. George's
University of London
London, United Kingdom

Paul Carter
St. George's
University of London
London, United Kingdom

Joel Coombs
St. George's
University of London
London, United Kingdom

Richard Dyball
University of Cambridge
Cambridge, United Kingdom

Najibullah Ghasemi
St. George's
University of London
London, United Kingdom

Valentina Gnoni
Kings College London
London, United Kingdom

Dhruv Gupta
St. George's
University of London
London, United Kingdom

Alan Hasanic
St. George's
University of London
London, United Kingdom

Chun Ho
St. George's
University of London
London, United Kingdom

Alina Humdani
St. George's
University of London
London, United Kingdom

Faris Hussein
St. George's
University of London
London, United Kingdom

Zahra Ismail
St. George's
University of London
United Kingdom

Hannah Katmeh
St. George's
University of London
United Kingdom

Adam Lebby
Ashford and St Peter's NHS Trust
Chertsey, United Kingdom

Sophie Leiner
St. George's
University of London
London, United Kingdom

Paros Loftus
St. George's
University of London
London, United Kingdom

Georga Longhurst
St. George's
University of London
London, United Kingdom

Thomas Marsh
Dorset County Hospital NHS Foundation
    Trust
Dorchester, United Kingdom

Hatidzhe Masteva
St. George's
University of London
London, United Kingdom

Aditya Mavinkurve
St. George's
University of London
London, United Kingdom

Emma J. Norton
University of Cambridge
Cambridge, United Kingdom

Parker O'Neill
St. George's
University of London
London, United Kingdom

Aditi Sinha
St. George's
University of London
London, United Kingdom

Ananya Sood
St. George's
University of London
London, United Kingdom

David Sunnucks
Queen Mary University
Malta

Vamsi Thammandra
St. George's
University of London
London, United Kingdom

Joanna Tomlinson
University of Otago
Otago, New Zealand

Leshanth Uthayanan
St. George's
University of London
London, United Kingdom

Meet Vaghela
Brighton and Sussex Medical School
Brighton, United Kingdom

John Ward
Royal Devon and Exeter NHS Foundation
  Trust
Exeter, United Kingdom

ARTISTS AND TECHNICAL SUPPORT

Chris Adds
Technical Support—Images
Brighton Metropolitan College
Brighton, United Kingdom

Ali Baker
Branding Arts
Sweden

Julian Bartholomew
Dhamecha Group Ltd
Croydon, United Kingdom

Gabriela Barzyk
University of Warwick Medical School
Coventry, United Kingdom

Amani Bashir
Plovdiv Medical University
Plovdiv, Bulgaria

Kathryn DeMarre
WellSpan York Hospital
York, Pennsylvania, USA

Neha Gadiyar
Croydon University Hospital
Croydon, United Kingdom

Calum Harrington-Vogt
St. George's
University of London
London, United Kingdom

Avni Kant
University of Southampton
Southampton, United Kingdom

Katie Michaels
Loughborough University
England, United Kingdom

Callum Moffitt
Northern School of Art
England, United Kingdom

Fallon O'Neill
University of Oxford
Oxford, United Kingdom

Xi Ming Zhu
Chelsea & Westminster Hospital
and
Imperial College Healthcare NHS Trust
London, United Kingdom

ACKNOWLEDGEMENTS (CLINICIANS WHO CONTRIBUTED IMAGES)

Abdel-Aziz Abdel-Ghany
Al Khazindara General Hospital
Cairo, Egypt

Mohammed H. Aldabbagh
Duhok Medical College
Kurdistan, Iraq

Maan L. Aldoori
Samaraa General Hospital
Samarra, Iraq

Munther I. Aldoori
Calderdale and Huddersfield Foundation
    Trust
Huddersfield, United Kingdom

Muthana Al Qassab
Medical College University of Baghdad
United Kingdom

Hamza Al Sabah
Baghdad Teaching Hospital
Baghdad, Iraq

Ahmed Alsagban
Al Diwanyia Teaching Hospital
Dewaniya, Iraq

Mohammed M. Altalal
Najaf Teaching Hospital
Iraq

Baqir A.A. Altemimi
Alkindy Teaching Hospital
Baghdad, Iraq

Walid M.G. El-Haroni
Military Medical Academy
Cairo, Egypt

Mohammed M. Habash
College of Medicine
University of Diyala
Diyala, Iraq

Ali Mohsin Hasan
Azadi Teaching Hospital
Kirkuk, Iraq

Mudhar Hassan
Danderyds University Hospital
Karolinska Institute
Stockholm, Sweden

Waleed M. Hussen
College of Medicine
University of Baghdad
Baghdad, Iraq

Salam Ismael
Robert Jones and Agnes Hunt
    Orthopaedic Hospital
Oswestry, United Kingdom

Omar Mudher Khalaf
Baquba Teaching Hospital
Baaqoba, Iraq

Dae Kim
St. George's Hospital NHS Trust
London, United Kingdom

Wan Khamizar
Hospital Sultanah Bahiyah
Setar Kedah, Malaysia

Aqeel Shakir Mahmood
College of Medicine
University of Baghdad
Baghdad, Iraq

Akram A. Najeeb
Gastroenterologist
Baghdad, Iraq

Sami Salman
College of Medicine
University of Baghdad
Baghdad, Iraq

Ahmed A. Shakir
Baghdad Teaching Hospital
Baghdad, Iraq

Rashide Yaacob
Hospital Sultan Abdul Haleem
Sungai Petani, Malaysia

LIST OF ABBREVIATIONS

ABG	Arterial blood gas	**JVP**	Jugular venous pressure
ACA	Anterior cerebral artery	**LAD**	Left anterior descending
ACL	Anterior cruciate ligament	**LD**	Latissimus dorsi
ADH	Anti-diuretic hormone	**LFT**	Liver function test
AICA	Anterior inferior cerebellar artery	**LSV**	Long saphenous vein
ABPI	Ankle brachial pressure index	**LOS**	Lower oesophageal sphincter
ACL	Anterior cruciate ligament	**LMN**	Lower motor neuron
A&E	Accident and emergency	**L**	Lumbar
AF	Atrial fibrillation	**MALT**	Mucosa-associated lymphoid tissue
ARDS	Acute respiratory distress syndrome	**MCA**	Middle cerebral artery
ASD	Atrial septal defect	**MI**	Myocardial infarction
ASIS	Anterior superior iliac spine	**MPD**	Main pancreatic duct
C	Cervical	**MPJ**	Metacarpophalangeal joint
CABG	Coronary artery bypass graft	**MRI**	Magnetic resonance imaging
CBD	Common bile duct	**MS**	Multiple sclerosis
CCA	Common carotid artery	**NICE**	National Institute for Clinical Excellence
CMC	Carpometacarpal	**OGD**	Oesophagogastroduodenoscopy
CN	Cranial nerve, for example, CN X for vagus nerve, CN V for the trigeminal nerve, CN V1 for the ophthalmic division, and so on	**PCA**	Posterior cerebral artery
		PCL	Posterior cruciate ligament
		PE	Pulmonary embolism
CNS	Central nervous system	**PEG**	Percutaneous endoscopic gastrostomy
COPD	Chronic obstructive pulmonary disease	**PNS**	Peripheral nervous system
COVID-19	Coronavirus disease 2019	**PICA**	Posterior inferior cerebellar artery
CSF	Cerebrospinal fluid	**RLN**	Recurrent laryngeal nerve
CT	Computed tomography	**S**	Sacral
CXR	Chest X-ray	**SAN**	Sinuatrial node
DIEP	Deep inferior epigastric perforator	**SMA**	Superior mesenteric artery
DVT	Deep venous thrombosis	**STI**	Sexually transmitted infection
ECG/EKG	Electrocardiogram	**SVC**	Superior vena cava
ERCP	Endoscopic retrograde cholangiopancreatography	**T**	Thoracic
ENT	Ear, nose, and throat	**TB**	Tuberculosis
GCS	Glasgow Coma Scale	**TIA**	Transient ischaemic attack
GIT	Gastrointestinal tract	**Triple A**	Abdominal aortic aneurysm
H. pylori	*Helicobacter pylori*	**TUR**	Transurethral resection
HPV	Human papilloma virus	**UMN**	Upper motor neuron
IBS	Inflammatory bowel disease	**USS**	Ultrasound scan
ICA	Internal carotid artery	**UTI**	Urinary tract infection
ICP	Intracranial pressure	**VF**	Ventricular fibrillation
IJF	Internal jugular vein	**VSD**	Ventricular septal defect
IMA	Inferior mesenteric artery	**WBC**	White blood cell
IVC	Inferior vena cava		

1A

NEUROANATOMY
Anatomy of the Brain

Reviewed by Richard Dyball

Learning Objectives

- Identify the major parts of the brain and their functions
- Understand the function and location of the diencephalon and its contents (thalamus, hypothalamus)
- Identify coverings of the brain and spinal cord (meninges) and their clinical significance
- Recall the blood supply of the brain and the spinal cord and its clinical significance
- Understand the function and location of the ventricular system and cerebrospinal fluid circulation

Introduction

This section covers basic concepts in neuroanatomy and is not meant to be comprehensive. This section only emphasises the anatomy relevant to common clinical problems.

The nervous system is composed of the central nervous system (CNS) and the peripheral nervous system (PNS). The CNS is made up of the brain and the spinal cord. The PNS is composed of afferent sensory and efferent motor nerve fibres. The afferent fibres carry sensory information to the CNS, and the efferent fibres carry motor and secretory signals to the muscles and glands.

The brain is composed of three major structures: the cerebrum, cerebellum, and brainstem.

Embryology of the Brain

The CNS originates from the neural tube, which is derived from the dorsal ectoderm of the embryo. The process by which the CNS and PNS form (neurulation) is discussed in the spinal cord section.

Cerebrum

The cerebrum consists of two halves, termed cerebral hemispheres, separated by a space called the longitudinal fissure. Each hemisphere controls the opposite, or contralateral, side of the body. Each half can be divided into **four anatomical lobes**: frontal, parietal, temporal, and occipital, and one functional limbic lobe, (or limbic system), and consists of structures from the aforementioned four anatomical lobes (**Figure 1.1**). The functionality of these is detailed in **Table 1.1**.

TABLE 1.1: Lobes of the brain

Lobe	Functions of This Lobe	Important Functional Regions within This Lobe	Examples of Dysfunctions Related with This Lobe
Frontal	• Cognitive reasoning • Planning and problem solving • Movement • Emotions and speech	• Primary motor cortex (M1) • Broca's area (usually in the left hemisphere)	• Non-fluent dysphasia (Broca's area) • Obsessive-compulsive disorder (orbitomedial prefrontal cortex)
Parietal	• Perception of stimuli, e.g., temperature, pain, pressure • Visuospatial representation of objects in extra personal space • Praxes (initiation of semi-automatic motor sequences)	• Primary somatosensory cortex (S1)	• Attentional problems, e.g., hemisensory neglect syndrome, anosognosia • Apraxia (but can also be caused by frontal lobe or frontal-parietal lobe white matter connections)
Temporal	• Hearing • Episodic memory and spatial navigation	• Primary auditory cortex (transverse temporal gyrus of Heschl) • Wernicke's area (left hemisphere only)	• Fluent dysphasia (Wernicke's aphasia) • Anterograde amnesia • Alzheimer's disease
Occipital	• Vision	• Primary visual cortex (found in calcarine sulcus)	• Visual field defects, e.g., homonymous hemianopia with macular sparing

DOI: 10.1201/9781003312895-1

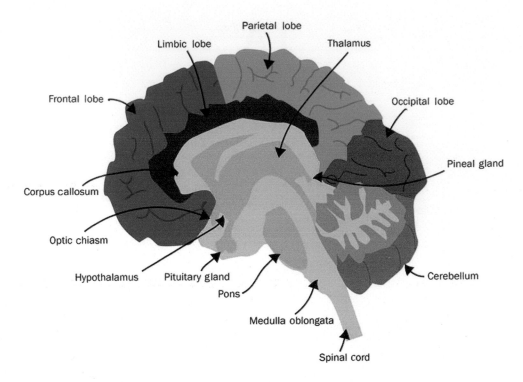

FIGURE 1.1 Sagittal view of the brain showing the positions of the major features. (Courtesy of Aditya Mavinkurve and John Ward.)

On the surface of each hemisphere, the folds of the brain are called **gyri** (singular is gyrus), and the grooves are called **sulci** (singular is sulcus). The lateral sulcus (also known commonly as the Sylvian fissure) separates the frontal, parietal, and temporal lobes. The central sulcus separates the frontal and parietal lobes as well as the M1 (primary motor cortex found in the precentral gyrus) and S1 (primary somatosensory cortex found in the postcentral gyrus). The parieto-occipital sulcus lies between the parietal and occipital lobes, as its name suggests.

The two halves of the cerebrum are connected by the **corpus callosum**, a large bundle of fibres which cross the midline. The corpus callosum is described as having several subdivisions (from rostral to occipital): rostrum, genu, body, isthmus (the thinnest part), and splenium (**Figure 1.2**).

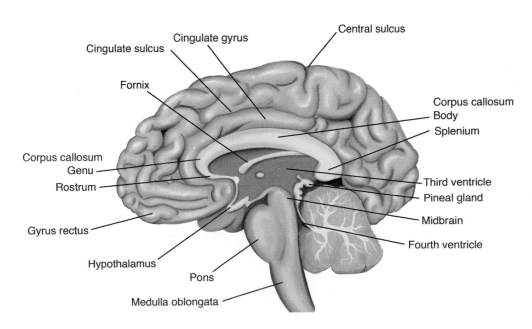

FIGURE 1.2 Sagittal section of the brain. (Courtesy of Kathryn DeMarre and John Ward.)

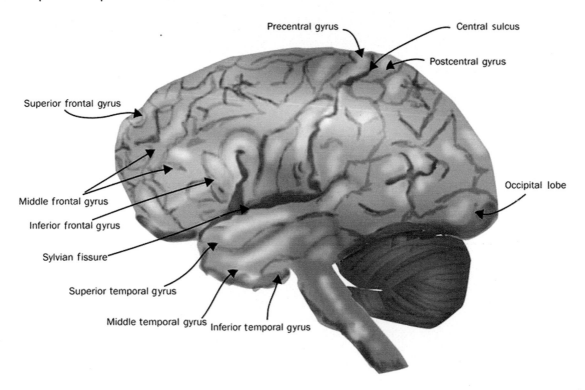

FIGURE 1.3 Lateral view of the cortex. (Courtesy of John Ward.)

Frontal Lobe

The frontal lobe is the anterior-most part of the cerebrum. The longitudinal gyri running parallel to the longitudinal fissure are termed superior, middle, and inferior frontal gyri. The **precentral gyrus**, found on the outer curvature of the brain at the posterior part of the frontal lobe, is responsible for the voluntary motor control of the body. The motor function of each body region is controlled by a corresponding area of this precentral gyrus. The lowest part controls the face, just above it is the region that controls the upper limb and hands, and the part that controls the feet and lower limb lies between the two hemispheres. Curiously, however, the face region is represented "the right way up". **Broca's area** is found in the posterior two-thirds of the inferior frontal gyrus (pars triangularis and pars opercularis), just superior to the Sylvian fissure. This is the centre for speech expression and is typically found in the left hemisphere (**Figure 1.3**).

CLINICAL NOTE

Broca's (non-fluent) aphasia is a condition that results in patients being unable to form fluent sentences, although they can still understand speech and know what they want to say.

The inferior aspect of the frontal lobe, also known as the **orbitofrontal cortex**, is an area of the brain that contains the optic and olfactory regions. The **olfactory sulcus** divides the orbitofrontal cortex into an optic and an olfactory region. The optic region can be found lateral to the olfactory sulcus. The olfactory tract can be seen running in a posterior direction from the olfactory sulcus. The area medial to the olfactory tract is the gyrus rectus (Latin, "straight gyrus").

The medial aspect of the frontal lobe is mostly responsible for motor control and personality. The dorsolateral prefrontal cortex can be found on the medial aspect superiorly. The medial prefrontal cortex can be found directly inferior to the dorsolateral prefrontal cortex. Lastly, the orbitofrontal cortex is found most inferiorly.

Temporal Lobe

The temporal lobe sits beneath the frontal lobe, separated from it by the lateral sulcus, or Sylvian fissure. It, like the frontal lobe, is divided into superior, middle, and inferior temporal gyri. It is the **main language centre of the brain**, allowing us not only to speak language but to also understand language from auditory cues.

In the posterior third of the superior temporal gyrus, in the left hemisphere, is **Wernicke's area** which is considered to be the centre for language comprehension.

CLINICAL NOTE

Wernicke's ("fluent/receptive") aphasia is the inability to understand language. Patients with this condition can often speak fluently and at a good rate.

CLINICAL NOTE

Conduction aphasia is caused by a lesion in the **arcuate fasciculus** which connects Broca's and Wernicke's areas. This presents as an inability to listen to a sentence and repeat it back to the instructor.

Parietal Lobe

The parietal lobe contains the **primary sensory strip (post-central gyrus)** which lies parallel and just posterior to the precentral gyrus. As the name suggests, the central sulcus divides these two gyri and marks the division between the frontal and parietal lobes. As with the motor cortex, the legs are represented superiorly and the upper limb inferiorly, although the face region is represented "the right way up" as it is in the motor cortex.

The parietal lobe is further divided into a superior and inferior parietal lobe. The superior parietal lobe is involved in spatial orientation, visual input, and sensory input from the hand. The inferior parietal lobe is involved in language, sensory analysis, and mathematical calculation.

Occipital Lobe

Located on the posterior aspect of the cerebrum, the occipital lobe **contains the primary visual cortex, responsible for visual perception**. The occipital lobe receives direct input from the eyes via the optic pathways (discussed in the eye subsection). **The primary visual cortex lies anatomically in the calcarine sulcus**. Interestingly, it is also the only functional area of the brain cortex which can be identified macroscopically because it contains the distinct stria of Gennari. (**Figure 1.4**).

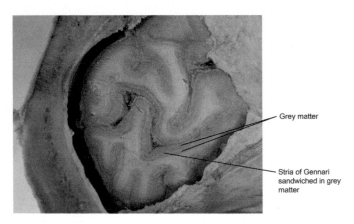

Grey matter

Stria of Gennari sandwiched in grey matter

FIGURE 1.4 Stria of Gennari. (Courtesy of Department of Anatomical Sciences, SGUL.)

Limbic System

The limbic system is defined by common functions: behaviour, emotion, and memory. Anatomically, it is formed of two gyri: the cingulate and parahippocampal gyri. The cingulate gyrus surrounds the corpus callosum on the medial aspect of the sagittal brain. It is separated from the frontal lobe by the **cingulate sulcus**, which extends posteriorly and superiorly to form the pars marginalis (marginal sulcus). The central sulcus can be identified using the pars marginalis as a visual landmark, with the central sulcus being the first sulcus directly anterior to the marginal sulcus, running on the convex surface of the cerebral cortex down to the lateral sulcus. The cingulate gyrus continues inferior to the splenium of the corpus callosum as the **parahippocampal gyrus**, which is bordered by the collateral sulcus. The

parahippocampal gyrus forms a region known as the **uncus**, as it curves upwards in the shape of a hook.

The limbic system also comprises several important structures, including the **hippocampus** and **amygdala**. The former is responsible for spatial navigation and episodic memory. It sits deep in the temporal lobe on the floor of the temporal horn of the lateral ventricle. The amygdala is responsible for attention, emotional memory (e.g., fear conditioning), and memory consolidation. The amygdala (from the Greek word *amygdale* meaning "almond" or "tonsil") is an almond-shaped structure found in the anterior temporal lobe on each side anterior to the hippocampus. The amygdala receives and projects pathways to the cortex, the thalamus, the hypothalamus, and the brainstem. The amygdala receives olfactory input and also has a central pathway of white matter called the **stria terminalis** which connects the amygdala to the brainstem. It has wide connections and seems to be important in the perception of emotions and the assessment of risks.

Cerebellum (Latin: "little brain")

The cerebellum consists of **two cerebellar hemispheres and a central area, the vermis** ("worm-like"). It lies in the posterior cranial fossa below the tentorium cerebelli and at the back of the brainstem. It is important to remember that each lobe of the cerebellum controls coordination on the ipsilateral side (same side). The cerebellum is also involved in motor learning, in conjunction with the basal ganglia. The cerebellum contains more neurons than the rest of the brain. The cerebellum controls fine motor actions (*vide infra*, the basal ganglia). Cerebellar pathologies result in problems with gait, equilibrium, and speech.

The cerebellum can be divided into 3 anatomical lobes. The anterior and posterior lobes are separated by the primary fissure. The cerebellar tonsils are part of the posterior lobe, and they flank the medulla. The cerebellum also has 2 flocculi inferiorly, alongside a nodule of the vermis, which forms the flocculonodular lobe (**Figure 1.5**).

Learning Point

Cerebellar tonsillar herniation can occur due to increased intracranial pressure (ICP). This condition leads to cardio-respiratory arrest and death, as it compresses the vital centres (particularly vagal nuclei) of the medulla oblongata.

Looking at a sagittal section of the cerebellum, the dentate nucleus can be seen centrally within the white matter (provides the primary outflow tract of the cerebellum). The white matter is branched (sometimes, because of its shape, it is called the ***arbor vitae*** meaning "tree of life"). The cerebellum is attached to the brainstem (covered in detail later in this subsection) via three cerebellar peduncles:

- *Superior cerebellar peduncle:* attached to the midbrain (contains input and output fibres from the cerebellum)
- *Middle cerebellar peduncle:* attached to the pons (contains input fibres from the pontine nuclei)
- *Inferior cerebellar peduncle:* attached to the medulla (mostly contains input fibres from the spinal cord and vestibular systems)

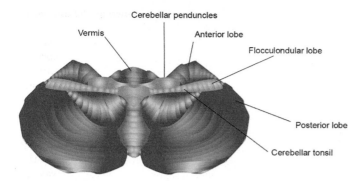

FIGURE 1.5 Anterior view of the cerebellum. (Courtesy of John Ward.)

Diencephalon

The diencephalon ("between brain") includes the **thalamus, hypothalamus**, and **pineal gland**. These structures sit lateral to the third ventricle (discussed later). The diencephalon contains the links between the nervous system and the endocrine system.

The **thalamus** is located dorsally within the diencephalon. In simple terms, it regulates the inputs to the cerebral cortex and directs them to the correct areas of the cerebrum.

The **hypothalamus** acts as a central regulator of homeostasis, including regulation of temperature, thirst, and cardiorespiratory functions and control of the autonomic nervous system, circadian rhythm, and limbic system. Its nuclei secrete chemical messengers, "releasing factors", that influence anterior pituitary (adenohypophysis) hormone secretion, in turn controlling growth, energy regulation, and reproductive function. Both the **supra-optic** and **paraventricular nuclei** produce antidiuretic hormone (ADH) and oxytocin; these pass via axons in the pituitary stalk to be stored at the posterior pituitary gland (neurohypophysis).

The **pituitary gland** has anterior (adenohypophysis) and posterior (neurohypophysis) parts. Each has a different embryological origin. The pituitary gland is situated in the hypophyseal fossa (part of the sella turcica) (**Figure 1.6**). The posterior pituitary secretes ADH and oxytocin, produced by the hypothalamus. The anterior pituitary develops as an outpouching of the roof of the pharynx. It is controlled by hypothalamic releasing factors via the hypophyseal portal circulation and produces:

- **ACTH** (adrenocorticotrophic hormone) which acts on the adrenal cortex to produce cortisol, sex hormones, and mineralocorticoids (see **Section 5**)
- **FSH** (follicle-stimulating hormone) and **LH** (luteinising hormone) which are responsible for puberty, the menstrual cycle, menopause, and sexual drive
- **Melanocyte-stimulating hormone** which stimulates melanin synthesis in melanocytes in the skin
- **GH** (growth hormone)
- **TSH** (thyroid-stimulating hormone) which regulates the thyroid gland to produce T3 and T4
- **Dopamine** which inhibits prolactin; prolactin initiates lactation and promotes growth of mammary glands and reproductive organs
- **Somatostatin** which inhibits the release of GH and TSH; also referred to as growth hormone–inhibiting hormone

Learning Point

The *trans-sphenoidal* approach is the most commonly used approach to remove tumours of the pituitary gland via the sphenoid sinus. Pituitary adenomas may be classified according to their size as macro-nodular (above 10 mm in size) or micro-nodular (below 10 mm) and as functional or non-functional, depending on whether they oversecrete a particular pituitary hormone.

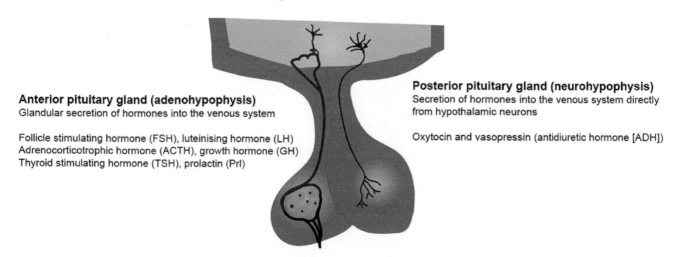

Hypothalamus
Relays endocrine signals to the anterior hypothalamus, and directly secretes into the posterior pituitary via magnocellular neurons

Anterior pituitary gland (adenohypophysis)
Glandular secretion of hormones into the venous system

Follicle stimulating hormone (FSH), luteinising hormone (LH)
Adrenocorticotrophic hormone (ACTH), growth hormone (GH)
Thyroid stimulating hormone (TSH), prolactin (Prl)

Posterior pituitary gland (neurohypophysis)
Secretion of hormones into the venous system directly from hypothalamic neurons

Oxytocin and vasopressin (antidiuretic hormone [ADH])

FIGURE 1.6 Diagrammatic representation of the hypothalamus, anterior pituitary, and posterior pituitary. (Courtesy of John Ward.)

Basal Ganglia

The basal ganglia are a group of nuclei (cell bodies) situated below the cortex of the cerebrum. Their main functions include motor control, cognition, and emotion.

Anatomically, the basal ganglia can be described as follows:

- The **lentiform nucleus** (shaped like a lens) is a cone-shaped structure which is divided into the putamen laterally and the globus pallidus (pale globe) medially. It sits just anterior to the thalamus. On a CT scan, the putamen appears dark, whereas the globus pallidus has a lighter tone. The globus pallidus may be subdivided into internal (globus pallidus internus) and external (globus pallidus externus) segments.
- The **caudate nucleus** is a C- or tadpole-shaped structure which curves over the lentiform nucleus. The caudate nucleus has a head (anterior), body, and tail (which sits near the hippocampus in the temporal lobe).
- The **subthalamic nucleus** sits, as its name suggests, inferior to the thalamus.
- The **internal capsule** is the name given to the bundles of white matter projection fibres that run between the basal ganglia nuclei. The **anterior limb** runs between the lentiform nucleus and caudate nucleus. The **genu**, or bend, sits at the point of the cone of the lentiform nucleus in line with the interventricular foramen of Monro (discussed later). The **posterior limb** runs between the lentiform nucleus and the thalamus, and notably contains descending motor fibres and ascending sensory fibres (**Figure 1.7a**).

Functionally, the basal ganglia form part of an extremely complex circuit of connections. Fibres project to the "input centres" of the basal ganglia, known as the **striatum**. This consists of the caudate nucleus, **nucleus accumbens** (a small area where the putamen and caudate fuse inferior to the internal capsule), and putamen. They then project to the "output areas" of the basal ganglia, known as the pallidum. This consists of the globus pallidus internus and externus. The internal pallidus inhibits the thalamus, preventing uncontrolled movements and allowing for precision and fine motor control.

The key neurotransmitter needed for the motor basal ganglia loops is **dopamine**. This is supplied by the *substantia nigra* ("black substance" in Latin) in the midbrain (**Figure 1.9b**). Movement is initiated by the "direct pathway", which involves disinhibition of the thalamus. The striatum stops pallidal inhibition of the thalamus, thereby increasing neuron firing from the thalamus. Movement is prevented by the "indirect pathway", in which the subthalamic nucleus stimulates pallidal inhibition of the thalamus. It puts a foot down on the brakes, preventing thalamic neurons firing. This is shown in **Figure 1.7b**.

The dopaminergic supply to the emotion loops of the basal ganglia comes from the ventral tegmental area of the midbrain. This supplies the nucleus accumbens, among other structures. This "mesolimbic" pathway is responsible for reward-based learning, including gambling and addiction.

Learning Point

Pathologies of the basal ganglia include Parkinson's disease and Huntington's disease. Degeneration of the dopaminergic neurons from the substantia nigra, the nigrostriatal tract, is associated with Parkinson's disease. Loss of the function of the direct pathway leads to poor initiation of movement and bradykinesia. In Huntington's disease, the indirect pathway's action is reduced. This correlates with motor symptoms, including chorea (abnormal involuntary movements).

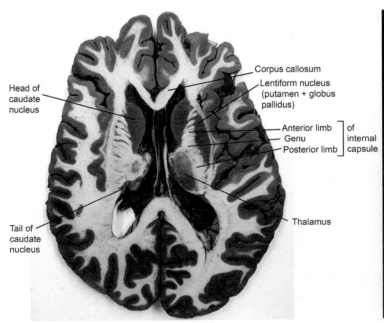
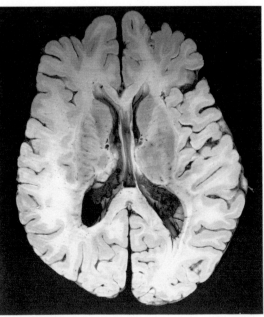

(a)

FIGURE 1.7a Transverse brain section showing basal ganglia, stained with Mulligan's stain (*left*); the unstained section is shown (*right*) for comparison. (Courtesy of Department of Anatomical Sciences, SGUL.)

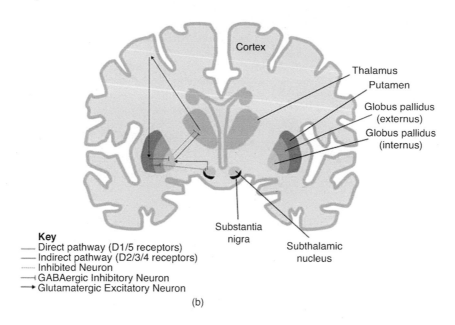

FIGURE 1.7b   Coronal brain slice showing the basal ganglia and thalamocortical circuits. (Courtesy of John Ward.)

Brainstem

The brainstem connects the cerebrum to the spinal cord and contains many long tracts projecting up and down. These are discussed in detail in the spinal cord section. Cardiac and respiratory centres found within the brainstem are necessary to maintain life (**Figure 1.8**).

The brainstem consists of 3 parts: midbrain, pons, and medulla oblongata.

Between them lies a space, termed the **interpeduncular fossa**, within which sit two round structures: the **mammillary bodies**. On the posterior aspect of the midbrain lie the paired **superior** and **inferior colliculi**, often referred to as the tectal plate. The four colliculi (superior and inferior) are concerned with visual and auditory reflexes, respectively. **Remember: Sight before sound – superior colliculus above inferior colliculus**.

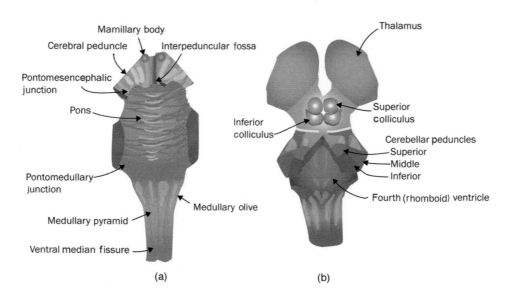

FIGURE 1.8   Brainstem (a) anterior (ventral) and (b) posterior (dorsal) view showing the main surface features. (Courtesy of John Ward.)

Midbrain

The midbrain is formed of two large cerebral peduncles anteriorly (*peduncle* is Latin for "small foot"). These contain descending nerve fibres responsible for motor control.

Looking at a transverse section of the midbrain, the area can be divided into 2 sections relative to the **cerebral aqueduct**, which runs within the midbrain on the dorsal side. The area dorsal to the cerebral aqueduct is known as the **tectum**. The tectum contains the four colliculi. The remaining area (ventral) is known as the **tegmentum**. The tegmentum contains a large black band known as the **substantia nigra** (see above, "Basal Ganglia") and the red nuclei, where fibres projecting up from the cerebellum synapse. Ventral to the substantia nigra lie the crura (singular: crus) cerebri which contain the descending motor fibres (**Figure 1.9**).

fissure. These contain the descending motor fibres (corticospinal and corticobulbar) that pass through the crus cerebri and anterior pons in turn. The **olives** are prominences which are located lateral to the pyramids. The medulla contains the vital centres for controlling blood pressure and oxygen and carbon dioxide saturation (see the baroreceptors, chemoreceptors and glossopharyngeal nerve, Head and Neck Section).

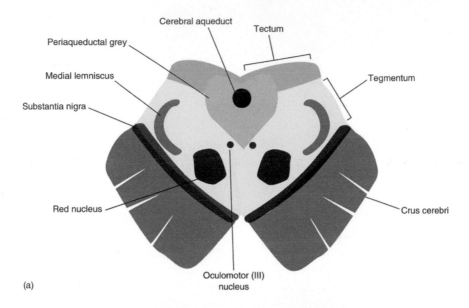

(a)

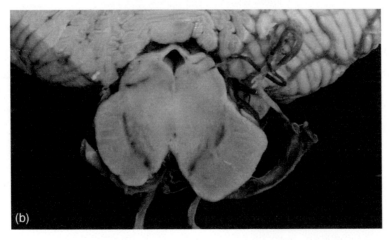

(b)

FIGURE 1.9   (a) Schematic cross-section of the brainstem at the level of the superior colliculi. (Courtesy of John Ward.) (b) Brainstem section shown for comparison; note the visible substantia nigra. (Courtesy of Department of Anatomical Sciences, SGUL.)

Pons

The pons contains fibres projecting vertically, as well as fibres crossing horizontally. The horizontal fibres decussate and enter the cerebellum via the middle cerebellar peduncle. This allows fibres from the left cerebrum to connect with the cerebellum on the right side and vice versa.

Medulla Oblongata

The medulla oblongata, or "medulla", is a direct continuation of the spinal cord above the foramen magnum, and it is about 3 cm in length. Close to the midline on the anterior surface of the medulla lie two **pyramids**, separated by the ventral median

Cranial Nerves

Collectively, the cranial nerves supply sensation to the head, face, and neck. There are 12 cranial nerves, which are usually denoted by Roman numerals: CN I–CN XII. The function and path of the cranial nerves is summarised in **Table 1.2**.

CLINICAL NOTE

CN I and CN II arise from the cerebral hemispheres; the rest come from the brainstem (**Figures 1.10** and **1.11**). This will be discussed later in this subsection.

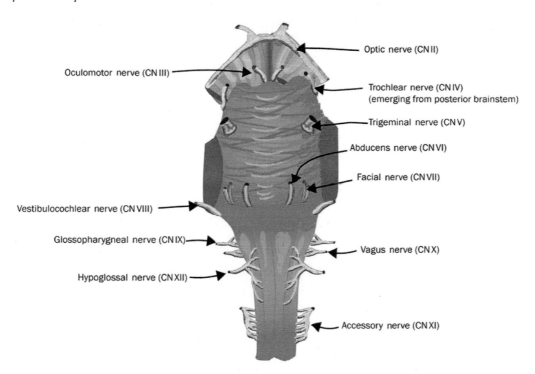

FIGURE 1.10 Cranial nerve roots II to XII emerging from the brainstem (ventral view). (Courtesy of John Ward.)

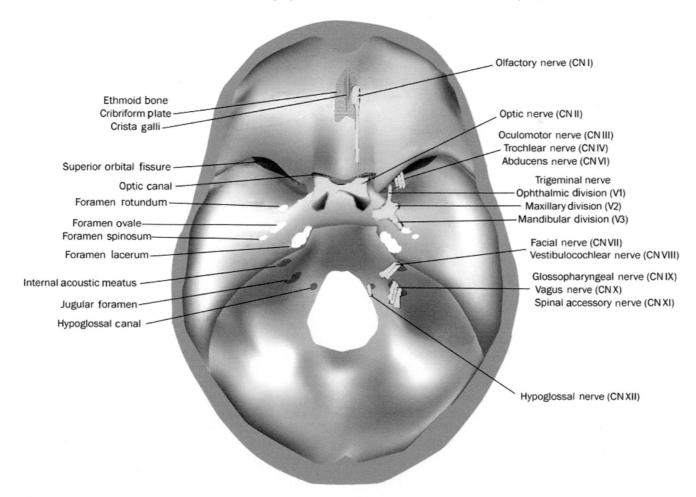

FIGURE 1.11 Internal view of the cranial cavity: the cranial nerves emerging through the skull base foramina. (Courtesy of John Ward.)

TABLE 1.2: Cranial nerves (2,3)

Cranial Nerve	Anatomical Path	Function
I. Olfactory	• Nerve receptors in the nasal mucosa, filaments pass through the cribriform plate of the ethmoid to the olfactory bulbs and then to the olfactory tracts, which divide into medial and lateral striae • The lateral stria connects to the olfactory cortex of the temporal lobe • The medial stria is connected to the hypothalamus and brainstem • The olfactory cortex is connected to the orbitofrontal cortex of the frontal lobe and to the amygdala	• Sensory – smell • Trauma to the skull base can cause anosmia • Other causes of anosmia include upper respiratory tract infections, Parkinson's disease, Alzheimer's disease, Huntington's disease, and COVID
II. Optic	• Arises from the retina and runs posterior to the eyeball through the optic canal • See further details in Section 2	• Sensory – vision • Lesions at different points in the visual pathway cause different defects
III. Oculomotor	• Arises from the interpeduncular fossa of the midbrain and exits the skull base through the superior orbital fissure	• Motor – superior/inferior/medial rectus, inferior oblique muscles, and levator palpebrae superioris (opens eyelids) • Lesions cause the eye to look down and out • Parasympathetic fibres of the short ciliary nerves are carried on the surface of the third cranial nerve to innervate the sphincter pupillae, causing pupil constriction and ciliary muscle contraction (responsible for accommodation)
IV. Trochlear	• Arises from the posterior part of the midbrain, below the inferior colliculi, decussates, and exits the skull base through the superior orbital fissure	• Motor – superior oblique muscle • Lesions cause the eyes to look upwards
V. Trigeminal	• Arises from the angle of the pons and the middle cerebellar peduncle • V1 (ophthalmic branch) exits through the superior orbital fissure, V2 (maxillary branch) through the foramen rotundum, and V3 (mandibular branch) through the foramen ovale	• Sensory – touch to the face. • Motor – muscles of mastication
VI. Abducens	• Arises from the junction of the pons and the medulla and exits through the superior orbital fissure	• Motor – lateral rectus muscle • Lesions cause the eyes to deviate medially
VII. Facial	• Arises from the cerebello-pontine angle, runs through the internal acoustic meatus, and exits the skull via the stylomastoid foramen	• Special sensory – taste from the anterior two-thirds of the tongue • Motor – muscles of facial expression, stapedius, and the posterior belly of the digastric muscle • Parasympathetic – supplies the submandibular and sublingual glands and the lacrimal and nasal mucosa to increase secretions
VIII. Vestibulocochlear	• Arises with CN VII from the cerebello-pontine angle and passes through the internal acoustic meatus	• Sensory – balance (vestibular division) and hearing (cochlear division)
IX. Glossopharyngeal	• Arises posterior to the olive of the medulla and passes through the jugular foramen of the skull base	• Sensory – taste from the posterior one-third of the tongue • Parasympathetic – parotid salivary gland • Motor – stylopharyngeus muscle • Sensory innervation of carotid body and carotid sinus
X. Vagus	• Arises posterior to the olive of the medulla and passes through the jugular foramen of the skull base	• Sensory and parasympathetic – larynx, aorta, thoracic, and abdominal viscera • Sensory innervation also includes the aortic body chemoreceptors and aortic arch baroreceptors • Motor innervation of pharynx, palatoglossus, larynx, oesophagus, and GIT down to the splenic flexure
XI. Accessory (spinal)	• Arises posterior to the olive of the medulla and passes through the jugular foramen of the skull base	• Motor – sternocleidomastoid and trapezius muscles
XII. Hypoglossal	• Arises anterior to the olive of the medulla and passes through the hypoglossal canal	• Motor – intrinsic muscles of the tongue, except palatoglossus, which is supplied by the vagus

Skull Base (See Head and Neck Section)

Meninges

The brain and spinal cord have 3 covering membranes. The outer membrane, the **dura mater**, is the toughest, and consists of 2 layers: a periosteal layer lining the inside of the skull, beneath which is the deep or meningeal layer. Key double folds of dura include:

- The **falx cerebri** (*falx*: latin, "sickle-shaped"): occupies the longitudinal fissure and separates the two cerebral hemispheres
- The **tentorium cerebelli** separates the occipital and temporal lobes from the cerebellum and brainstem. Its posterior margin is fixed to the occipital bone and contains the transverse venous sinus
- The **diaphragma sellae**: roofs the sella turcica of the sphenoid bone and is attached to the anterior and posterior clinoid processes. The pituitary stalk passes through it

The venous sinuses are spaces within the dura that collect blood from the brain. The anatomical layout of the sinuses is shown in **Figure 1.13**.

The second covering is the **arachnoid mater** (Greek: *arachne*, "spider"). It attaches to the inside of the dura. The innermost layer is the **pia mater**, which is a very thin layer that covers the brain and spinal cord. The space between the pia mater and the arachnoid mater is the **subarachnoid space** and is filled with cerebrospinal fluid (CSF).

Learning Point

Meningitis is inflammation of the meninges, which cover the brain and the spinal cord, which can be caused by bacteria, e.g., meningococci, or viruses such as Coxsackie. It can be a life-threatening condition. The diagnosis is based on interpretation of the symptoms (severe headache, fever, fits, and vomiting) and signs, such as neck rigidity, in addition to the spinal tap (CSF examination).

Intracranial bleeding is characterised by where the blood is collecting in relation to the dural layers (**Table 1.3**).

An **intracerebral aneurysm** is an artery supplying the brain that is dilated to more than 50% of its original diameter, often following the formation of atheromatous plaques that weaken the wall. It commonly occurs where arteries branch (especially due to hypertension) and in the circle of Willis (congenital berry aneurysms). They produce few symptoms until the artery eventually ruptures, which is a medical emergency.

CSF Circulation and the Ventricular System

The ventricular system comprises four chambers, or **ventricles** (**Figure 1.13**). CSF is formed from the **choroid plexus**, a vascular structure sitting within the lateral ventricles. The fluid then drains through the ventricular system and out into the subarachnoid space, where it bathes the brain. CSF drains

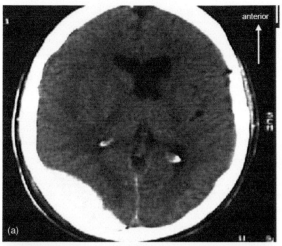
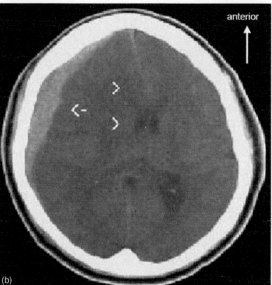
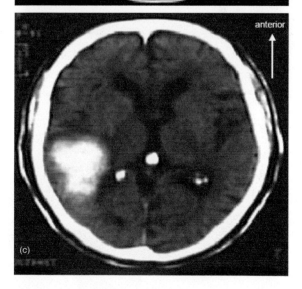

FIGURE 1.12 (a) CT scan of head showing an acute extradural haematoma caused by damage to a posterior branch of the middle meningeal artery. (b) CT scan of the head showing acute right subdural haematoma. There is significant mass effect and midline shift to the left. (c) CT scan of acute intra-parenchymal haemorrhage in left parietal lobe. (Courtesy of Abdel-Aziz Abdel-Ghany.)

TABLE 1.3: Types of intracranial bleed

Type of Bleed	Causes	Characteristic Presentation	Image
Extradural (between the dura and the inner table of the skull)	Trauma to pterion lacerates the middle meningeal artery	Loss of consciousness followed by a "lucid interval" (typically hours); remember the story of the footballer who collapsed in the changing room after being hit on the side of his head while playing.	See **Figure 1.12a**
Subdural (between dural and arachnoid)	Brain atrophy with age or alcoholism puts tension on the bridging veins, which then shear more easily upon the impact of a fall, for example	Disorientation, confusion, gradual loss of consciousness; can present acutely or chronically	See **Figure 1.12b**
Subarachnoid (between arachnoid and pia)	Ruptured arterial aneurysms, arteriovenous malformations, or trauma	Thunderclap headache, with a sudden decrease in consciousness	
Intracerebral (within the brain tissue)	Trauma or, commonly, hypertensive bleeds	Focal neurological symptoms of a haemorrhagic stroke	See **Figure 1.12c**

from the subarachnoid space through arachnoid granulations in the superior sagittal sinus, where it enters the venous system.

Paired lateral ventricles sit within each cerebral hemisphere. They extend into the hemispheres of the brain and are described as having frontal, temporal, and occipital horns. These horns join at the atrium. The CSF in the lateral ventricles drains into the **third ventricle** via the interventricular foramina of Monro. The third ventricle sits in the midline of the brain, between the hypothalami and thalami. It drains into the **fourth ventricle** via the cerebral aqueduct. The fourth ventricle sits posterior to the brainstem but anterior to the cerebellum. It has foramina through which CSF drains into the cisterna magna: the median foramen of Magendie and the two lateral foramina of Luschka.

CLINICAL NOTE

Hydrocephalus is an abnormal accumulation of CSF, which could be caused by obstruction of CSF flow due to pathologies such as infections and brain tumours.

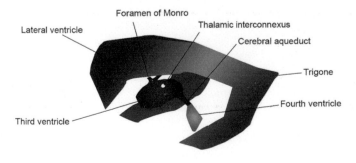

FIGURE 1.13 The isolated ventricular system. (Courtesy of John Ward.)

Arterial Vasculature of the Brain

The brain accounts for only 2.5% of body weight but requires one-sixth of the cardiac output.

The blood supply of the brain originates from two sets of paired arteries: the vertebral and internal carotid arteries on each side. They anastomose to form the **circle of Willis**, which gives branches to supply the brain (**Figures 1.14** and **1.15**).

The anterior circulation of the brain arises from the internal carotid arteries. The common carotid arteries branch from the brachiocephalic trunk and the arch of the aorta on the right and left, respectively. Each common carotid artery (CCA) travels up the neck in the carotid sheath with the internal jugular vein and the vagus nerve. It bifurcates into the internal and external carotid arteries at the level of the fourth cervical vertebra/upper border of thyroid cartilage (C4). The internal carotid arteries (ICAs) enter the cranium through the carotid canals in the temporal bone. They run in the cavernous sinus, with the cranial nerves coursing towards the orbital cavity, before turning upwards and backwards (a feature known as the carotid siphon). They terminate in the circle of Willis. The internal carotid artery has four parts:

- Cervical (within the carotid sheath)
- Petrous (within the petrous part of the temporal bone)
- Cavernous (at the lateral wall of the cavernous sinus with CN III, IV, V1, V2, and VI)
- Cerebral (within the cranial subarachnoid space)

The posterior circulation arises from the vertebral arteries. Each vertebral artery stems from the first part of the subclavian artery and travels up the neck in the transverse foramina of the cervical vertebrae (all but C7), entering the cranium via the foramen magnum. The two vertebral arteries unite to form the basilar artery. As the vertebral arteries ascend, they give off the paired posterior spinal artery, posterior inferior cerebellar artery (PICA), and singular anterior spinal artery. The basilar artery runs within the pontine cistern (within the central groove of the pons) and gives off the pontine arteries, anterior inferior cerebellar arteries (AICAs), and superior cerebellar arteries (**Figure 1.15**). The basilar artery divides into the posterior cerebral arteries, which form the posterior part of the circle of Willis and connect with the anterior circulation via the posterior communicating arteries and supply the inferior surface of the brain and occipital lobes (**Figure 1.14**).

In the circle of Willis, the internal carotid artery on each side (anterior circulation) continues as the middle cerebral artery (MCA) (80% of blood flow), which supplies the lateral surface of each cerebral hemisphere. It also gives origin to the anterior cerebral artery (ACA), which supplies the medial parts of each hemisphere except the occipital lobes. Both ACAs are connected by the very short anterior communicating artery.

Learning Point

Stroke is when an area of the brain does not receive sufficient blood flow, resulting in the death of the cells in that area and neurological defects.

Common causes of stroke are:

*   *Thrombosis:* occlusion from a locally formed blood clot.
*   *Embolism:* occlusion from a distally formed blood clot that travelled to the arteries supplying the brain (often originating from a fibrillating left atrium to form a thrombosis).
*   *Hypoperfusion:* brain doesn't receive adequate blood supply, e.g., low blood pressure while in shock.
*   *Haemorrhage:* bleeding inside the cranial cavity, e.g., traumatic blow to the head ruptures blood vessels. The blood outside the vessels takes up space in the cranial cavity but outside the brain and so reduces the blood supply of the capillaries within the brain.

Approximately 85% of strokes are ischaemic strokes (thromboembolic, primary occlusion of intracerebral arteries), with the remaining 15% haemorrhagic strokes.

Learning Point

Symptoms of an MCA stroke include:
*   **Sensory loss on the contralateral (opposite) side of the body**
*   **Motor loss, hemiparesis, or hemiplegia of the muscles on the contralateral side of the body**
*   **Visual loss as the optic radiations passes through the parietal, temporal, and frontal lobes**
*   **Speech disturbance if the language-dominant hemisphere is affected**
*   **Visuospatial disturbance, such as hemi-spatial neglect, if the non-language-dominant hemisphere is affected**

Venous Vasculature of the Brain

The dural venous sinuses carry venous blood and CSF away from the brain. They are located between the periosteal and meningeal layers of the dura mater, and unlike other veins, they are valveless (which allows bidirectional flow) and do not travel alongside any arteries.

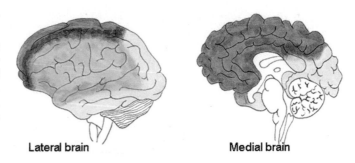

FIGURE 1.14 Arterial supply to the brain (Pink: anterior cerebral artery; Green: middle cerebral artery; Yellow: posterior cerebral artery). (Courtesy of Calum Harrington-Vogt.)

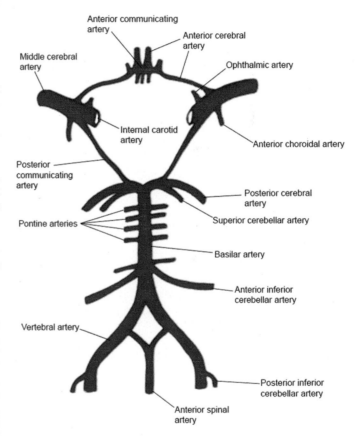

FIGURE 1.15 Circle of Willis; schematic view seen from anterior and inferior. (Courtesy of Calum Harrington-Vogt.)

The superior sagittal sinus (SSS) runs in the upper edge of the falx cerebri, while the inferior sagittal sinus runs within the lower edge. The great cerebral vein of Galen (from the deep structures of the brain) joins the inferior sagittal sinus to form the straight sinus. The SSS joins the straight sinus at the confluence of sinuses to form the transverse sinus, which continues as the sigmoid (S-shaped) sinus, and this finally becomes the internal jugular vein (IJV), which leaves the cranial cavity at the jugular foramen.

The cavernous sinus lies on either side of the sella turcica. Both ophthalmic veins drain into the anterior aspect of the cavernous sinuses. The internal carotid artery runs through the sinus (**Figure 1.16**).

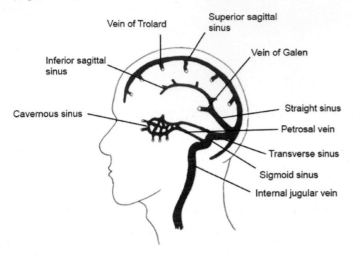

FIGURE 1.16 Venous drainage of brain, schematic lateral view. (Courtesy of Calum Harrington-Vogt.)

Learning Point

Cavernous sinus thrombosis can be caused by infections in the "dangerous triangle" of the face. Infection within the nose, ear, and face (which drain to the cavernous sinus) can spread to the cavernous sinus. The causative organism is usually *Staphylococcus aureus*. Cranial nerves III, IV, V1, and V2 and VI travel through the cavernous sinus and are therefore affected and potentially paralysed. This is characterised by severe systemic signs, periorbital swelling, and protrusion of the eyeball (exophthalmos). It should be urgently treated with IV antibiotics.

1B

NEUROANATOMY
Anatomy of the Spinal Cord

Reviewed by Valentina Gnoni

Introduction

The spinal cord is part of the central nervous system (CNS) and extends from the foramen magnum, as a continuation of the medulla oblongata, to the level of the first or second lumbar vertebra. This structure is contained within the spinal canal and acts as a conduit for multiple nerve pathways ascending and descending to or from the brain. This section sheds light upon the development, function, and clinical conditions associated with the spinal cord.

Learning Objectives

- Understand the development of the spinal cord and central nervous system
- Recall the gross anatomy of the spinal cord and its coverings
- Recall the important ascending tracts and descending tracts, their anatomy, and clinical relevance
- Recall the blood supply to the spinal cord
- Understand the anatomy and pathophysiology of common spinal cord pathologies

Development of the Spinal Cord

Early Development and Gastrulation

Development begins following the fusion of the male and female pronuclei to form the diploid zygote nucleus. The zygote undergoes a series of cellular divisions to form the blastocyst, a ball of cells that travel along the fallopian tube to implant in the lining of the uterine cavity.

The blastocyst is composed of an inner cell mass surrounded by a second group of cells called the trophectoderm. Upon implantation, the inner cell mass differentiates into two layers of cells, epiblast and hypoblast, collectively referred to as the bilaminar disc.

The hypoblast layer forms the extraembryonic tissue, placenta, and placental cord (umbilical cord), which support the growing embryo. During the third week of development, the epiblast layer gives rise to three germ layers, ectoderm, mesoderm, and endoderm, in a process called gastrulation. These germ layers give rise to all the structures within the body, including the future CNS (**Table 1.4**).

Neural Tube

Neural tube formation, shown in **Figure 1.17**, follows gastrulation. The mesoderm layer gives rise to a rod-like structure called the notochord. Axial mesodermal cells within the notochord

cause a patch of ectodermal cells to differentiate into the neural plate (neuroectoderm) by releasing chemical mediators, including Sonic hedgehog protein. A groove forms within the neural plate to produce neural folds that fuse at the midline to form a hollow, fluid-filled neural tube. This tube gives rise to the CNS.

Fusion of the neural tube begins at the midline and continues in a zipper-like fashion in both rostral and caudal directions. Free edges, known as neuropores, are the last to close during this process.

Fusion of the neural folds also causes neural crest cells to disconnect from the epidermis. These cells migrate to their adult position to give rise to structures that form the peripheral nervous system. The hollow, fluid-filled cavity within the neural tube (neural canal) later forms the ventricular system of the brain. The notochord degenerates and persists as the nucleus pulposus of the intervertebral discs.

Alar and Basal Plates

The developing spinal cord consists of an alar plate and a basal plate, separated by a longitudinal groove known as the sulcus limitans. The basal plate forms the ventral aspect of the developing spinal cord, whilst the alar plate forms the dorsal dimension. This arrangement is modified in the brainstem, as the fourth ventricle displaces the alar plate region laterally, changing the direct dorsal-ventral arrangement. This is demonstrated by the distribution of sensory and motor cranial nerve nuclei in the floor of the fourth ventricle, the rhomboid fossa, as shown in **Figure 1.18**.

The basal plate consists of anterior horn cells, which develop into motor neurons. Axons project out of the basal plate to form the ventral nerve roots. In contrast, sensory neurons arise from the alar plate. Axons entering this region form the dorsal nerve roots.

TABLE 1.4: Anatomical structures within the adult that develop from the respective germ layers

Germ Layer	Adult Structures
Ectoderm	• Epidermis • Nervous system
Mesoderm	• Muscles • Dermis • Cartilage • Vertebral body plan • Blood vessels
Endoderm	• Epithelial lining of the digestive tract and its associated organs, along with respiratory, urinary, and reproductive tracts • Glands (thymus, thyroid, and parathyroid glands)

DOI: 10.1201/9781003312895-2

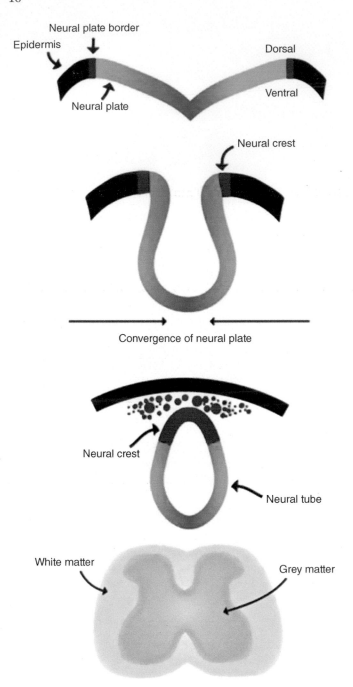

FIGURE 1.17 Formation of the neural tube. (Courtesy of John Ward.)

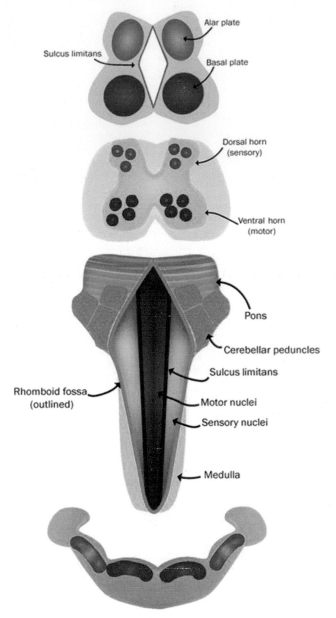

FIGURE 1.18 Alar and basal plates. A depiction of how the developing alar (sensory, blue) and basal (motor, red) plates map onto the grey matter of the adult spinal cord, rhomboid fossa, and a cross-section of the caudal pons. (Courtesy of John Ward.)

CLINICAL NOTE

Neural tube defects: spina bifida

Spina bifida arises following the failure of the caudal neuropore to close, leaving an abnormal opening within the vertebrate body plan of the individual. Three distinct forms of spina bifida have been identified: occulta, meningocoele, and myelomeningocoele (**Figure 1.19**).

Spina bifida occulta is the mildest and most common form of the condition. It is characterised by the presence of skin covering the surface of the vertebral opening. The layer of skin prevents the communication of spinal nerves and meninges with the external environment. As a result, patients remain unaffected and are usually unaware of their condition. The defect can be identified by tufts of hair or dimples within the skin at the site of the defect.

Meningocoele is less common but is a more severe form of the condition. It is characterised by the herniation of meninges and cerebrospinal fluid (CSF) across the defect, with little to no involvement of nervous tissue. As a result, the child does not suffer from any neurological problems.

Myelomeningocoele is the most severe form of the condition, involving the protrusion of the spinal cord and its coverings. Children with this defect suffer from severe neurological problems below the level of the lesion, including motor paralysis, loss of sensation, and bladder and bowel problems. In extreme cases, the upper extremities are also involved.

Primary prevention is regular folic acid supplementation before conception or during pregnancy. Surgery can be carried out to close the vertebral opening and remove the cyst that has herniated posteriorly.

emerge at increasingly oblique angles and travel further to exit the vertebral canal. The mixed spinal nerve then divides again into a ventral primary ramus supplying the anterior trunk, limbs, and viscera, and a dorsal primary ramus supplying the skin of the back and the vertebral muscles (**Figure 1.21**). Each spinal nerve carries motor neurons (α to skeletal muscle; γ to muscle spindle fibres), sensory (myelinated and unmyelinated), and autonomic fibres (see "Autonomic Nervous System and the Spinal Cord").

The adult spinal cord ends at the level of the L1/L2 vertebrae. The distal bulbous part is called the **conus medullaris**, and its tapering end continues as a fibrous cord, the **filum terminale**, which extends towards the bottom of the vertebral canal, stabilising the spinal cord and anchoring it to the coccyx. Below the

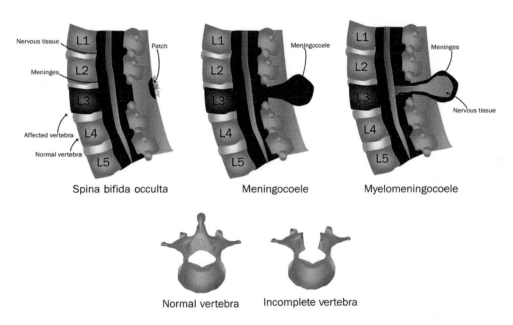

FIGURE 1.19   Spina bifida. (Courtesy of John Ward.)

Gross Anatomy of the Spinal Cord

The spinal cord is non-uniform in structure, 40 to 50 cm long, and consists of four regions: cervical, thoracic, lumbar, and sacral. There are two enlargements, cervical and lumbar, which correspond to the regions of the nerve plexuses which innervate the upper and lower limbs.

The **spinal cord is organised into 31 segments**, defined by 31 pairs of spinal nerves extending from both sides of the spinal cord, travelling towards the periphery via the intervertebral foramina. The spinal nerves are divided into 8 cervical, 12 thoracic, 5 lumbar, 5 sacral, and 1 coccygeal nerve. As there are eight pairs of cervical nerves and seven cervical vertebra, C1–C7 nerves exit the vertebral column above their corresponding vertebra, whilst **C8 nerves exit below the seventh cervical vertebra**. The remaining pairs of spinal nerves exit below their corresponding vertebra (**Figure 1.20**).

Each nerve emerges via two short roots: the anterior (motor) root and the posterior (sensory) root. Spinal nerves are formed from the union of these roots, and emerge through the intervertebral foramina. As you descend the cord, the spinal nerves

conus medullaris, the vertebral canal contains only the roots of the spinal nerves, which are collected in the **cauda equina** (Latin, "horse's tail", named after its distinctive appearance).

Coverings of the Spinal Cord

The spinal cord and part of the spinal nerve roots are sheathed and protected by three layers of meninges (pia mater, arachnoid mater, and dura mater). The dura extends along the nerve roots as the epineurium. The space between the dura and the internal surface of the vertebral canal is called the epidural space. The subarachnoid space is formed between the arachnoid and the pia mater, with the latter closely covering the external surface of the spinal cord. The **subarachnoid space, which extends to the level of the second sacral vertebra, contains the CSF** in which the nerve roots of the cauda equina are bathed. The pia mater is the innermost meningeal layer of the spinal cord. Thickenings of the pia mater, collectively known as the **denticulate ligaments** (tooth-like projections), are found on either side of the spinal cord. Their function is to suspend the spinal cord in the midline by attaching the spinal cord to the dura. The meningeal coverings of the spinal cord are shown in **Figure 1.22**.

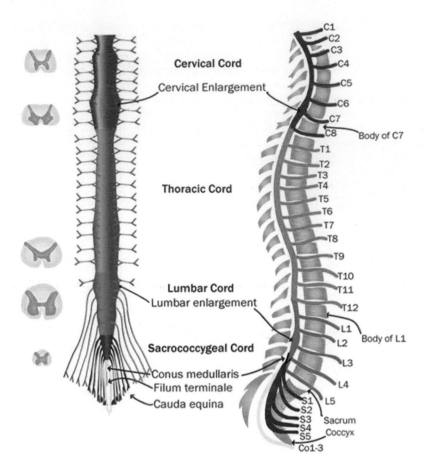

FIGURE 1.20 Gross anatomy of the spinal cord. (Courtesy of John Ward.)

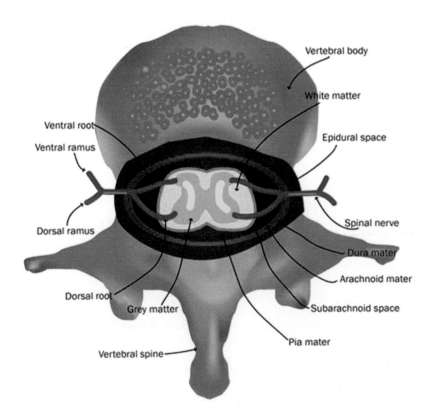

FIGURE 1.21 Bony covering of the spinal cord. (Courtesy of John Ward.)

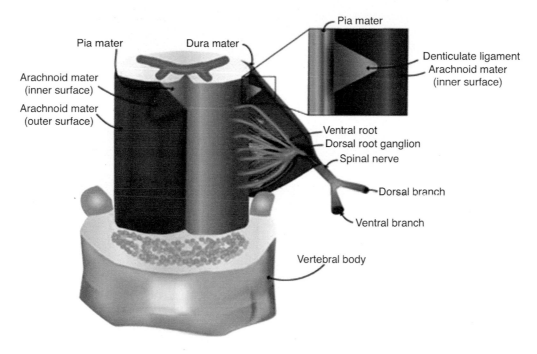

FIGURE 1.22 Meningeal covering of the spinal cord. (Courtesy of John Ward.)

Cross-Section of the Developed Spinal Cord

A cross-section of the spinal cord shows a central body of grey matter, shaped like an H or a butterfly, with its anterior and posterior wings (anterior and posterior horns) containing cell bodies and fibres and peripheral white matter, which contains only nerve fibres. The grey matter "wings" are connected by a transverse tract, the grey commissure, where the central or ependymal canal is located. In front of the grey commissure lies the anterior white commissure, where a bundle of white fibres crosses the midline.

Within the white matter surrounding the central grey matter, ascending tracts transmit sensory information to the brain, whilst descending tracts relay motor information from the brain to skeletal muscles. Key ascending and descending tracts have been highlighted in **Figure 1.23**.

Autonomic Nervous System and the Spinal Cord

The autonomic nervous system innervates smooth and cardiac muscles, secretory glands, and metabolic organs via a two-neuron chain. Pre-ganglionic fibres, with cell bodies in the brainstem or spinal cord, exit in the ventral ramus of the spinal nerve to ganglia (a ganglion is structure outside the CNS containing neuronal cell bodies. NB: the term "ganglion" can also refer to a cystic lesion related to a muscle tendon). This is the location of the cell body of post-ganglionic fibres, which then continue to visceral targets. The autonomic nervous system is subdivided into the sympathetic nervous system (SNS) and parasympathetic nervous system (PSNS).

The SNS outflow is described as thoracolumbar (T1–L2) and comes from the intermediolateral cell column or lateral horn – a lateral protuberance of the crossbar of the H of grey

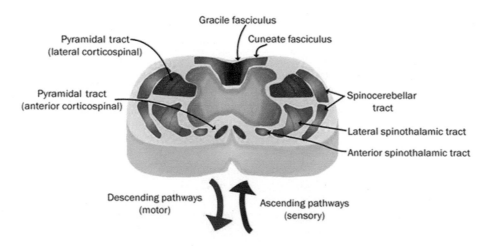

FIGURE 1.23 Key ascending (*blue*) and descending (*red*) tracts of the spinal cord. (Courtesy of John Ward.)

matter. Pre-ganglionic fibres enter the sympathetic chain as white (myelinated) *rami communicantes*, and post-ganglionic fibres exit as grey (unmyelinated) *rami communicantes* (singular: ramus communicans). Nerve plexuses surrounding the aorta (coeliac, superior mesenteric, and inferior mesenteric) also form a target for pre-ganglionic sympathetic nerves.

The PSNS outflow is described as craniosacral and is composed of the parasympathetic pre-ganglionic fibres which run with cranial nerves (III, VII, IX, X) and the interomediomedial sacral cord (S2–S4). Named ganglia associated with the PNS include:

- Ciliary ganglion (fibres from the Edinger-Westphal nucleus with the oculomotor nerve)
- Pterygopalatine ganglion (fibres within the facial nerve to supply the lacrimal gland)
- Submandibular ganglion (via the facial nerve to supply the submandibular salivary gland)
- Otic ganglion (via the glossopharyngeal nerve to the parotid gland) (see **Section 2**)
- **The vagus nerve (CN X) provides parasympathetic supply to most viscera and synapses in ganglia close to the target structures** (see **Sections 2, 4,** and **5** for more details)

The autonomic nervous system aims to maintain homeostasis of the body's internal environment. The effect of the SNS is commonly described as "fight or flight" and, conversely, the effect of the PSNS as "rest and digest". A comparison of sympathetic and parasympathetic effects is provided in **Table 1.5**.

TABLE 1.5: Opposing effects of the sympathetic and parasympathetic nervous systems

Body System	Sympathetic Effect	Parasympathetic Effect
Cardiovascular	Increased heart rate and force of contraction, peripheral vasoconstriction	Decreased heart rate and force of contraction, peripheral vasodilation
Respiratory	Dilation of bronchi	Constriction of bronchi
Digestive	Decreased motility	Increased motility
Excretory	Reduced salivation, reduced lacrimation, increased sweat gland secretion	Increased salivation, increased lacrimation
Thermoregulatory	Contraction of erector pili muscles	
Visual	Pupil dilation and ciliary muscle relaxation	Pupil constriction and ciliary muscle contraction

CLINICAL NOTE

Sensory examination
A dermatome is an area of skin supplied by sensory (afferent) nerve fibres from a single spinal nerve. Their exact distribution varies between individuals, so common landmarks are used during clinical neurological examination (see **Table 1.6** and **Figure 1.24**).

TABLE 1.6: Commonly examined dermatomes

Spinal Nerve	Landmark
C2	Posterior skull, lateral to the occipital protuberance
C3	Supraclavicular fossa
C4	Acromioclavicular joint
C5	Radial (lateral) aspect of the distal upper arm, just proximal to the elbow
C6	Dorsal surface of the base of the thumb
C7	Dorsal surface of the base of the middle finger
C8	Dorsal surface of the base of the little finger
T4	Level of the nipples (fourth intercostal space)
T6	Level of the xiphoid process
T10	Level of the umbilicus
L2	Anteromedial thigh
L3	Level of the knee (medial epicondyle of the femur)
L4	Medial malleolus
L5	Dorsum of the foot (except the lateral aspect)
S1	Lateral aspect of the foot
S2	Popliteal fossa

Note: C1 has no dermatome.

CLINICAL NOTE

Motor examination
A myotome is a group of muscles innervated by a spinal nerve. Neurological examination should assess the strength (power) of muscle groups. Power is recorded using the Medical Research Council (MRC) grading: 0 – total paralysis, 1 – a flicker of movement, 2 – active movement with gravity eliminated, 3 – normal movement against gravity but not against additional resistance, 4 – movement against both gravity and resistance but still overcome, and 5 – normal power (**Table 1.7**).

TABLE 1.7: Spinal nerves associated with commonly tested movements

Action	Spinal Segment Tested
Upper Limb	
Shoulder abduction	C5, C6 (axillary nerve)
Elbow flexion	C5, C6 (musculocutaneous nerve)
Elbow extension	C7, C8 (radial nerve)
Wrist/finger flexion	C7, C8, T1
Wrist/finger extension	C6, C7
Finger abduction	C8, T1 (ulnar nerve)
Lower Limb	
Hip flexion	L2, L3
Hip extension	L4, L5
Knee flexion	L5, S1 (sciatic nerve)
Knee extension	L3, L4 (femoral nerve)
Ankle dorsiflexion	L4, L5 (deep peroneal nerve)
Ankle plantarflexion	S1, S2
Hallux extension	L5, S1
Anal tone	S2, S3, S4

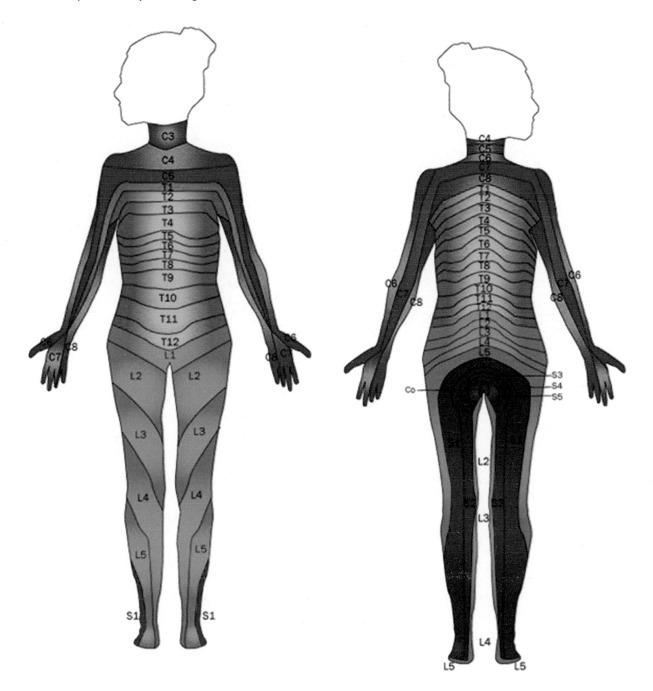

FIGURE 1.24 Dermatome map. (Courtesy of John Ward.)

Reflexes

Reflexes are involuntary responses to a stimulus. Stretch or tendon reflexes assess the integrity of a two-neuron reflex arc: an afferent (sensory) neuron and an efferent (motor) neuron. When a muscle is stretched – for example, by tapping on the attached tendon – groups of sensory proprioceptors (intrafusal muscle fibres) called muscle spindles are stimulated. They trigger a reflex arc instructing the muscle to contract (via extrafusal fibres). Relaxation of the antagonistic muscle group also occurs via inhibitory interneurons (**Table 1.8**).

TABLE 1.8: Commonly examined deep tendon reflexes

Tendon Reflex	Spinal Segment Tested
Biceps reflex	C5, C6
Brachioradialis reflex	C5, C6, C7
Triceps reflex	C6, C7, C8
Quadriceps reflex (Knee jerk)	L3, L4
Gastrocnemius reflex (Ankle jerk)	S1, S2
Plantar reflex	Integrity of the corticospinal tract

A normal response to testing the plantar reflex is a downward movement of the great toe; an upward movement is termed *Babinski's sign.*

Ascending Tracts

Ascending tracts transmit sensory information coming from the peripheral receptors to the brain. Sensory information can be processed consciously or subconsciously.

Subconsciously processed information is transmitted by tracts which do not follow a three-neuron sequence. These tracts transmit proprioceptive information from the skeletal muscles to the cerebellum. Anatomy of these tracts is beyond the scope of this chapter.

Consciously processed information is transmitted by ascending tracts that follow a three-neuron sequence. Two examples of tracts following this neuronal sequence and carrying consciously processed sensory information are the dorsal column and spinothalamic tracts.

Dorsal Column and Spinothalamic Tracts

The dorsal column pathway transmits tactile (fine touch), proprioception (joint position sense), and vibration sensation. First-order neurons enter the spinal cord through the dorsal root and ascend ipsilaterally as the ***fasciculus gracilis*** and ***fasciculus cuneatus***, the dorsal columns. The medial fasciculus gracilis carries information from below T6, and the fasciculus cuneatus carries information from above T6. In the medulla oblongata, first-order neurons synapse with second-order neurons, which then cross the midline as arcuate fibres (forming the "**great sensory decussation**") and twist up the brainstem, akin to a ribbon, as the **medial lemniscus**. Third-order neurons arise in the ventral posterior nucleus of the thalamus and traverse the posterior limb of the internal capsule to **terminate primarily in the postcentral gyrus, the somatosensory cortex**.

The spinothalamic tract transmits crude touch and pressure (anterior spinothalamic) and pain and temperature sensation (lateral spinothalamic). The first-order neurons of the spinothalamic tract travel through the dorsal root and synapse with second-order neurons in the grey matter of the spinal cord. The second-order neurons decussate in the anterior white commissure and then ascend contralaterally in the anterolateral white matter of the cord. The majority of fibres project to the thalamus and synapse onto third-order neurons, which follow the same path as those in the dorsal column pathway.

Pain triggers a polysynaptic "nociceptive flexion reflex" which can be seen clinically. Afferent sensory neurons stimulate interneurons in the spinal cord that result in almost instantaneous contraction of muscle flexors, moving your hand off a hot stove, for example (and relaxation of the opposite group of extensor muscles). The sensation of pain is described in two waves corresponding to two types of afferent neurons. Fast-onset, sharp, localised pain is mediated by A-delta neurons, and slower-onset, dull, poorly localised pain is mediated by C fibres.

It is important to note that the first-order neurons of the dorsal column pathway are large and myelinated, whilst the first-order neurons of the spinothalamic tract are small and thinly myelinated in nature. Therefore, the transmission of sensory information is faster across the dorsal column pathway than the spinothalamic tract.

The anatomy of the key ascending tracts is summarised in **Table 1.9** and **Figure 1.25**.

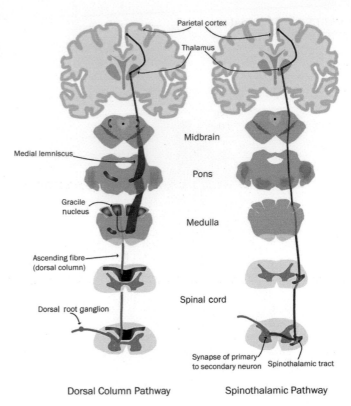

FIGURE 1.25 Anatomy of the dorsal column and spinothalamic pathways. (Courtesy of John Ward.)

CLINICAL NOTE

Lesions to the principal ascending tracts (see **Tables 1.10** and **1.11**).

Descending Tracts

Descending tracts transmit motor signals from the cortex to the motor neurons of the spinal cord (and brainstem) which innervate skeletal muscles. These tracts are involved in the regulation of motion (voluntary and involuntary), muscle tone, posture, and muscle reflexes. These tracts can be categorised into two groups depending on whether they pass through the medullary pyramids: the pyramidal tracts involved in the voluntary control of the muscles, and the extrapyramidal tracts involved in the involuntary control of the muscles, e.g., tone, posture, and balance.

This section will focus on the key pyramidal tracts, which include the corticospinal tract and the corticobulbar tract.

Corticospinal Tract

The corticospinal tract arises from several regions within the brain, mainly from the motor regions of the brain, including the primary motor cortex (precentral gyrus), supplementary motor area, and premotor cortex and from the somatic sensory cortex, parietal lobe, and cingulate gyrus. The tract projects ipsilaterally through the corona radiata, posterior limb of the internal capsule, crus cerebri, pons, and medulla. In the medulla, the

TABLE 1.9: Neuronal arrangement of the key ascending pathways

	First-Order Neuron	Second-Order Neuron	Third-Order Neuron
Dorsal column pathway	The cell body is found in the dorsal root ganglion	The cell body is found within the nucleus cuneatus and nucleus gracilis in the posterior medulla oblongata	The cell body is found in the ventral posterolateral nucleus of the thalamus
	Ascends ipsilaterally in the dorsal aspect of the spinal cord (via fasciculus gracilis and fasciculus cuneatus)	Decussates in the medulla oblongata ("great sensory decussation") and ascends contralaterally as the medial lemniscus	Ascends through the posterior limb of the internal capsule
	Synapses with second-order neurons in the medulla oblongata	Synapses with third-order neurons in the ventral posterolateral nucleus of the thalamus	Ends in the somatosensory cortex of the brain (postcentral gyrus of the parietal lobe)
Spinothalamic tract	The cell body is found in the dorsal root ganglion	The cell body is found in the spinal cord	The cell body is found in the ventral posterolateral nucleus of the thalamus
	Descend or ascend one or two vertebral levels within the spinal cord	Decussates in the anterior white commissure and ascends in the anterolateral spinal cord	Ascends through the posterior limb of the internal capsule
	Synapses with second-order neurons in the substantia gelatinosa of Rolando of the spinal cord	Synapses with third-order neurons in the ventral posterolateral nucleus of the thalamus	Terminates in the somatosensory cortex of the brain (postcentral gyrus of the parietal lobe)

corticospinal tract, together with the corticobulbar tract, form the pyramids. When the tract reaches the inferior boundary of the medulla, at the lower limit of the pyramids, it separates into two tracts: the lateral corticospinal tract and the anterior corticospinal tract.

The lateral (crossed) corticospinal tract decussates at the inferior margin of the medulla, while the anterior corticospinal tract continues to descend ipsilaterally into the cervical/thoracic region of the spinal cord before decussating at the respective segment. **Roughly 10% of corticospinal tract fibres continue without decussation at the level of the foramen magnum as the anterior (uncrossed) tract**.

The corticospinal tracts are formed of a two-neuron chain. Upper motor neurons (UMNs) that form the lateral corticospinal tract synapse with the lower motor neurons (LMNs) that supply all the skeletal muscles involved in controlling the movement of the limbs. In contrast, UMNs that form the anterior corticospinal tract synapse with LMNs that supply all the skeletal muscles involved in producing axial movement of the trunk. The axons of the LMNs leave the spinal cord to synapse with muscle fibres at the neuromuscular junction (NMJ).

The lateral (crossed) corticospinal tract is depicted in **Figure 1.26**.

Corticobulbar Tract

Corticobulbar tract fibres originate mainly from the primary motor cortex, but also the somatosensory cortex and the middle frontal gyrus.

The tract follows a similar path to the corticospinal tract and is also formed of a two-neuron chain. It descends ipsilaterally through the corona radiata and the genu of the internal capsule into the brainstem to synapse with LMNs of the cranial nerves (trigeminal, facial, vagus, spinal accessory, and hypoglossal). The LMNs usually receive a bilateral innervation (ipsilateral and contralateral) except for the lower facial and hypoglossal nuclei. LMNs arise from these nuclei and synapse with muscle fibres found within the face, head, and neck.

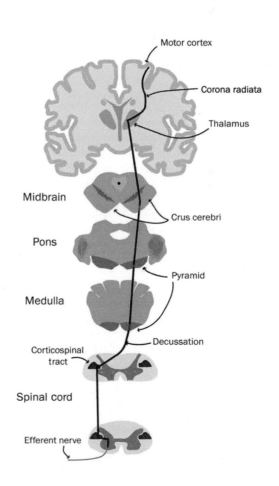

Corticospinal Pathway

FIGURE 1.26 Anatomy of the corticospinal pathway. (Courtesy of John Ward.)

Each facial nucleus is separated into an upper and lower compartment, supplying muscles of facial expression in the respective upper and lower segments of the face. **The upper facial nucleus receives bilateral innervation, whereas the lower facial nucleus receives contralateral innervation only. The hypoglossal nucleus receives contralateral innervation only.** This has clinical implications.

crying (pseudobulbar affect), dysarthria, dysphagia and slowness of speech, and hyperreflexia.

Blood Supply

The spinal cord is supplied by both vertical and segmental arteries.

TABLE 1.10: Dorsal column pathway lesions

Site of Lesion	Symptoms Presented by the Patient	Common Causes	Sensory Testing
Above the point of decussation (e.g., internal capsule)	Contralateral loss of vibration, proprioception, and tactile sensation below the level of the lesion	Causes include subacute combined degeneration (vitamin B_{12} deficiency), multiple sclerosis, trauma, neurosyphilis, space-occupying lesions including tumours, cysts syringomyelia, paraneoplastic, and genetic diseases	The best way to test for this pathway is by using a low-frequency tuning fork (128 Hz) (vibration) and to test position sense (proprioception); positive Romberg's sign
Below the point of decussation (e.g., spinal cord)	Ipsilateral loss of sensory sensation below the level of the lesion		

TABLE 1.11: Spinothalamic tract lesions

Site of Lesion	Symptoms Presented by the Patient	Common Causes	Sensory Testing
Spinothalamic tract	Contralateral loss of pain and temperature, pressure, and light touch sensation below the level of the lesion	Common causes include multiple sclerosis, space-occupying lesions, and penetrating injuries	The best way to test for this pathway is by using a pin prick to induce pain
Anterior white commissure	Bilateral loss sensation at the level of the lesion		

CLINICAL NOTE

Lesions to the principal descending tracts
UMN and LMN lesions present differently in different clinical settings. Patients with UMN lesions present with muscle weakness (pyramidal weakness), hyperreflexia, hypertonia, spastic paralysis with clasp-knife spasticity, and Babinski's sign. Patients with LMN lesions present with muscle weakness, muscle atrophy, fasciculations, hyporeflexia, hypotonia, and flaccid paralysis (**Table 1.12**).

TABLE 1.12: Corticospinal tract lesions

Site of Lesion	Clinical Presentation
UMN lesion above the point of decussation (above the level of the foramen magnum)	Symptoms associated with an UMN lesion on the contralateral side of the body
UMN lesion below the point of decussation	Symptoms associated with an UMN lesion on the ipsilateral side of the body
LMN lesion	Symptoms associated with a LMN lesion on the ipsilateral side of the body

Pseudobulbar Palsy (Corticobulbar Tract)
Pseudobulbar palsy is a medical condition that arises when both sides of the corticobulbar tract become injured. Patients with this condition present with uncontrollable episodes of laughing and

Vertical Arteries
Vertical arteries run longitudinally along the length of the spinal cord. There are three vertical arteries: the anterior spinal artery and the paired posterior spinal arteries.

The anterior spinal artery originates from the vertebral artery and passes through the ventral median fissure, supplying the anterior two-thirds of the spinal cord.

The paired posterior spinal arteries originate from the vertebral artery or the posterior inferior cerebellar artery (PICA) and run along the posterolateral aspect of the spinal cord, supplying the posterior one-third of the spinal cord.

The anterior and posterior vertical arteries are joined by an anastomosis through the pia mater called the arterial vasocorona, which encircles the spinal cord, supplying the lateral aspect. Inferiorly, the descending vertical arteries anastomose again to form the cruciate anastomosis of the conus medullaris, supplying the distal aspect of the spinal cord.

Segmental Arteries
The blood supply provided by the vertical arteries is reinforced by segmental arteries that enter the spinal cord at each segmental level. Segmental arteries at different levels of the spinal cord have different origins, e.g., vertebral arteries, PICAs, ascending cervical arteries, deep cervical arteries, posterior intercostal arteries, lumbar arteries, and lateral sacral arteries.

In the thoracic region, each segmental artery gives rise to an anterior and posterior radicular artery. In addition, at some vertebral levels, the segmental artery gives rise to segmental medullary arteries, which join the anterior spinal artery and the paired posterior spinal arteries. The artery of Adamkiewicz is the largest segmental medullary artery, originating from the aorta at the level of T9–L2, supplying the lower half of the spinal cord (**Figure 1.27**).

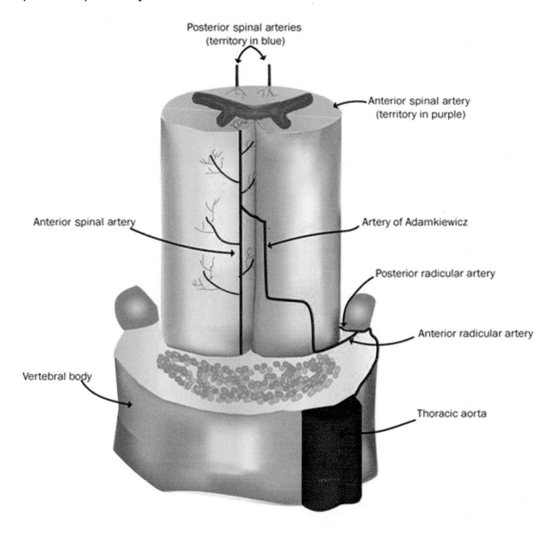

FIGURE 1.27 Blood supply to the spinal cord. (Courtesy of John Ward.)

Venous Drainage

The spinal cord is drained by three anterior and three posterior spinal veins, which run along the length of the spinal cord, receiving blood from radicular veins. This network of spinal veins drains into the internal and external vertebral plexuses, which drain into the systemic circulation. The internal vertebral plexus also communicates superiorly with the dural venous sinuses, and inferiorly, in the male, with the prostatic plexus.

CLINICAL NOTE

Spinal cord ischaemia
Spinal cord segments T3–T7 are most vulnerable to ischaemia, as these regions receive the smallest amount of arterial input from radicular arteries.

Spinal Cord Pathologies

Several factors can contribute to pathologies within the spinal cord, including developmental issues, trauma, infection, inflammatory disease, autoimmune attacks, vascular dysfunction, nutrient deficiency, and genetic predisposition. The following segments of this section focus on a variety of clinical disorders that are associated with the spinal cord. These conditions have been stratified as traumatic, compressive, or non-traumatic, with respect to aetiology.

Traumatic Causes of Spinal Cord Damage

Brown-Séquard Syndrome

Brown-Séquard syndrome is a rare spinal disorder characterised by a hemisection of the spinal cord. Commonly caused by penetrating trauma (e.g., a stab wound), the condition causes the individual to present with ipsilateral UMN signs below the level of the lesion (corticospinal tract lesion) and ipsilateral LMN signs at the level of the lesion (flaccid paralysis). Sensory deficits, including ipsilateral loss of vibration, pressure, touch, and proprioceptive sense (dorsal columns lesion), as well as contralateral (spinothalamic tract) loss of temperature and pain sensations, are also seen below the level of the lesion. If the hemisection involves the oculosympathetic pathway, the patient will also present with symptoms associated with Horner's syndrome, including miosis, partial ptosis, and anhidrosis.

In clinical practice, a complete hemisection of the spinal cord is rare; therefore, patients typically present with some motor, sensory, and autonomic deficits representing damage to certain tracts within the spinal cord.

Central Cord Syndrome

Central cord syndrome is the most common form of incomplete spinal cord injury (SCI). The injury is commonly cervical in nature, and patients present with a characteristic cape-like distribution of pain and temperature sensory loss, as well as greater levels of muscle weakness in their upper limbs than their lower limbs and bladder dysfunction. This condition arises following trauma and falls in young patients or hyperextension of the cervical spine in the elderly.

Anterior Cord Syndrome

Anterior cord syndrome is an incomplete cord syndrome characterised by interruption of blood flow (ischaemia of the anterior spinal artery), resulting in damage to the anterior two-thirds of the spinal cord.

As the spinothalamic and corticospinal tracts are found within this region, patients present with sensory deficits, such as loss of crude touch, pressure, pain, and temperature sensation. These patients may become paralysed below the level of the lesion and may present with bladder/bowel, autonomic (e.g., hypotension), and sexual dysfunction.

following a lesion to the dorsal column pathway. The lesion follows as a result of direct trauma to the spinal cord, or the interruption of blood flow through the posterior spinal arteries (**Figure 1.28**).

Epidemiology of Spinal Cord Injuries

The annual incidence of traumatic SCIs varies worldwide. Among developed regions, the incidence of traumatic SCI is higher in North America (39 cases per million individuals) than in Australia (16 cases per million individuals) or Western Europe (15 cases per million individuals), owing to higher rates of violent crime and self-harm (Ahuja et al., 2017).

Cervical spine injury comprises about half of these cases, with motor vehicle accidents, falls, and sport-related as the most common reasons for injury. SCIs are an economic burden on modern society, with estimated lifetime costs of £1.12 million per case in the United Kingdom (McDaid et al., 2019). These injuries are debilitating for the individual and require long-term care. Improvement in patients' function varies, depending on the severity of the injury; however, the regenerative capacity of the CNS is minimal. Current academic research aims to identify ways to regenerate neurons that have become damaged during the injury process and to restore connectivity in order to re-establish functionality (National Institute for Health and Care Excellence [NICE], 2016).

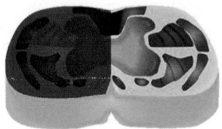

Brown Sequard Syndrome

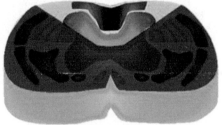

Anterior Cord Syndrome

Central Cord Syndrome

Posterior Cord Syndrome

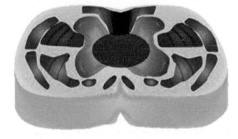

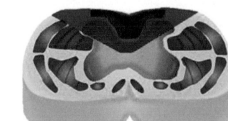

FIGURE 1.28 Traumatic spinal cord pathology. (Courtesy of John Ward.)

Proprioceptive and vibratory sensations remain intact within these patients, as the dorsal column pathway resides in the posterior third of the spinal cord.

Posterior Cord Syndrome

Posterior cord syndrome is an incomplete cord syndrome characterised by the loss of proprioceptive and vibratory sensations

Compressive Causes of Spinal Cord Injury/Defect

Spinal Cord and Nerve Root Compression

Spinal cord compression can be caused by an array of pathologies. Common examples include intervertebral disc disease, tumours, infection, haematomas, cysts, or pathological fractures (fractures that occur in diseased vertebrae commonly due to secondary cancer spread from prostate, breast, and lung cancers). Clinically, one should check for UMN signs, sensory loss, sphincter control, and signs of infection (the latter may indicate an extradural abscess).

Whilst compression of the cord itself produces UMN signs due to corticospinal tract damage, compression of the emerging spinal nerves produces LMN signs. **This is commonly caused by herniation of an intervertebral disc, which classically protrudes posterolaterally.**

Cauda Equina Syndrome

Cauda equina syndrome is a collection of signs and symptoms caused by the compression of lumbar and sacral nerves below the end of the spinal cord, most commonly due to the herniation of intervertebral discs of the lumbar vertebrae. Patients present with an acute onset of lower back pain, saddle anaesthesia, sciatica, hyporeflexia, and bladder, bowel, and sexual dysfunction, as well as a reduction in anal tone. This condition is a medical emergency because of the possibility of paralysis of the lower limbs, as well as permanent damage to the bladder and bowels. This condition needs urgent neurosurgical referral.

Learning Point

The cauda equina is composed of L2–L5, S1–S5, and coccygeal nerve spinal roots within the dural sac.

Non-Traumatic Causes of Spinal Cord Injury/Defect

Non-traumatic SCI can result from many causes. Notable causes, not discussed in detail here, include infections and inflammation, which present variably depending on their location and the spinal segments involved.

Degenerative Changes

Spinal stenosis most commonly occurs due to spinal degeneration occurring with age. The facet joints enlarge as they become arthritic, osteophytes protrude into the spinal canal, and the supportive ligaments stiffen and thicken, all contributing to encroachment upon the spinal cord. Compressive symptoms include backache, pain radiating down the buttocks and calves, and pins and needles in the legs and feet. Symptoms classically arise with long periods of standing or walking, and improve upon spine flexion.

Learning Point

In contrast to patients with vascular claudications, patients with spinal canal stenosis have normal pulses and ABPI on both sides. The straight-leg-raise test (SLR) is restricted on both sides.

Syringomyelia

The cape-like distribution of pain and temperature loss seen in central cord syndromes can also be caused by syringomyelia, a cystic collection of CSF within the central canal. As with central cord syndromes, an inverse paraplegia is also seen where motor weakness is seen predominantly in the upper limbs. This condition has a strong association with Chiari malformation – the protrusion of the cerebellar tonsils through the foramen magnum.

Acute Poliomyelitis

Acute poliomyelitis is an infectious disease caused by poliovirus. The virus enters the CNS by either crossing the blood–brain barrier or by transport via a peripheral nerve.

Patients with this disease present with muscle weakness and muscle atrophy as a result of damage to the anterior motor neurons within the spinal cord and the brainstem.

The disease is relatively rare, with a low incidence in the UK. This is attributable to the introduction of the polio vaccine as part of the childhood immunisation programme.

Multiple Sclerosis

Multiple sclerosis (MS) is a progressive neurodegenerative disorder characterised by demyelination, where the immune system attacks the myelin protective sheath that covers the nerve cells in the brain and spinal cord. This damage disrupts communication between neurons. Immune cells attack oligodendrocytes and myelin sheaths to disrupt communication between adjacent neurons. Lesions can occur anywhere within the CNS; therefore, symptoms vary widely amongst different patients.

Transverse Myelitis

Transverse myelitis is a condition characterised by the inflammation of whole spinal cord segment(s) involving the entire width of the spinal cord, with subsequent demyelination and disruption of electrical signals passing through the spinal cord. The exact aetiology of the condition remains to be elucidated, but it can arise following infections, autoimmune attacks (e.g., MS), and other inflammatory disorders. Treatment relies on the underlying causes of the disease, with anti-microbials, corticosteroids, and immunosuppressants often used as therapies for treating these patients.

Guillain-Barré Syndrome

Guillain-Barré syndrome (GBS) affects the peripheral rather than central nervous system but is of significant clinical importance. It is a rare autoimmune condition triggered by an upper respiratory tract infection or a gastrointestinal infection. Patients experience an "ascending paralysis", sensory deficits, and absent deep tendon reflexes. If the paralysis extends up to the muscles of respiration, the condition becomes life-threatening.

Lumbar Puncture (Spinal Tap)

A lumbar puncture is a medical procedure that involves the percutaneous aspiration of CSF from the subarachnoid space of the spinal cord for diagnostic purposes (commonly for the diagnosis of meningitis or encephalitis). It can also be performed for therapeutic purposes, including drainage of CSF when pressure is high, intrathecal injection of local anaesthetic (spinal anaesthesia, *vide infra*), or chemotherapy. This procedure is usually performed below the L2 level, at the level of L3/L4 or L4/L5, to avoid the conus medullaris. To locate this region, one must palpate for the iliac crests, usually while the patient is seated (see **Section 6**, Pelvis and Perineum). A lumbar puncture must not be performed in a patient with raised intracranial pressure for fear of coning of the brainstem through the foramen magnum.

Epidural versus Spinal Anaesthesia

Spinal anaesthesia is a medical procedure involving the administration of anaesthetic drugs into the subarachnoid space. The substances injected take immediate effect (within

5 minutes), as substances need to diffuse only a short distance towards the nerves of the cauda equina.

Epidural anaesthesia involves the administration of anaesthetics into the epidural space of the spinal cord. It is usually carried out in patients undergoing labour to alleviate pain associated with uterine contractions. However, it can also be performed in individuals undergoing major thoracic or abdominal surgery to continue postoperative pain control by topping up with opioids. The level of anaesthesia can be varied to suit the surgical indication; there is more flexibility than spinal anaesthesia, as the needle lies outside the coverings of the spinal cord. The analgesia takes a longer time to take effect, as the anaesthetic needs to diffuse through the meningeal layers before affecting nervous tissue within the spinal cord.

The most important side effect of spinal and epidural anaesthesia is hypotension. This side effect is more pronounced in patients undergoing spinal anaesthesia. Headaches can also follow lumbar puncture or spinal anaesthesia. There is a risk of spinal haematoma in patients undergoing anticoagulant therapy, and the coagulation status should be well optimised before embarking on spinal or epidural anaesthesia and until the epidural catheter is removed (**Figure 1.29**).

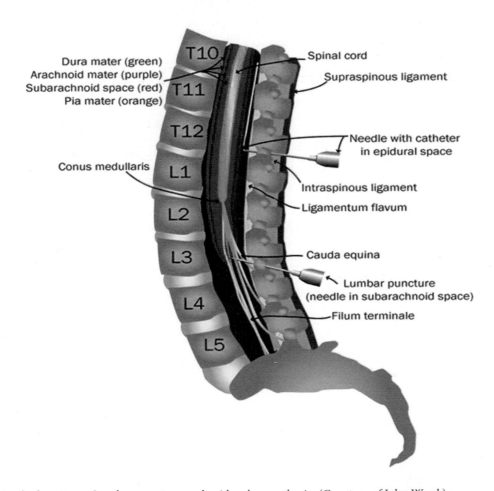

FIGURE 1.29   Applied anatomy: Lumbar puncture and epidural anaesthesia. (Courtesy of John Ward.)

Revision Questions

Written Questions

Q1. Where do the internal carotid arteries enter the skull?

Q2. Which arteries anastomose to connect the circle of Willis, and where do they branch from?

Q3. What are the four main mechanisms of stroke?

Q4. If the lateral part of the cerebral hemisphere appears ischaemic, which artery is most likely to be occluded?

Q5. Why do most strokes affect the lateral part of the cerebral hemisphere?

Q6. At how many weeks gestation does the neural tube form, and which germ layer is it formed from?
   a. 3 weeks gestation, ectoderm
   b. 3 weeks gestation, mesoderm
   c. 3 weeks gestation, endoderm
   d. 12 weeks gestation, ectoderm
   e. 12 weeks gestation, mesoderm

Q7. The developing basal plate gives rise to neurons with which function in the adult spinal cord?
   a. Sensory neurons
   b. Motor neurons
   c. Autonomic neurons
   d. Rami communicantes
   e. Mixed spinal nerve

Q8. How many pairs of nerves emerge from the spinal cord?
   a. 27: C7, T12, L5, S2, Co1
   b. 29: C7, T12, L5, S2, Co3
   c. 29: C8, T12, L5, S3, Co1
   d. 31: C8, T12, L5, S5, Co1
   e. 31: C8, T10, L5, S5, Co3

Q9. In which parts of the spinal cord do the two enlargements corresponding to plexuses innervating the limbs lie?
   a. Cervical and thoracic
   b. Thoracic and lumbar
   c. Lumbar and sacral
   d. Thoracic and sacral
   e. Cervical and lumbar

Q10. Which meningeal layer thickens to form the denticulate ligament?
   a. Pia
   b. Arachnoid
   c. Dura
   d. Arachnoid and dura
   e. Pia and arachnoid

Q11. What best describes the outflow of the sympathetic nervous system (SNS)?
   a. Cranio-sacral (S2–S4)
   b. Sacral only (below S2)
   c. Thoracolumbar (T1–L5)
   d. Thoracolumbar (T1–L2)
   e. All levels of the spinal cord

Q12. Where does the spinothalamic tract decussate?
   a. The great sensory decussation
   b. The anterior white commissure
   c. The arcuate fibres
   d. The caudal medullary pyramids
   e. It runs ipsilaterally

Q13. How many neurons form the corticospinal tract?
   a. *Two-neuron chain:* greater motor neuron, lesser motor neuron
   b. *Two-neuron chain:* afferent motor neuron, efferent motor neuron
   c. *Two-neuron chain:* upper motor neuron, lower motor neuron
   d. *Three-neuron chain:* primary order, secondary order, tertiary order
   e. *Three-neuron chain:* first order, second order, third order

Q14. From which parent vessel does the artery of Adamkiewicz arise and at which spinal level?
   a. Vertebral artery, C5–C7
   b. Vertebral artery, C1–C3
   c. Anterior spinal artery, T9–L2
   d. Aorta, T5–T7
   e. Aorta, T9–L2

Q15. Which ascending/descending pathway(s) run in the territory supplied by the posterior spinal artery?
   a. Dorsal columns
   b. Dorsal columns and spinothalamic pathway
   c. Spinothalamic pathway
   d. Anterior corticospinal and spinothalamic
   e. Medial lemniscus

Spotter Questions

Q1. Which of the following best describes the fibre bundle indicated by the arrow?

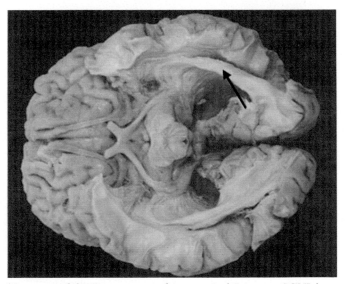

(Courtesy of the Department of Anatomical Sciences, SGUL.)

   a. Anterior commissure
   b. Corpus callosum
   c. Crus cerebri
   d. Fornix
   e. Optic radiation

Q2. Which of the following functions will be impaired by damage to the fibre bundle indicated by the arrow?
   a. Balance
   b. Hearing
   c. Olfaction
   d. Taste
   e. Vision

Q3. Which of the following best describes the feature indicated by the arrow?

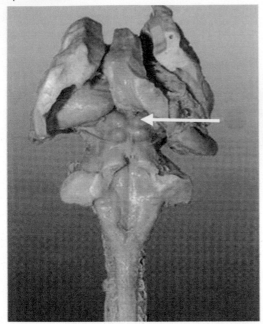

(Courtesy of the Department of Anatomical Sciences, SGUL.)

   a.   Inferior cerebellar peduncle
   b.   Inferior colliculus
   c.   Pulvinar
   d.   Superior cerebellar peduncle
   e.   Superior colliculus

Q4. Which of the following best describes the function of the feature indicated by the arrow?
   a.   Control of balance
   b.   Control of hearing
   c.   Control of visual reflexes
   d.   Processing of touch sensation
   e.   Processing of vision

Q5. Which of the following best describes the feature indicated by the arrow?

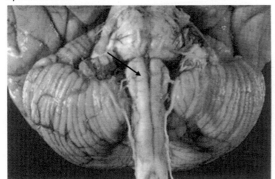

(Courtesy of the Department of Anatomical Sciences, SGUL.)

   a.   Flocculus
   b.   Olive
   c.   Pons
   d.   Pyramid
   e.   Tonsil

Q6. Which of the following best describes the function of the feature indicated by the arrow?
   a.   It is a source of an important input to the cerebellum from the cerebral cortex
   b.   It is made up of fibres carrying spinal input to the thalamus
   c.   It is made up of fibres carrying spinal input to the cerebellum
   d.   It is made up of fibres carrying vestibular input to the cerebellum
   e.   It is made up of fibres projecting from the motor cortex to the spinal motor neurons

Q7. Which of the following best describes the region of grey matter indicated by the arrow?

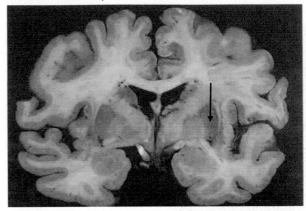

(Courtesy of the Department of Anatomical Sciences, SGUL.)

   a.   Caudate nucleus
   b.   Globus pallidus
   c.   Insula
   d.   Putamen
   e.   Thalamus

Q8. Which of the following describes the role of the region of grey matter indicated by the arrow?
   a.   Cognitive function
   b.   Endocrine regulation
   c.   Episodic memory
   d.   Motor function
   e.   Sensory regulation

Q9. Which of the following best describes the structures indicated by the arrow?

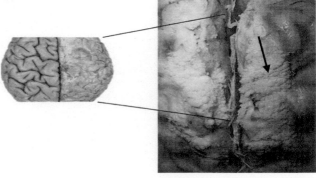

(Courtesy of the Department of Anatomical Sciences, SGUL.)

a.   Arachnoid granulations
b.   Falx cerebri
c.   Inferior sagittal sinus
d.   Superior sagittal sinus
e.   Tentorium cerebelli

Q10.   Which of the following best describes the function of the structures indicated by the arrow?
a.   Reabsorption of CSF from the subarachnoid space
b.   Formation of CSF
c.   Secretion of neurohormones
d.   Stabilisation of the brain within the cranial cavity
e.   Transfer of blood from the cerebral cortex to the superior sagittal sinus

Q11.   Which structure is indicated by the arrow?

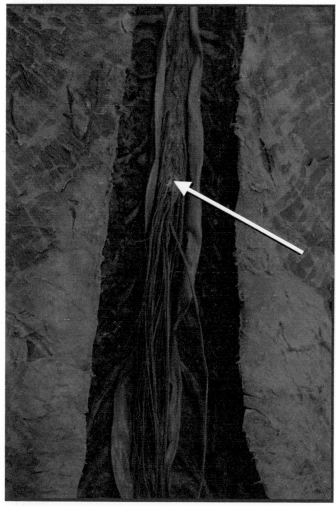

(Courtesy of the Department of Anatomical Sciences, SGUL.)

a.   Cauda equina
b.   Conus medullaris
c.   Denticulate ligament
d.   Filum terminale
e.   Pia mater

Q12.   At which vertebral level does this structure taper off?
a.   T11/T12
b.   L1/L2
c.   L2/L3
d.   L3/L4
e.   L4/L5

Q13.   Which structure is indicated by the arrow?

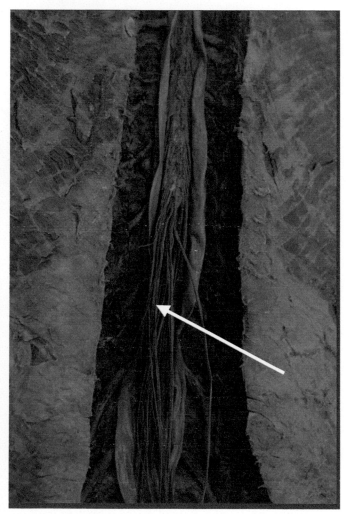

(Courtesy of the Department of Anatomical Sciences, SGUL.)

a.   Conus medullaris
b.   Cauda equina
c.   Filum terminale
d.   Arachnoid mater
e.   Dura mater

Q14.   Which nerves make up this structure?
a.   C1–C4
b.   C5–C8
c.   T1–T6
d.   T7–T12
e.   Lumbosacral nerves

Q15. Which of the following functions would be impaired by damage to the region indicated by the arrow?

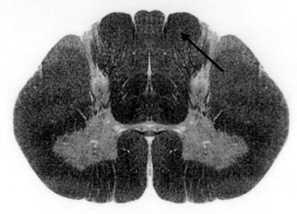

(Courtesy of the Department of Anatomical Sciences, SGUL.)

a. Control of upper limb flexors
b. Fine touch perception
c. Pain perception
d. Temperature perception
e. Control of lower limb extensors

Q16. Which of the following best describes the level of the spinal cord section shown in the image?
a. C4
b. L1
c. L5
d. T1
e. T7

Answers

Written Questions

A1: The internal carotid arteries enter the middle cranial fossa through the carotid canal (through temporal bone).

A2: The anterior communicating artery connects the two anterior cerebral arteries. On each side, the anterior cerebral artery branches from the internal carotid artery, which is connected to the posterior communicating artery. The posterior communicating artery connects to the posterior cerebral artery, completing the circle of Willis.

A3: The four main causes of stroke are thrombosis, embolism, hypoperfusion, and haemorrhage.

A4: The middle cerebral artery is most likely to be occluded because it supplies the lateral portions of the cerebrum. The middle cerebral arteries are branches of the internal carotid arteries.

A5: Most strokes affect the lateral part of the cerebral hemisphere, as the middle cerebral arteries are a continuation of the internal carotid arteries, which carry about 80% of the blood supply to the brain.

A6:	a	A11:	d
A7:	b	A12:	b
A8:	d	A13:	c
A9:	e	A14:	e
A10:	a	A15:	a

Spotter Questions

A1:	e	A9:	a
A2:	e	A10:	a
A3:	e	A11:	b
A4:	c	A12:	b
A5:	d	A13:	b
A6:	e	A14:	e
A7:	d	A15:	b
A8:	d	A16:	a

Further Reading

Age of Fontanelles/Cranial Sutures Closure | Carta. 2017. Carta.anthropogeny.org. [cited 10 October 2017]. Available from: https://carta.anthropogeny.org/moca/topics/age-closure-fontanelles-sutures

Ahuja CS et al., *Nat Rev Dis Primers*. 2017. 27(3):17018. DOI: 10.1038/nrdp.2017.18. PMID: 28447605.

Middle Cerebral Artery Stroke Causes, Symptoms & Treatments Middle Cerebral Artery Stroke Causes, Symptoms & Treatments [Internet]. 2017. New Health Advisor [cited 15 August 2017]. Available from: http://www.newhealthadvisor.com/middle-cerebral-artery-stroke.html

Johns Hopkins Medicine Health Library [Internet]. 2017. Cerebral Venous Sinus Thrombosis(CVST)Hopkinsmedicine.org.[cited16July2017].Availablefrom: https://www.hopkinsmedicine.org/healthlibrary/conditions/nervous_system_disorders/cerebral_venous_sinus_thrombosis_134,69

Johns, P. 2014. Clinical Neuroscience. Elsevier, Edinburgh: Churchill Livingstone.

McDaid et al. 2019. *Spinal Cord* 57(9):778–788. DOI:10.1038/s41393-019-0285-1

National Institute for Health and Care Excellence (NICE). 2016. Spinal injury: Assessment and initial management [Internet]. [London]: NICE. (Clinical guideline [NG41]). Available from: https://www.nice.org.uk/guidance/ng41/evidence/full-guideline-2358425776

National Spinal Cord Injury Strategy Board (NSCISB). 2012. The Initial Management of Adults with Spinal Cord Injuries [Internet]. MASCIP. Available from: https://www.mascip.co.uk/wp-content/uploads/2015/03/The-Initial-Management-of-Adults-with-SCI.-NSCISB.pdf

Strigenz T. 2014. Cauda equina syndrome. *J Pain Palliat Care Pharmacother.* 28(1):75–7.

2

ANATOMY OF THE HEAD AND NECK

Reviewed by Qassim F. Baker, David Sunnucks, and Georga Longhurst

Learning Objectives

- Scalp
- Bones of the skull, cranial fossae, and foramina
- Eye and orbit
- Infratemporal fossa
- Ear
- Nose and paranasal sinuses
- Cranial nerves
- Oral cavity, tongue, and palate
- Salivary glands: parotid and submandibular glands
- Cervical vertebrae
- Fascia and nerves of the neck, along with the suprahyoid and infrahyoid muscles
- Triangles of the neck and their contents
- Blood supply of the head and neck: carotid arteries, subclavian vessels, and jugular veins
- Hyoid bone, larynx, and trachea
- Thyroid and parathyroid glands
- Lymphatic drainage of the head and neck
- The clinical approach to the diagnosis of neck swellings
- Pharynx and cervical oesophagus

The Scalp

The scalp is the area of the head that extends from the forehead to the superior nuchal line of the occipital bone and extends laterally to the zygomatic arch. It consists of the following five layers, which are easy to memorise using the mnemonic SCALP:

S: skin, which has abundant sebaceous glands and hair follicles, so it is a common site for sebaceous cysts.

C: connective tissue, which has a rich blood supply, therefore scalp lacerations bleed profusely.

A: aponeurosis (epicranial) of the **occipitofrontalis** muscle.

The occipitofrontalis muscle is supplied by the facial nerve and functions to move the scalp on the skull and to raise the eyebrows during the expression of surprise (one of the clinical tests to examine the facial nerve).

The anterior frontal belly originates from the subcutaneous tissues of the eyebrows and nose, in addition to the zygomatic arch.

The posterior occipital belly originates from the superior nuchal line of the occipital bone.

Both bellies insert into the epicranial aponeurosis, which is attached laterally to the temporal fascia.

L: loose connective tissue, where fluids, such as pus and blood, can collect.

P: periosteum (pericranium), which adheres to the sutures of the calvaria.

Arterial Supply of the Scalp

The arterial supply of the scalp is profuse and arises from branches of the internal carotid artery via the supratrochlear and supraorbital arteries arising from the ophthalmic artery and the external carotid artery via the superficial temporal, posterior auricular, and occipital arteries.

- *Supratrochlear artery:* supplies the medial region of the forehead
- *Supraorbital artery:* supplies the lateral region of the forehead
- *Superficial temporal artery:* supplies the frontal and temporal regions of the scalp
- *Posterior auricular artery:* supplies the region superior and posterior to the ear
- *Occipital artery:* supplies the posterior scalp

Venous Drainage of the Scalp

The anterior aspects of the scalp and forehead are drained by the supratrochlear and supraorbital veins, which unite to form the facial vein. The posterior aspect of the scalp is drained by the occipital vein, which forms the suboccipital venous plexus. Laterally, the scalp is drained by the superficial temporal vein. This unites with the maxillary vein to form the retromandibular vein. All of the veins of the scalp eventually drain into the external jugular vein, which joins the subclavian vein at the root of the neck.

Note that there are anastomoses of the veins of the scalp and the diploic veins of the cortical bone with the intracranial venous plexuses, through emissary veins. This is of clinical significance, as infection can spread from the scalp to intracranial structures.

Innervation of the Scalp

Sensory supply is by the trigeminal nerve (CN V) and cervical plexus.

Anteriorly, the scalp is supplied by the divisions of the trigeminal nerve:

- Supratrochlear and supraorbital nerves arise from the ophthalmic division (CN V1)
- Zygomaticotemporal nerve arises from the maxillary division (CN V2)
- Auriculotemporal nerve arises from the mandibular division (CN V3)

Posteriorly, the scalp is supplied by branches from the greater (dorsal ramus of C2) and lesser occipital nerves (ventral ramus of C2), which arise from the cervical plexus.

DOI: 10.1201/9781003312895-3

Bones of the Skull

The skull contains 22 bones (8 form the neurocranium, plus 14 facial bones or viscerocranium) (**Figure 2.1**).

The bones of the neurocranium are one frontal, one occipital, two parietal, two temporal, one ethmoid, and one sphenoid.

The bones of the facial skeleton are one vomer, two nasal conchae, two nasal bones, two maxillae, one mandible, two palatine bones, two zygomatic bones, and two lacrimal bones.

The neurocranium may be divided into the calvaria (cranial vault) and cranial base. The bones of the calvaria are mostly flat and consist of outer and inner tables with cancellous marrow in between them (the diploë, or diploic bone).

Sutures: the joints between the bones of the skull are called sutures. These are fibrous joints that allow only a small amount of movement. Premature closure of sutures is called craniosynostosis, which clinically may manifest as increased intracranial pressure, with or without hydrocephalus and mental retardation.

Four major sutures are described:

- Sagittal suture between the parietal bones
- Coronal suture between the frontal and parietal bones
- Lambdoid suture between the occipital and parietal bones
- Squamous suture (lateral suture) between the parietal and temporal bones

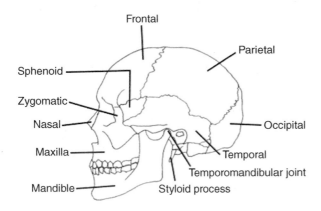

FIGURE 2.1 Lateral view of skull showing the positions of the skull bones. (Courtesy of Calum Harrington-Vogt.)

Learning Point

The *pterion* is the point on lateral side of the skull where four bones (sphenoid, temporal, frontal, and parietal) meet. The bone is thin here, so this is the weakest part of the bony skull. Blunt trauma may thus fracture the pterion, resulting in laceration of the anterior branch of the middle meningeal artery that lies deep to it, causing an extradural haematoma between the bone and dura. Its surface anatomy is two finger-breadths superior to the zygomatic arch and one thumb-breadth lateral to the side of the orbit.

The **fontanelles** are soft regions between the cranial bones of the infant skull. They are important because they allow the skull to deform during birth (known as caput moulding), and they stretch to accommodate the growing brain. There are two major fontanelles in the new-born. The anterior fontanelle is the largest and lies between the frontal suture (frontal bones are separate in the new-born) and the parietal bones (at the junction of the frontal, coronal, and sagittal sutures). The posterior fontanelle lies between the parietal bones and the occipital bone (the junction between the sagittal and lambdoid sutures).

The posterior fontanelle closes (ossifies) 2 to 3 months after birth, whilst the anterior fontanelle closes between 18 and 24 months after birth. In some individuals (prevalence varies according to race) the frontal suture fails to close, leaving a persistent metopic suture in the adult.

CLINICAL NOTE

Anterior and posterior fontanelles are important clinically because they allow clinicians to undertake ultrasound imaging of the fetal brain to look for pathology (e.g., hydrocephalus), because the unossified cartilage fontanelles act as acoustic windows and do not absorb much ultrasound energy.

A bulging fontanelle may indicate increased intracranial pressure (before closure of the fontanelles) and is seen in conditions such as encephalitis, meningitis, and hydrocephaly. Sunken fontanelles are a sign of dehydration. Additionally, a cerebrospinal fluid (CSF) drain can be placed percutaneously into a fontanelle to relieve an acute hydrocephalus.

QUIZ QUESTION

Q. Name the bones that form the calvaria.

Base of the Skull

The base of the skull is described as having three fossae (**Figure 2.2**):

- Anterior cranial fossa
- Middle cranial fossa
- Posterior cranial fossa

The contents of each fossa are shown in **Table 2.1**.

CLINICAL NOTE

HEAD TRAUMA

Head trauma can be an isolated injury or part of trauma to other body regions. Following paramedic assessment, all head trauma patients should be clinically assessed in A&E following a special head injury chart, including the Glasgow Coma Scale (GCS), to assess the level of consciousness, and is not only applied to head trauma patients but to other acutely ill patients, in addition to CN and pupil examination. All severe head injury patients should be assumed to have an associated cervical spine injury. For this reason, applying a cervical collar is an important part of resuscitation.

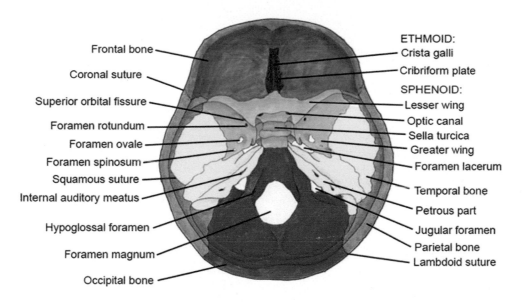

Frontal bone
Coronal suture
Superior orbital fissure
Foramen rotundum
Foramen ovale
Foramen spinosum
Squamous suture
Internal auditory meatus
Hypoglossal foramen
Foramen magnum
Occipital bone

ETHMOID:
Crista galli
Cribriform plate
SPHENOID:
Lesser wing
Optic canal
Sella turcica
Greater wing
Foramen lacerum
Temporal bone
Petrous part
Jugular foramen
Parietal bone
Lambdoid suture

FIGURE 2.2 Cranial fossae with calvaria removed and seen from above. (Courtesy of Calum Harrington-Vogt.)

TABLE 2.1: Contents of the cranial fossae

Fossa	Contents	Cranial Bones Are Formed By
Anterior cranial fossa	• Frontal lobes, cribriform foramina in cribriform plate (part of ethmoid bone) to transmit the fibres of CN I (olfactory) • Optic canal for optic nerve and ophthalmic artery	• Frontal and ethmoid bones and lesser wings of sphenoid
Middle cranial fossa	Temporal lobes, foramen rotundum, foramen ovale, foramen spinosum, foramen lacerum, sella turcica (where the pituitary gland is situated), and superior orbital fissure	Greater wings and body of sphenoid and the anterior aspect of the petrous temporal bones
Posterior cranial fossa	• The occipital lobe is positioned above the tentorium cerebelli • The brainstem and the cerebellum sit beneath the tentorium cerebelli • It contains the foramen magnum (within the occipital bone), jugular foramen, internal acoustic meatus, and the hypoglossal canal	Posterior aspect of the petrous temporal bone, the squamous and mastoid of temporal bones, and the occipital bone

Skull Fractures

Skull fractures can be linear, depressed, or compound, where there are scalp or facial wounds, or both (**Figure 2.3**).

Note that most fractures occur at the anterior cranial fossa (about 70%) and may be associated with the following:

• CSF can escape through the nose (rhinorrhoea), and this has a risk of meningitis, as the meninges are torn
• Bruising around the eyes (raccoon or panda eyes)
• There is risk of infection if the frontal sinus is involved, due to its communication with the nasal cavity
• Anosmia (loss of smell sensation) can follow fractures of the anterior cranial fossa due to damage to the filaments of the olfactory nerve

Basal fractures of the petrous temporal bone may be associated with leakage of CSF from the ears (otorrhoea) and Battle's sign (bruising behind the ear over the mastoid process).

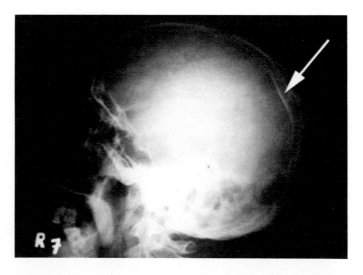

FIGURE 2.3 Lateral skull X-ray showing a compression fracture (*arrowed*). (Courtesy of Qassim F. Baker.)

Skull fractures are serious when they are complicated by intracranial bleeding, injury to the brain and CNs, and risk of infection when associated with scalp/facial wounds or connected to a cavity such as the pharynx and the nasal sinuses. Axial CT scan is the imaging of choice.

Foramina and Their Contents
As mentioned in **Table 2.1**, many foramina can be found at the base of the skull. **Table 2.2** highlights structures which pass through these foramina.

Note that the foramen lacerum is not a true foramen, but a gap which transmits the pterygoid (Vidian) nerve and vessels.

TABLE 2.2: Foramina of the skull

Foramen	Structures Passing Through
Cribriform foramina of cribriform plate (of ethmoid bone)	Olfactory nerve fibres (CN I)
Optic foramen	Optic nerve (CN II), ophthalmic artery (branch of the internal carotid artery before it divides into the MCA and ACA)
Superior orbital fissure	Oculomotor nerve (CN III), trochlear nerve (CN IV), ophthalmic branch of trigeminal nerve (CN V1), abducens nerve (CN VI), superior and inferior ophthalmic veins, sympathetic fibres from the internal carotid plexus
Foramen rotundum	Maxillary branch of trigeminal (CN V2)
Foramen ovale	Mandibular branch of trigeminal (CN V3)
Foramen spinosum	Middle meningeal artery and veins, meningeal branch of mandibular nerve (CN V3)
Internal auditory meatus	Facial nerve (CN VII), vestibulocochlear nerve (CN VIII), nervus intermedius and labyrinthine vessels
Jugular foramen	Internal jugular vein, glossopharyngeal nerve (CN IX), vagus nerve (CN X), accessory nerve (CN XI)
Foramen magnum	Spinal cord, vertebral arteries, lowest part of brainstem
Hypoglossal canal	Hypoglossal nerve (CN XII)

The Orbit and Eye

The Orbit
The orbit is a pyramidal cavity of the skull, with the base anteriorly and the apex posteriorly (**Figure 2.4**). It contains the following:

- Eyeball (globe, or bulbus oculi)
- *Nerves:* optic, abducens, oculomotor, branches of CN V1 and V2, ciliary ganglion
- *Muscles:* extraocular muscles (*vide infra*)
- Ophthalmic vessels
- Nasolacrimal apparatus

The boundaries of the orbit are:

- *Roof:* orbital plate of the frontal bone (separating the orbit from the anterior cranial fossa) and lesser wing of the sphenoid
- *Floor:* orbital plate of the maxilla (forming the roof of the maxillary sinus) and orbital process of palatine bone and zygomatic bone
- *Medial wall:* ethmoid bone, frontal bone, and lacrimal and sphenoid bones. The nasolacrimal canal is located anteriorly within the medial wall. It drains tears to the inferior meatus of the nasal cavity
- *Lateral wall (the thickest wall of the orbit):* the zygomatic and greater wing of the sphenoid bone and the zygomatic process of the frontal bone
- *Apex:* located at the opening of the optic canal
- *Base:* opens anteriorly into the face and is bound by the eyelids
- The orbital margin is formed by the frontal bone superiorly, the frontal and zygomatic bones laterally, the zygomatic and maxilla bones inferiorly, and the maxilla and frontal bones medially

Foramina of the Orbit
The foramina include the optic canal and the superior orbital fissure, both of which allow structures to enter and leave the orbit.

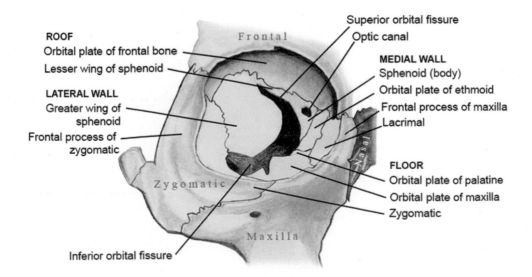

FIGURE 2.4 Boundaries of the right orbit. (Courtesy of Aditya Mavinkurve.)

Superior Orbital Fissure

The superior orbital fissure is a slit-like opening located between the greater and lesser wings of the sphenoid. From superior to inferior, it transmits the:

- *Lacrimal nerve* (branch of CN V1), which supplies the skin of the upper eyelid
- *Frontal nerve* (branch of CN V1), which divides into supratrochlear and supraorbital nerves to supply the skin of the forehead
- *Ophthalmic veins*, which drain into the cavernous sinus
- *Trochlear nerve* (CN IV), which innervates the superior oblique muscle
- *Oculomotor nerve* (CN III), which innervates all the extrinsic muscles of the eye except for the superior oblique and lateral rectus
- *Nasociliary nerve* (branch of CN V1), which gives rise to the long ciliary nerve, which carries sympathetic fibres to the dilator pupillae muscle
- *Abducens nerve* (CN VI), which innervates the lateral rectus

The inferior orbital fissure (**Figure 2.4**) lies within the floor of the orbit and transmits the infraorbital nerve (from CN V2) and artery (from the maxillary artery) and vein, in addition to the zygomatic nerve (from CN V2) and branches from the pterygopalatine ganglion.

Optic Canal

The optic canal is located within the lesser wing of the sphenoid. It transmits the following structures:

- Optic nerve (CN II), which transmits visual information from the retina to the occipital lobe of the brain
- Ophthalmic artery, which supplies the structures of the orbit

Eyelids

The eye is protected by the upper and lower eyelids. The palpebral fissure is the opening between the two eyelids. Closure of the eyelids results from contraction of orbicularis oculi, which is supplied by the facial nerve (CN VII), and opening results from contraction of the levator palpebrae superioris, which is supplied by the oculomotor nerve (CN III). The superior tarsal muscle is a smooth muscle that raises the upper eyelids and is supplied by sympathetic nerves (paralysis of this muscle is one of the features of Horner's syndrome).

The conjunctiva is the mucous membrane that lines the inside of the eyelids (palpebral conjunctiva) and is continuous with the conjunctiva over the globe (bulbar conjunctiva).

Arterial Supply

The eyelid receives a rich blood supply from the lateral and medial palpebral arteries (branches of the ophthalmic artery), the facial artery (via the angular branch), and the superficial temporal artery (via the transverse facial artery).

Venous Drainage

The medial eyelid drains via the medial palpebral vein into the angular and ophthalmic veins. The lateral eyelid drains via the lateral palpebral vein into the superficial temporal vein.

Innervation

The trigeminal nerve (CN V) provides sensory innervation to the eyelid; eyelid muscle innervation is discussed in more detail later. The supraorbital branch of the ophthalmic nerve (CN V1) innervates the upper lid, and the infraorbital branch of the maxillary nerve (CN V2) supplies the lower lid.

The Eye

The eye consists of the eyeball and the optic nerve. The eyeball is the globe-shaped structure located within the bony orbit that contains the optical apparatus. The optic nerve (CN II) is the cranial nerve responsible for vision, while the oculomotor (CN III), trochlear (CN IV), and abducens (CN VI) are responsible for eye movements.

Layers of the eyeball (**Figure 2.5**) include the following:

1. *Fibrous layer:* contains the sclera and cornea, which are continuous with each other and provide shape to the eyeball. The sclera is the white part of the eyeball and provides attachment for extraocular muscles. The cornea is

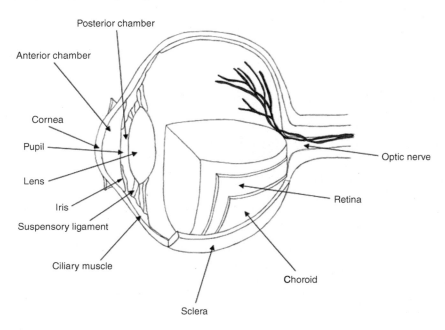

FIGURE 2.5 Layers of the eye. (Courtesy of Calum Harrington-Vogt.)

the transparent part of the eyeball and is located anteriorly; it functions to refract light entering the eye so that it is focused on the retina. The cornea has a stronger refractory power than the lens; however, only the lens can change shape and therefore is responsible for accommodation. The cornea is avascular and is dependent on the aqueous humour for nourishment. If the cornea becomes damaged due to disease or trauma, corneal grafting (transplant) can provide definitive treatment. It involves surgically replacing the damaged cornea with a healthy donor's cornea.

2. *Vascular layer:* consists of the choroid, iris, and ciliary body. The choroid is a layer of connective tissue that is highly vascularised to support and nourish the retina. The iris is a group of smooth muscles that change the diameter of the pupil in response to light stimuli. The ciliary body attaches to the lens through the ciliary processes (**Figure 2.5**). Contraction of the ciliary muscle relaxes the pull on the lens. This results in the lens forming a more rounded shape and moving slightly anterior. The lens is a biconvex, transparent structure which is situated posterior to the iris. Similar to the cornea, it is completely avascular and is dependent on the aqueous humour for nourishment.

3. *Inner layer:* contains the retina, which can be divided into neural and pigmented layers. The neural layer is located on the lateral and posterior surfaces of the eye. It contains photoreceptors which detect light. The pigmented layer does not contain any photoreceptors, but instead is connected to the choroid layer. This helps to support and nourish the neural layer and is continuous throughout the inner eyeball. The centre of the retina is called the macula and is located posteriorly in the eyeball. The central point of the macula is termed the fovea (meaning a small hole or depression) and can be viewed during ophthalmoscopy (**Figure 2.6**). The macula is responsible for central (focused) vision and most

of coloured vision, as a high density of photoreceptor cells are located here. Photoreceptors are divided into rods and cones. Rods are responsible for vision in low-light environments and have low acuity. Cones, on the other hand, are for high-light environments and have high acuity as well as colour receptors. The fovea contains only cone photoreceptors, while the macula contains mostly cone cells with a few rod cells.

Innervation of the Eye

Optic Nerve

The optic nerve (CN II) arises as an outpouching of the diencephalon (optic stalks) during embryonic development. Light enters the retina through the optic disc and relays visual information to the brain. The optic nerve runs through the optic canal to the optic chiasma (partial decussation) and continues as the optic tract (posterior to the chiasma) to the lateral geniculate nucleus (relay centre in the thalamus for the visual pathway). It then travels to the pretectal nuclei and superior colliculus of the midbrain. The visual fibres continue from the lateral geniculate body to the optic radiation and terminate in the occipital cerebral cortex. The optic nerve is encased by the meningeal layers (pia, arachnoid, and dura) along its course, until it pierces the sclera, where it subsequently fuses with all three layers. The central retinal artery (first branch of the ophthalmic artery) enters within the nerve and runs to the retina (**Figure 2.7**).

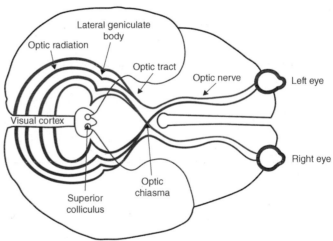

FIGURE 2.7   Visual pathways. (Courtesy of Parker O'Neill.)

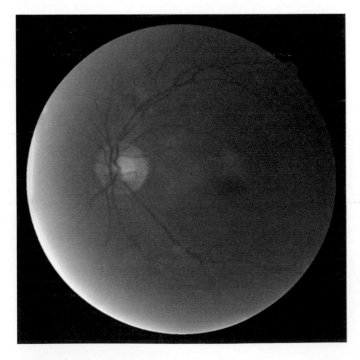

FIGURE 2.6 Ophthalmoscopy showing the optic disc (the yellow spot) and the radiating retinal vessels. (Courtesy of Qassim F. Baker.)

Oculomotor Nerve (CN III)

Through its superior and inferior divisions, it supplies motor branches to all the extrinsic ocular muscles (except the superior oblique and lateral rectus) and the levator palpebrae superioris.

The oculomotor nerve carries parasympathetic branches from the Edinger-Westphal nucleus in the brainstem, via the ciliary ganglion, to the sphincter pupillae muscle and the ciliary muscle.

Pupillary Light Reflex

Light shone in one eye will cause consensual pupil constriction of both eyes. The light is detected in the retina and sends a signal through the optic nerve (CN II) to the pretectal nucleus in the midbrain, which activates the bilateral Edinger-Westphal nuclei and causes bilateral pupil constriction (parasympathetic stimulation).

Accommodation Reflex

The accommodation reflex changes the shape of the lens (through the ciliary body) and pupil (through the iris) to adjust vision for short and long distances. It is controlled by the optic nerve (afferent limb of reflex) and the oculomotor nerve (efferent limb of reflex, which stimulates the ciliary body to contract).

Ciliary Ganglion

The ciliary ganglion is a small ganglion which is located near the apex of the orbit. It is traversed by sensory fibres (from the nasociliary nerve, which conveys sensation from the cornea), sympathetic fibres (from the internal carotid plexus), and parasympathetic fibres, which travel with the oculomotor nerve and synapse at the ganglion, to supply the sphincter pupillae and the ciliary muscle.

Aqueous Humour Chambers

There are two aqueous humour chambers of the eyeball. The anterior chamber is located between the cornea and the iris, while the posterior chamber is located between the iris and the ciliary processes (**Figure 2.5**). The chambers are filled with aqueous humour, a clear fluid that functions to protect and nourish the eye. It flows through the pupil from the posterior chamber to the anterior chamber and is drained via the trabecular meshwork into the canal of Schlemm at the angle between the iris and the cornea.

Arterial Supply of the Eye

The eye is supplied by the ophthalmic artery, which is the first branch of the internal carotid artery. The ophthalmic artery gives rise to the central artery of the retina, which supplies its internal surface. Other branches that supply the eye include the supraorbital, lacrimal, and anterior and posterior ethmoidal arteries. The terminal branches are the supratrochlear and dorsal nasal arteries.

Venous Drainage of the Eye

The eyeball is drained by the superior and inferior ophthalmic veins, as well as the central retinal vein, all of which drain into the cavernous sinus.

Lymphatics of the Eye

The eyeball (including the cornea, lens, iris, ciliary body, retina, choroid, and sclera) do not contain any lymphatics. However, the majority of the surrounding tissue (including the eyelid, lacrimal gland, and conjunctiva) do contain lymphatics. Lymphatic drainage is to the submandibular nodes (medial) and pre-auricular nodes (lateral).

> ### CLINICAL NOTE
>
> Occlusion of the retinal artery is an ophthalmic emergency, as it can lead to blindness. It is recognised by sudden unilateral vision impairment. Common causes of retinal artery occlusion include diabetes mellitus and atherosclerosis.

Infections can spread into the cavernous sinus from the face (cavernous sinus thrombosis) and can lead to congestion and protrusion of the eyes (exophthalmos). Exophthalmos is an important sign of thyroid gland hyperactivity (thyrotoxicosis) (**Figure 2.8**).

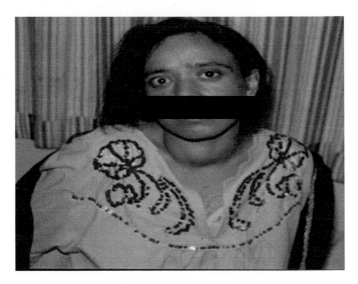

FIGURE 2.8 Right exophthalmos in a patient with toxic goitre. (Courtesy of Qassim F. Baker.)

Extraocular Muscles

There are six extraocular muscles which function to move the eyes and three extraocular muscles that move the eyelids (**Table 2.3**, **Figure 2.9**).

The recti muscles originate from the tendinous ring, which surrounds the optic canal and part of the superior orbital fissure.

The four recti move the eye in different directions in accordance with their names:

- Superior rectus moves the eye upwards
- Inferior rectus moves the eye downwards
- Lateral rectus moves the eye outwards away from the midline
- Medial rectus moves the eye inwards towards the midline

The superior oblique muscle rotates the eyeball downwards and laterally (for example, when looking downstairs), and the inferior oblique rotates the eyeball upwards and laterally.

The levator palpebrae superioris elevates the upper eyelid to open the eye.

The superior tarsal muscle (smooth muscle) assists the levator palpebrae superioris in elevating the upper eyelid to open the eye.

The orbicularis oculi muscle has three distinct parts, each with its own function:

- *Palpebral:* gently closes eyelids
- *Orbital:* tightly closes eyelids
- *Lacrimal:* drains tears

Innervation of the extraocular muscles is as follows:

- *Oculomotor nerve (CN III):* levator palpebrae superioris, superior rectus, medial rectus, inferior rectus, and inferior oblique
- *Trochlear nerve (CN IV):* superior oblique (SO4)
- *Abducens nerve (CN VI):* lateral rectus (LR6)
- *Facial nerve (CN VII):* orbicularis oculi

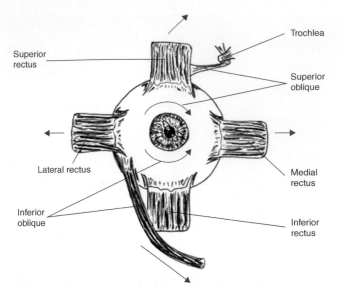

Superior rectus

Trochlea

Superior oblique

Lateral rectus

Medial rectus

Inferior oblique

Inferior rectus

FIGURE 2.9 Extraocular muscles of the right eye. (Courtesy of Alina Humdani.)

Intrinsic Muscles

The intrinsic muscles of the eye are smooth muscles which are supplied by autonomic nerves. The parasympathetic fibres of the oculomotor nerve (CN III) innervate the sphincter pupillae of the iris (which constricts the pupil for near vision) and the ciliary muscles (which control the shape of the lens). The dilator pupillae dilates the pupil and is supplied by the sympathetic branches of the long ciliary nerve (CN V1).

CLINICAL NOTE

Lesions to the oculomotor nerve will cause the eyes to move and remain in a "down and out" position, since the superior oblique and lateral rectus muscles will not be antagonised.

Lacrimal Gland

The lacrimal gland (one for each orbit) is an exocrine gland located laterally in the lacrimal fossa of the frontal bone. It secretes serous fluid, commonly known as tears, which contains

TABLE 2.3: Extraocular muscles

Muscle	Origin	Insertion	Action	Innervation
Superior rectus	Common tendinous ring	Sclera	Elevates, adducts, and laterally rotates eyeball	Oculomotor nerve (CN III)
Medial rectus	Common tendinous ring	Sclera	Adducts eyeball	Oculomotor nerve (CN III)
Inferior rectus	Common tendinous ring	Sclera	Depresses, adducts and medially rotates eyeball	Oculomotor nerve (CN III)
Lateral rectus	Common tendinous ring	Sclera	Abducts eyeball	Abducens nerve (CN VI)
Superior oblique	Body of sphenoid bone	Sclera	Abducts, depresses and medially rotates eyeball	Trochlear nerve (CN IV)
Inferior oblique	Floor of orbit	Sclera	Abducts, elevates and laterally rotates eyeball	Oculomotor nerve (CN III)
Levator palpebrae superioris	Lesser wing of sphenoid bone	Superior tarsal plate and skin of the upper lid	Elevates upper eyelid	Oculomotor nerve (CN III)
Superior tarsal muscle	Underside of levator palpebrae superioris	Superior tarsal plate	Elevates upper eyelid	Post-ganglionic sympathetic fibres from the superior cervical ganglion
Orbicularis oculi	Medial orbital margin, medial palpebral ligament, nasal part of the frontal bone and the lacrimal bone	Superior and inferior tarsal plates and the skin around the orbit	Closes eyelids and drains tears	Facial nerve (CN VII), via the temporal and zygomatic branches
Corrugator supercilii	Supraorbital ridge	Skin of the forehead medial to the eyebrow	Wrinkling of the forehead and assists in closing the eyeball	Temporal branch of the facial nerve

immunoglobulin A, lipocalin, lysosomal enzymes, and other constituents similar to plasma, via the lacrimal ducts. These ducts open into the superior fornix of the conjunctiva, and the secretions are drained inferiorly to the lacrimal sac and through the nasolacrimal duct into the lacrimal groove. The nasolacrimal duct then descends through the nasolacrimal canal of the maxilla to the inferior nasal meatus, where it is partially covered by a fold of mucous membrane (the plica lacrimalis). The serous fluid prevents the eye from drying out and protects it from harmful

environmental factors, such as dust. The glands are supplied by the lacrimal arteries (branches of the ophthalmic arteries) and are drained by the superior ophthalmic veins.

Sensory innervation is through the lacrimal nerve (branch of CN V1), and it is supplied with parasympathetic secretomotor nerves from the facial nerve, synapsing at the pterygopalatine ganglion, which accompany the zygomatic and lacrimal branches of the maxillary division of the trigeminal nerve (CN V2).

CLINICAL NOTES

ORBITAL BLOWOUT FRACTURE

This is caused by large blunt objects impacting the orbit. Common causes include road traffic accidents and sporting injuries; hence patients tend to be young males. The most common sites for fractures are the medial and inferior walls of the orbit, as they are the weakest. Symptoms include swelling, pain, and diplopia (double vision) due to swelling of the ocular muscles or entrapment in the fracture; numbness around the orbit, cheek, and/or teeth, due to injury of the infraorbital nerve; and inferior displacement of the eyeball. Diagnosis is aided with a CT scan, and the fractures are usually treated with surgery.

CONJUNCTIVITIS

Conjunctivitis (inflammation of the conjunctiva) is a common clinical occurrence, usually caused by adenovirus. Other causes include *Staphylococcus aureus* and allergens in atopic patients. It is characterised by hyperaemia (bloodshot eye) and watery discharge.

RETINOBLASTOMA

Retinoblastoma (cancer of the retina) can be detected by failure to elicit the normal red-light reflex during fundoscopy. Instead, the retina will appear white during examination. Retinoblastoma is the most common intraocular tumour in children.

RETINAL DETACHMENT

The inner layer of the retina becomes detached from the choroid layer. If not promptly treated, it can cause permanent loss of vision. Symptoms include patients describing "a black curtain progressively lowering over my vision" or they report "floaters" (*muscae volitantes*: literally "flying flies" in Latin) that obscure their vision.

CATARACTS

Cataracts are the result of opacification of the lens, which distorts the lens's refractive power, leading to loss of visual acuity. Cataracts are quite common, with half of the population over 75 years old suffering from them (National Eye Institute, 2019). Common causes include old age, diabetes, and smoking.

OPTIC NEURITIS

Optic neuritis is inflammation of the optic nerve, which leads to temporary unilateral vision loss with pain. It is commonly linked to multiple sclerosis (MS), as it can be the first clinical manifestation of the disease.

PITUITARY ADENOMA

Tumours of the pituitary gland can compress the optic chiasma and cause bitemporal hemianopia (loss of vision laterally in both visual fields).

GLAUCOMA

Glaucoma is a disease of the optic nerve caused by increased intraocular pressure and is one of the leading causes of blindness in people over the age of 60. There are many types of glaucoma, but they generally fall within two categories:

- Open angle glaucoma is a chronic condition where the outflow of aqueous humour becomes impaired leading to a slow increase in intraocular pressure. This leads to a slow loss of peripheral vision
- Acute closed angle glaucoma is an ophthalmologic emergency caused by a rapid increase in intraocular pressure due to occlusion of the anterior chamber angle (between the iris and the cornea) leading to impaired drainage of the aqueous humour. This condition can lead to irreversible vision loss if not treated within hours

DACRYOADENITIS

Dacryoadenitis is inflammation of the lacrimal gland. The presentation can be acute or chronic. The acute presentation has a rapid onset (hours/days), with severe pain and pressure in the supratemporal region of the orbit. The chronic presentation has a slow onset (months), with painless enlargement of the lacrimal gland. It can result from viral infections or secondary causes such as Graves' disease, Sjögren's syndrome, and sarcoidosis.

Sjögren's syndrome is a chronic autoimmune disease which decreases lacrimal and salivary gland activity through lymphocytic infiltration. Symptoms include dry mouth, eyes, and skin. Females are more commonly affected than males, and the normal age of onset is 40 to 60 years old.

REVISION QUIZ ON THE EYE

Q1. What are the three layers of the eye? List the major components and function of each layer.

Q2. What does the ophthalmic artery supply, and where does it originate from?

Q3. What are the differences between open and closed angle glaucoma?

Answers are at the end of the section.

The Ear

External Ear

- The externally visible part of the ear is formed by the auricle (or pinna) and external acoustic meatus
- The auricle captures and transfers sound waves to the tympanic membrane via the external acoustic meatus. The auricle is composed of elastic cartilage (except for the lobule), which is covered by skin
- The outer lateral curvature and the inner medial prominence of the auricle are termed the helix and anti-helix, respectively. The anti-helix bifurcates into the superior and inferior crura (**Figure 2.10**)

- The concha is a shallow depression which is located in the middle of the auricle and is continuous with the external acoustic meatus
- The tragus is a small projection over the external acoustic meatus. It partially covers the concha, as does the infero-lateral anti-tragus (*tragus*, Gr: "goat", because of its resemblance to a goat's beard in elderly men)

Ear Canal

- The external acoustic meatus (ear canal) continues for approximately 2.5 cm as a sigmoid-shaped canal, which terminates at the tympanic membrane.
- The outer one-third of the ear canal is composed of elastic cartilage, whereas the inner two-thirds is composed of bone.
- The ceruminous glands are modified sweat glands that secret ear wax as a protective mechanism against foreign bodies. Ear wax can accumulate and block the external ear, causing conductive deafness.
- The tympanic membrane, colloquially known as the eardrum, forms the boundary between the external and middle ear.

Blood Supply of the External Ear

The arterial supply of the external ear arises from the:

- Posterior auricular artery (branch of the maxillary artery)
- Superficial temporal artery (terminal branch of the external carotid artery)

The venous draining of the ear is through corresponding veins.

Innervation of the External Ear

The external ear is innervated by the:

- Great auricular nerve (C2–C3).
- Auriculotemporal nerve (branch of CN V3).
- Auricular branch of the vagus nerve (CN X); the meatal side of the tympanic membrane is supplied by the auriculotemporal nerve and the vagus.

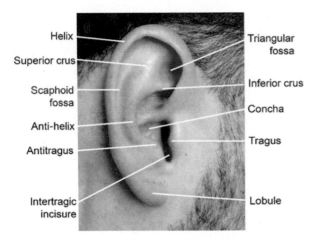

FIGURE 2.10 The auricle or pinna. (Photograph courtesy of Philip J. Adds.)

CLINICAL NOTE

EXTERNAL EAR INJURY

Injury to the pinna from trauma and sports such as rugby can result in pinna haematoma. Blood collects between the perichondrium and the auricular cartilage causing loss of auricular contour. If not aspirated or evacuated the haematoma enlarges, diminishing blood supply to the cartilage resulting in a "cauliflower ear" (**Figure 2.11**).

Acute Otitis Externa

Otitis externa is inflammation of the external auditory canal. It is a very painful condition caused by bacteria such as *Pseudomonas aeruginosa*, *Proteus mirabilis*, and *S. aureus*. Fungal causes include *Candida albicans* or *Aspergillus*. It may follow ear syringing for removal of wax.

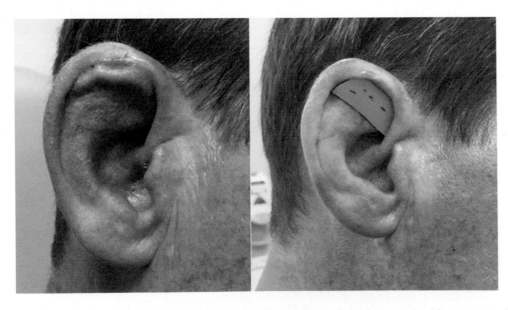

FIGURE 2.11 Recurrent pinna haematoma pre– and post–incision and drainage with anterior and posterior splinting to prevent re-accumulation of blood under the perichondrium. (Courtesy of Asha Ali.)

Middle Ear

The middle ear is an air-filled cavity which begins at the tympanic membrane and is located within the petrous part of temporal bone. The function of the middle ear is to convert sound waves into vibrations, which travel via the auditory ossicles to the inner ear. It is continuous posteriorly with the mastoid antrum and mastoid air cells.

Tympanic Membrane

The tympanic membrane is orientated obliquely and is mainly composed of the pars tensa and pars flaccida, the latter of which is located above the manubrium of the malleus. Both parts are composed of an epidermal layer (which is continuous with the skin of the external auditory meatus), a fibrous layer (composed of radial and circular fibres), and an inner mucosal layer.

The tympanic membrane is supplied by branches from the external carotid artery (*vide infra*). As the internal carotid artery also supplies the hypothalamus, the core body temperature regulator (through the thermoregulatory centre), the ear acts as an easily accessible and convenient way of measuring core body temperature.

Sound waves travel through the external acoustic meatus to the tympanic membrane and cause it to vibrate. This transfers the sound waves into mechanical vibrations. As the amplitude

Auditory Ossicles

The three bones of the middle ear are the smallest bones in the body and are known as the auditory ossicles: the malleus ("hammer"), incus ("anvil"), and stapes ("stirrup") (**Figure 2.12**). The auditory ossicles articulate successively to connect the tympanic membrane to the oval window (fenestra ovalis) of the cochlea.

The malleus, the largest and most lateral of the auditory ossicles, is bound to the tympanic membrane via its manubrium. The head of the malleus articulates with the anvil-shaped incus bone. The incus is held in place by the posterior incudal ligament and articulates with the stapes. The stapes is the smallest and most medial of the three auditory ossicles. The footplate of the stapes is connected to the oval window of the cochlea in the inner ear.

An easy way to remember the bony connections is that the *m*anubrium of the *m*alleus connects to the tympanic *m*embrane and that the *s*tapes is *s*tirrup-*s*haped.

Muscles of the Middle Ear

The two muscles of the middle ear are the **tensor tympani** and the **stapedius**. When the tensor tympani contracts, it pulls the malleus medially, thereby stretching the tympanic membrane inwards. The tensor tympani is innervated by the mandibular branch of the trigeminal nerve (CN V3).

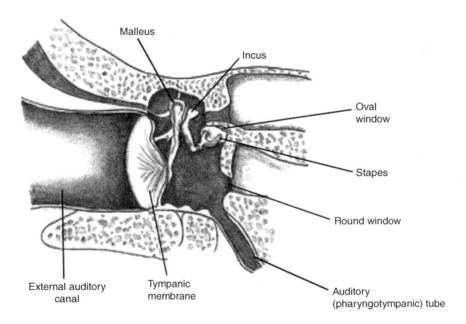

FIGURE 2.12   Middle ear. (Courtesy of Amani Bashir.)

of the sound waves increases, the magnitude of deflection of the tympanic membrane increases. Similarly, as the frequency of the sound waves increases, the rate of vibration increases.

The tympanic membrane is supplied mainly by the auriculotemporal nerve.

CLINICAL NOTE

The tympanic membrane is visually examined with an otoscope (auroscope). A healthy tympanic membrane is a translucent pale grey colour. It can rupture from barotrauma, blast, and direct injuries (e.g., when cleaning the ears with cotton buds).

The stapedius, the smallest skeletal muscle in the body, acts to stabilise the stapes. The stapedius is innervated by the facial nerve (CN VII).

Auditory Tube (Eustachian or Pharyngotympanic Tube)

The middle ear communicates with the lateral wall of the nasopharynx via the auditory tube, which is composed of bony and cartilaginous elements and which is normally closed. Contraction of the tensor veli palatini muscle (e.g., when swallowing) opens up the eustachian tube, which helps to equalise the pressure between the external and middle ear in order to prevent damage to the tympanic membrane. It also drains the mucus secreted in the middle ear.

Blood Supply of the Middle Ear

The main blood supply comes from branches of the maxillary artery (from the external carotid artery) and from the stylomastoid artery (which originates from either the posterior auricular or the occipital branches of the external carotid artery).

Venous drainage is via the pterygoid venous plexus and the superior petrosal sinus.

Innervation of the Middle Ear

The middle ear, including the mucosal side of the tympanic membrane, is innervated by the glossopharyngeal nerve (CN IX), with a contribution from the vagus nerve (CN X).

CLINICAL NOTE

ACOUSTIC REFLEX

The middle ear muscle reflex, also known as the acoustic reflex, helps to protect against high-intensity, low-frequency sounds. When this stimulus is present, the tensor tympani and stapedius contract, causing the malleus to pull the tympanic membrane medially and the stapes to move away from the oval window. This reduces the transmission of mechanical vibration to the cochlea, thereby having a protective effect.

Otic barotrauma occurs when the eustachian tube fails to equalise the pressure of the middle ear with the atmospheric pressure. This can occur upon an aeroplane's ascent or descent or during deep-sea diving.

Middle Ear Infections

Middle ear infections are often caused by upper respiratory infections. Infection of the middle ear is known as otitis media and may be followed by discharge from the ear after perforation of the tympanic membrane. Otitis media is more common in children because the eustachian tube is much shorter and less vertical, meaning that fluid is more likely to build up. "Glue ear" is the colloquial name for the accumulation of glue-like fluid in the middle ear that can cause deafness.

Complications of otitis media can include labyrinthitis (inflammation of the inner ear) and, very rarely, facial nerve paralysis, meningitis, brain abscesses, and mastoiditis (inflammation of the mastoid air cells).

Mastoiditis

Mastoiditis, a complication of acute otitis media, is characterised by inflammation of the mastoid antrum and air cells. There is a classical anterolateral displacement of the pinna due to a post-auricular abscess. The infection may spread superiorly into the middle cranial fossa, causing osteomyelitis of the tegmen tympani (the roof of the tympanic cavity).

QUIZ QUESTION

Q. When draining pus from the mastoid air cells in cases of suspected mastoiditis, which of the following nerves is at most risk of being damaged? (The answer is at the end of the section.)

a. *Vestibulocochlear nerve*
b. *Great auricular nerve*
c. *Auricular branch of vagus nerve*
d. *Facial nerve*
e. *Auriculotemporal nerve*

Inner Ear

The inner ear, also known as the labyrinth, is involved in both hearing and balance, and therefore consists of the cochlea and vestibular systems, respectively. The cochlea functions to convert the mechanical vibrations from the middle ear into nerve impulses, which the brain perceives as sound.

Vibrations from the middle ear reach the cochlea and cause the basilar membrane to vibrate. The sensory hair cells of the organ of Corti, located on the basilar membrane, convert these vibrations into nerve impulses, via perilymph. (Cochlea is from the Greek *cochlos*, meaning "snail".)

The inner ear is located within the temporal bone and consists of the bony labyrinth and the membranous labyrinth (also known as the cochlear duct). The bony labyrinth consists of the bony structures of the inner ear, whereas the membranous labyrinth is located within the bony labyrinth.

In contrast to the middle ear, the inner ear is filled with fluid. Perilymph flows between the bony and membranous labyrinths, whereas endolymph flows within the membranous labyrinth. The endolymphatic system is separated from the perilymphatic system by the basilar and Reissner's membranes (**Figure 2.13**).

The cochlea, a spiral cavity, is composed of three separate cavities:

- Scala tympani
- Scala media
- Scala vestibuli

The basilar membrane separates the scala media and scala tympani, whereas the Reissner's membrane separates the scala vestibuli from the scala media. Note that the scala vestibuli and scala tympani contain perilymph, but the scala media contains endolymph.

The scala vestibuli is connected to the oval window, whereas the scala tympani is connected to the round window. A passage connecting the scala vestibuli and scala tympani, the helicotrema, acts to equalise pressure in response to low frequencies. The perilymphatic aqueduct, located at the vestibular end of the inner ear, connects to the CSF surrounding the brain.

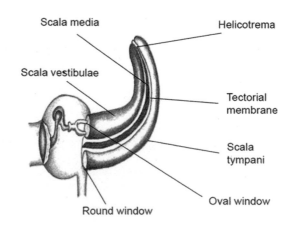

FIGURE 2.13 The inner ear (schematic). (Courtesy of Amani Bashir.)

Innervation of the Inner Ear

The vestibulocochlear nerve (CN VIII) innervates the inner ear and bifurcates into the vestibular nerve and the cochlear nerve. It originates at the cerebello-pontine angle within the posterior cranial fossa and enters the internal acoustic meatus together with the facial nerve (CN VII), the nervus intermedius, and the labyrinthine vessels.

Stimulated hair cells of the organ of Corti send afferent nerve impulses via the cochlear nerve to the brainstem. The two types of hair cells, outer hair cells and inner hair cells, both contain stereocilia. The outer hair cells are tightly adherent to the tectorial membrane, whereas the inner hair cells are loosely bound, if at all, to the tectorial membrane.

Equilibrium (balance) is due to the relationship between the visual system, the vestibular system, and proprioception via impulses in the posterior column of the spinal cord. However, only the vestibular system shall be considered here. The vestibular system consists of the semi-circular canals and the utricle and saccule, all of which contain vestibular receptors.

There are three semicircular canals (anterior, lateral, and posterior) in each ear, which contain endolymph. The canals are perpendicular to one another and detect head movement and acceleration via the movement of the endolymph. The dilated terminal ends of each canal are termed the ampullae. As the head moves, endolymph in the semicircular canals moves the hair cells of the ampullae, thereby stimulating them. As a result, nerve impulses are sent to the brain via the vestibular branch of the vestibulocochlear nerve (**Figure 2.14**).

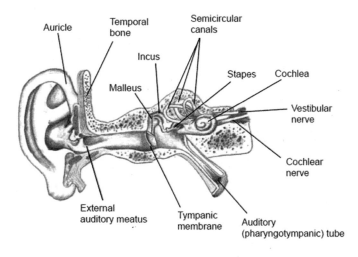

FIGURE 2.14 Anatomy of the parts of the ear. (Courtesy of Amani Bashir.)

A region known as the macula is present in each utricle and saccule. Maculae are found perpendicular to each other. The maculae have an otolithic membrane which contains calcium carbonate crystals. Otoliths and hair cells lie underneath this membrane. As the head moves, so does the otolithic membrane, causing stimulation of the underlying hair cells. This creates action potentials, causing nerve impulses to travel via the vestibular nerve.

Arterial Supply of the Inner Ear

The main blood supply of the inner ear is from branches of the labyrinthine artery, a branch of the anterior inferior cerebellar (AICA) or basilar artery. The stylomastoid branch of the posterior auricular artery or the occipital artery also supplies the semicircular canals.

CLINICAL NOTES

DEAFNESS (HEARING LOSS)

Conductive hearing loss occurs when sound waves are not efficiently transferred from the external acoustic meatus to the tympanic membrane and auditory ossicles. This can be caused by otitis media with effusion; accumulation of cerumen (ear wax), which is easily diagnosed; or by disruption of the tympanic membrane, for example, due to otic barotrauma.

Sensorineural hearing loss occurs due to malfunction of the cochlea or the cochlear nerve, which may be age-related (presbycusis). Hearing aids such as cochlear implants can sometimes be used to treat this condition. Cochlear implants are fitted surgically and bypass the external and middle ear, causing nerve impulses to be sent via the cochlear nerve. Therefore, the cochlear nerve must still be functional if cochlear implants are to be used.

Meniere's disease is a clinical condition characterised by attacks of vertigo, tinnitus, and sensorineural hearing loss.

Acoustic neuroma is a slowly growing benign tumour of the Schwann cells of the vestibular division of the vestibulocochlear nerve (CN VIII) within the inner ear, although if large it may extend to the cerebello-pontine angle. The main clinical features are gradual hearing loss, tinnitus, vertigo, and sometimes weakness of the facial muscles, due to the proximity of the facial nerve to CN VIII.

The Nose

The nose is a pyramidal-shaped structure, with variability in size and shape, and is the beginning of the respiratory tract. The main functions of the nose are to warm, humidify, and filter inspired air, along with containing olfactory receptors (CN I) to detect smells. The external and visible aspect of the nose protrudes from the face. The nasal cavity, separated by the nasal septum, extends from the external openings (nares or nostrils) to the oval-shaped posterior openings (the choanae) into the nasopharynx. The piriform aperture can be observed with removal of the external nose.

External Part

The external nose consists of a bony and cartilaginous skeleton. The skeletal (bony) part consists of the two nasal bones, and the cartilaginous part consists of major and minor alar cartilages in addition to the midline septal cartilage and its lateral processes.

Muscles of the Nose

The nasal muscles are grouped according to their function (**Table 2.4**).

TABLE 2.4: Muscles of the nose

Muscle	Main Function
Procerus (Latin, "tall, extended")	"Frowning" of the nose or concentration muscle
Nasalis in two parts: the compressor and dilator	Narrowing or widening of nares
Depressor nasi septi	Multiple actions, helps pull tip of nose downward
Levator labii superioris alaeque nasi (from the maxilla to the skin of the alar cartilage and the upper lip)	The "Elvis muscle" Widens nares and elevates the nose and the upper lip (in homage to Elvis Presley)

These muscles are supplied by branches of the facial nerve (CN VII), both zygomatic and buccal. All these muscles help facilitate facial expression and respiration.

Blood Supply

The skin of the nose and nasal muscles receive their arterial blood supply via branches from the:

- Facial artery
- Ophthalmic artery (dorsal nasal branch)
- Infraorbital branch of the maxillary artery

Venous return is via the facial veins and ophthalmic veins. Lymphatic drainage is mainly to the submandibular group of lymph nodes.

Cutaneous innervation is via the external nasal and infratrochlear nerve (CN V1) and infraorbital nerve (CN V2).

Boundaries of the Nasal Cavity and Internal Parts (Table 2.5)

Roof: nasal spine of the frontal bone, nasal bones, and cribriform plate of the ethmoid, which separates the nasal cavity from the floor of the anterior cranial fossa and the body of the sphenoid (**Figure 2.15**).

Floor: palatine processes of the maxilla and horizontal plates of the palatine bones (forming the hard palate).

TABLE 2.5: Parts of the nasal cavities

Vestibule	• The area just inside the nostril • Lined by stratified squamous epithelium, (keratinized) skin, and hair follicles • Its main function is to trap and remove pathogens which enter the nose during inspiration
Respiratory	• Largest part of the nasal cavity • Lined with pseudostratified ciliated columnar epithelium and flask-shaped goblet glands, which secret mucus to trap foreign bodies • Contains apertures for drainage from the paranasal sinuses and submucous venous plexuses to warm and humidify inspired air
Olfactory	• Located on the superior aspect of the nose, above the superior concha, for the detection of smells • It is lined by olfactory epithelium and consists of olfactory receptors which continue with the filaments of the olfactory nerve (*fila olfactoria*) passing through the cribriform plate of the ethmoid bone

Medial wall: consists of a bony and cartilaginous septum (**Figure 2.15**)

- Anteriorly the nasal septum is composed of cartilage (the quadrangular cartilage), which meets the bony part posteriorly.
- *Bony:* vomer, perpendicular plate of ethmoid, plus the crests of the maxilla and the palatine, which unite with the inferior border of the vomer (**Figure 2.15**).

Lateral wall: three shelf-like structures called the turbinate bones (conchae) and the three meatuses, inferior to each concha (**Figure 2.16**).

Conchae and Meatuses (Figure 2.16)

The **inferior conchae** are the largest turbinate bones. They run horizontally along the entire length of the lateral nasal wall and **are separate bones**. The opening for the nasolacrimal canal is located approximately midway along the inferior concha, which allows drainage of tears from the lacrimal gland. The middle and superior conchae are lateral projections of the ethmoid.

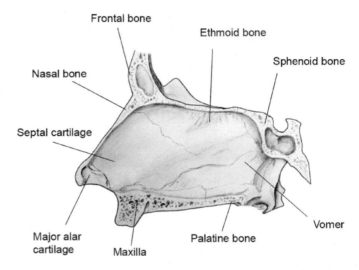

FIGURE 2.15 Structure of the nasal septum. (Courtesy of Kathryn DeMarre.)

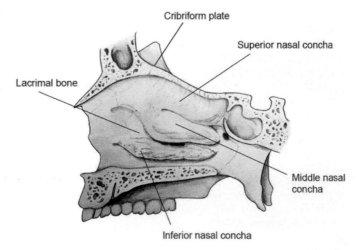

FIGURE 2.16 Turbinate bones of the nose. (Courtesy of Kathryn DeMarre.)

The superior, middle, and inferior meatuses are located inferior and lateral to each respective concha. Incoming air passes posteriorly through the meatuses and collects briefly at the posterior choanae.

Their function is the regulation of airflow direction, temperature and nasal resistance, and protection.

The nasal mucosa lines the nasal cavity, a post-vestibular space, and is lined with pseudostratified ciliated epithelium which has a rich blood supply and contains many goblet cells for mucus secretion.

CLINICAL NOTES

- *Inferior turbinate hypertrophy* is chronic swelling of the inferior turbinate bone. It is commonly caused by allergic reactions, upper respiratory tract infections, sinusitis, pregnancy, hormonal changes, and septal deviation. Symptoms include snoring, nosebleeds, nasal congestion, difficulty breathing, and sinusitis.
- *Nasal septum deviation* can be congenital or caused by trauma. Common symptoms include nasal congestion, sinusitis, epistaxis, dyspnoea, snoring, sleep apnoea, facial pain, and headaches. Symptoms usually arise when a large deviation is seen.
- *Trapped foreign bodies* are commonly observed in children (**Figure 2.17**).
- *Allergic rhinitis* (hay fever) is inflammation of the mucosa of the nasal cavity when a patient becomes exposed to an allergen, most commonly pollen. Symptoms include sneezing, itching, and a runny nose. Many patients often present with other immunological conditions, such as atopic dermatitis and allergic conjunctivitis.

Blood Supply of the Nasal Cavity

Blood Supply of the Septum

The septum receives its blood supply from the internal and external carotid arteries. The ophthalmic artery is the only branch of the internal carotid artery which supplies the nasal septum.

The ophthalmic artery gives rise to two main arteries which supply the superior aspect of the nasal septum: the anterior ethmoidal and posterior ethmoidal arteries.

The external carotid artery gives rise to two branches which supply the inferior portion of the nasal septum: the maxillary and facial arteries (**Figure 2.18**).

- The posterior inferior portion of the nasal septum is supplied by the sphenopalatine and greater palatine arteries (branches of the maxillary artery).
- The septal branches of the superior labial artery (from the facial artery) supply the anterior inferior portion of the nasal septum.
- **Kiesselbach's plexus** is an anastomosis of several arteries present at the anterior inferior aspect of the nasal septum. These arteries include the anterior and posterior ethmoidal arteries, sphenopalatine artery, greater palatine artery, and septal branch of the superior labial artery. The site at which Kiesselbach's plexus forms is referred to as **Little's area**, Kiesselbach's triangle, or Kiesselbach's area.

Blood Supply of the Lateral Walls and Floor

The superior aspect of the lateral wall is supplied by the anterior and posterior ethmoidal arteries (branches of the ophthalmic artery). The anterior inferior aspect of the lateral wall is supplied by the septal branches of the superior labial artery (from the facial artery). The sphenopalatine artery, from the maxillary artery, supplies the turbinate bones and meatuses and is the main blood supply to the nasal mucosa.

Blood supply of the floor of the nasal cavity is from the greater palatine and superior labial arteries.

Venous Drainage of the Nose

The superior region of the nose is drained by the anterior and posterior ethmoidal veins which drain into the ophthalmic veins, which finally drain into the cavernous sinus (see **Section 1A**).

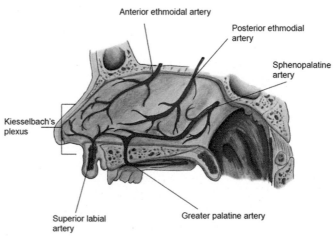

FIGURE 2.18   Blood supply of the nose. (Courtesy of Kathryn DeMarre.)

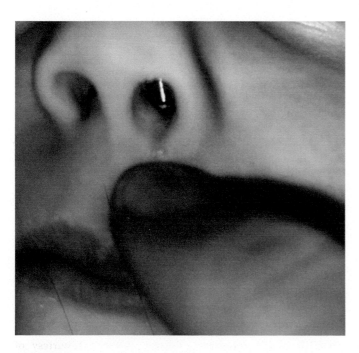

FIGURE 2.17   Foreign body in the nose. (Courtesy of Asha Ali.)

The anterior inferior region of the nose is drained by the angular vein, which drains into the facial vein. The facial vein drains into the internal jugular vein.

The central region of the nose is drained by the sphenopalatine and greater palatine veins, which drain into the maxillary vein.

The maxillary vein drains into the pterygoid plexus, located in the infratemporal fossa.

CLINICAL NOTES

- Little's area is a common site for epistaxis (nosebleed). The most common causes of epistaxis are picking and hard blowing of the nose. Other causes include allergic and non-allergic rhinitis. However, uncontrolled arterial hypertension can present as epistaxis.
- The danger triangle of the face refers to the area between the corners of the mouth and the bridge of the nose. Infection at this triangle can spread via the ophthalmic veins into the brain through the cavernous sinus. This can lead to conditions such as cavernous sinus thrombosis, meningitis, or brain abscess.

Innervation of the Nasal Cavity

Innervation of the nasal cavity can be divided into special and general sensory innervation (**Table 2.6**).

TABLE 2.6: Innervation of the nasal cavity

Special Sensory Innervation	General Sensory Innervation
Detection of smell Cranial nerve CNI – olfactory nerve Autonomic innervation: a. Post-ganglionic sympathetic fibres supply vasomotor branches to the nasal mucosa b. Pre-ganglionic parasympathetic (greater petrosal nerve) fibres synapse at the pterygopalatine ganglion in the pterygopalatine fossa, to supply secretomotor innervation to the nasal mucosa	The ophthalmic and maxillary divisions of the trigeminal nerve (CN V) provide general sensory innervation to skin, subcutaneous tissue, and mucosa of the nose and paranasal sinuses through: • The nasociliary nerve (branch of CNV1), which also supplies the skin of the external nose and part of the nasal septum • The nasal branches of the greater palatine nerve (CN V2) (posterior part of the lateral wall, roof, and floor of the nasal cavity) • The infraorbital nerve (CN V2) supplies the vestibule of the nose • The nasopalatine nerve (branch of CN V2) supplies the central six upper teeth, in addition to the inferior part of the mucous membrane of the nasal septum • The anterior superior alveolar nerve also supplies the anterior parts of the septum and lateral wall

Lymphatic Drainage of the Nasal Cavity

- The anterior part of the nasal cavity (vestibule) is drained by the submandibular nodes.
- The posterior part of the nasal cavity drains into the retropharyngeal and superior deep cervical lymph nodes.

Paranasal Sinuses

These air-filled chambers interconnect and communicate with the nasal cavity (**Table 2.7, Figures 2.19, 2.20, and 2.21**). They are lined with pseudostratified ciliated columnar epithelium. Paranasal sinuses play an important role in humidifying inspired air and provide protection, facilitate vocal resonance, and decrease the overall weight of the skull.

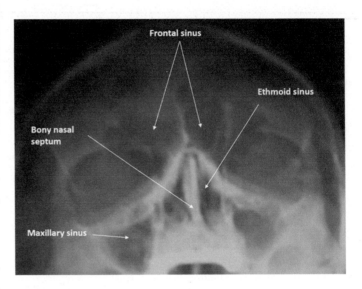

FIGURE 2.19 X-ray of the nasal sinuses. (Courtesy of Baqir Altimimi.)

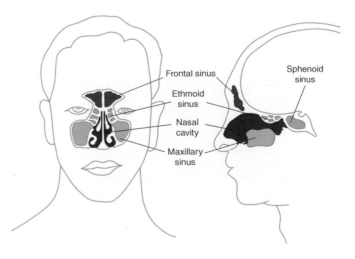

FIGURE 2.20 Paranasal sinuses. (Courtesy of Calum Harrington-Vogt.)

TABLE 2.7: The paranasal sinuses

Sinus	Location	Drainage
Frontal	*Frontal:* triangular in shape Varied morphology	Middle meatus
Maxillary	• Largest of the sinuses, within the maxilla • Its roof is the orbit, its floor is the part of the maxilla which holds the roots of the premolar and molar teeth • Lateral to the nasal cavity	Middle meatus, through the maxillary ostium (opening)
Ethmoidal	Within the ethmoidal bone, upper lateral aspect of nasal cavity three parts:	
	1. Anterior	Middle meatus
	2. Middle	*Middle meatus:* drain on or above the ethmoidal bulla (rounded swelling formed by the middle ethmoidal air cells)
	3. Posterior	Superior meatus
Sphenoidal	Body of the sphenoid	Sphenoethmoidal recess above the superior concha

CLINICAL NOTES

Inflammation of the sinuses and nasal cavity may follow upper respiratory tract infections. Causes can be infective, both bacterial and viral, or allergic. Around 98% are viral in origin. Common symptoms include toothache, sinus headache, and halitosis (bad breath). The condition can be both acute and chronic in nature.

MAXILLARY SINUSITIS

Maxillary sinusitis is the most common site of sinusitis due to the narrowness and position (high on the lateral nasal wall) of the ostium. This prevents adequate drainage, resulting in fluid build-up and infection (**Figure 2.21**). Dental pathology such as tooth root abscesses and oro-antral fistulas can occasionally lead to maxillary sinusitis, usually unilateral.

ORO-ANTRAL FISTULA

Oro-antral fistula is an abnormal communication between the maxillary sinus and the oral cavity.

PITUITARY TUMOUR REMOVAL

The pituitary gland is situated superior to the sphenoid sinus, housed in the sella turcica of the sphenoid bone. Pituitary tumours (commonly adenomas) can be accessed via a trans-sphenoidal approach by passing through the nasal cavity to the sphenoid sinus.

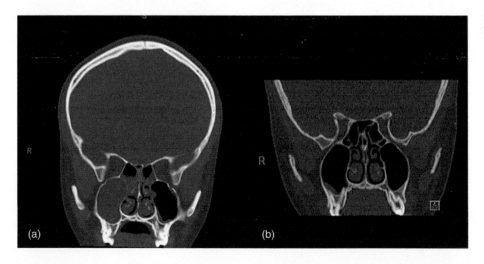

FIGURE 2.21 Coronal CT scan of paranasal sinuses (a) before and (b) after treatment of acute sinusitis. Note marked improvement of fluid/mucosal thickening within the right maxillary antrum. Following treatment, the maxillary antrum is almost completely aerated. (Courtesy of Asha Ali.)

Cranial Nerves (See Section 1)

Olfactory Nerve (CN I)
The shortest of the cranial nerves and can regenerate after damage; see **Table 1.2** in Section 1A.

Optic Nerve (CN II)
See earlier in this chapter. Note that the olfactory and optic nerves are the only cranial nerves which do not originate from the brainstem.

Oculomotor (CN III)

The oculomotor nerve arises from the third nerve nucleus in the midbrain. It traverses the lateral wall of the cavernous sinus (along with CN IV, VI, and V1 and V2, in addition to the internal carotid artery). It emerges from the skull through the supraorbital fissure (see above).

Trochlear (CN IV)

The trochlear nerve contains the fewest number of axons but has the longest intracranial course, as it is the only cranial nerve to arise from the dorsal aspect of the brainstem. It supplies the contralateral superior oblique muscle.

QUIZ QUESTIONS

Q1. *How do you clinically examine the function of the trochlear nerve?*

Q2. *Why has the trochlear nerve been named as such?*

Trigeminal (CN V)

The trigeminal nerve has three divisions, the ophthalmic (V1), maxillary (V2), and mandibular (V3) nerves, and is therefore the largest cranial nerve (**Figure 2.22**). It supplies sensory fibres to the skin of the face and mucous membrane of the nose, mouth, and nasal sinuses. It leaves the pons as two roots (large sensory and small motor). The Gasserian ganglion contains the sensory cell bodies of the three divisions. The motor root passes under the ganglion to join the sensory division of the mandibular nerve and exits the skull through the foramen ovale.

Ophthalmic Nerve (CV V1)

Contains sensory fibres for the scalp, forehead, cornea, conjunctiva and upper eyelid, nasal mucosa, and frontal sinus. It leaves the skull through the superior orbital fissure after passing through the cavernous sinus. Subsequently, it divides into the frontal, lacrimal, and nasociliary branches.

Maxillary Nerve (CN V2)

Contains sensory fibres for the buccal area, lower eyelid, nasal cavity, palate, pharynx, gums, and upper teeth and leaves the skull through the foramen rotundum to enter the pterygopalatine fossa. It then enters the infraorbital canal as the infraorbital nerve to emerge via the infraorbital foramen. It supplies sensory branches to the side of the nose (nasopalatine nerve), palate (greater and lesser palatine nerves), upper gingiva and mucosa (posterior, middle, and anterior superior alveolar nerves), medial part of the skin of the cheek and upper lip, skin, and conjunctiva of the lower eyelid (zygomatic and infraorbital nerves), and the nasopharynx (pharyngeal nerve). Two branches connect the maxillary nerve to the pterygopalatine ganglion.

Mandibular Nerve (CN V3)

The largest division and contains both sensory and motor fibres. Leaves the skull through the foramen ovale. It carries sensory fibres for the intrabuccal area, including the anterior two-thirds of the tongue, lower teeth, and gums, and motor fibres to the muscles of mastication, mylohyoid, tensor veli palatini, tensor tympani, and anterior belly of the digastric muscle. The mandibular nerve divides into anterior and posterior divisions. The anterior division supplies:

- Motor innervation to the temporalis, lateral pterygoid, and masseter muscles. The medial pterygoid muscle is supplied by the main trunk before division.
- The buccal nerve carries sensory fibres for the skin and mucous membrane of the cheek (the buccal branch of the facial nerve carries motor fibres to the buccinator muscle).

The posterior division gives rise to the following branches:

- *Auriculotemporal nerve:* supplies the skin of the external ear, meatal surface of the tympanic membrane and temporomandibular joint, and carries parasympathetic and sympathetic branches to the parotid gland.
- *Lingual nerve:* supplies sensory fibres to the floor of the mouth and anterior two-thirds of the tongue (the chorda tympani from the facial nerve accompanies this nerve and supplies secretory parasympathetic and taste sensation to the anterior two-thirds of the tongue). It traverses the floor of the mouth as it crosses the submandibular duct. It can therefore be injured during operations to remove stones from the duct or during removal of the submandibular salivary gland.
- *Inferior alveolar:* a mixed nerve which passes into the mandibular foramen (an opening into the mandibular canal on the medial aspect of the ramus of the mandible), giving branches to the roots of the lower teeth. It terminates by exiting through the mental foramen to give sensory innervation to the anterior vestibular gingiva and the skin of the lower lip and chin through its two terminal branches: the mental and incisive nerves. In addition, it supplies motor branches to the mylohyoid and anterior belly of the digastric muscle (via the nerve to the mylohyoid).

CLINICAL NOTES

- *Inferior alveolar nerve anaesthesia* is one of the most common injection techniques in dentistry. Dentists often block the inferior alveolar nerve before it enters the mandibular canal by injecting local anaesthetic solution to numb the ipsilateral lower teeth. The skin and mucosa of the lower lip, labial alveolar mucosa, and gingiva and skin of the chin are also anaesthetised because they are supplied by the mental branch of this nerve.
- *Trigeminal neuralgia* (tic douloureux) is characterised by intermittent attacks of unilateral intense facial pain. The majority of cases are idiopathic.

QUIZ QUESTION

Q. *How do you clinically test for trigeminal nerve function (remember that it has sensory and motor divisions)?*

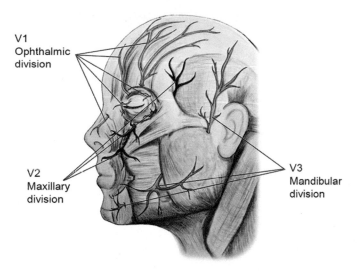

FIGURE 2.22 The distribution of the trigeminal nerve. (Courtesy of Kathryn DeMarre.)

Abducens Nerve (CN VI)

The abducens nerve originates from the abducens nucleus in the pons and emerges at the junction between the pons and medullary pyramids. It passes within the cavernous sinus and enters the orbit through the superior orbital fissure to supply the lateral rectus muscle. The lateral gaze results from a combination of contraction of the ipsilateral lateral rectus muscle and contralateral medial rectus muscle (supplied by CN III). This causes both eyes to fixate or track an object.

Facial Nerve (CN VII)

The facial nerve emerges with the vestibulocochlear nerve (CN VIII) at the ventrolateral aspect of the ponto-medullary junction (intracranial part) and enters the internal auditory meatus (intratemporal part), accompanied by the sensory root. Within the temporal bone (facial canal), it gives rise to the greater petrosal nerve, which joins the deep petrosal nerve to form the nerve of the pterygoid canal (Vidian nerve) and motor fibres to the stapedius.

It leaves the cranial cavity at the stylomastoid foramen (extratemporal part) and passes through the parotid gland (bisecting it into superficial and deep lobes). Therefore, the facial nerve should be examined as part of the examination of parotid swellings. Note that the facial nerve does not supply the parotid gland. The sensory root (the intermediate nerve or nervus intermedius) supplies part of the skin of the external auditory meatus and a small area posterior to the ear (thereby supplementing CN V3). The chorda tympani leaves the facial nerve before it emerges from the stylomastoid foramen to enter the tympanic cavity and passes within the substance of the tympanic membrane. It exits the skull at the petrotympanic fissure to join the lingual nerve.

The facial nerve contains special sensory fibres which supply taste sensation for the anterior two-thirds of the tongue and the hard and soft palate, as well as visceral secretomotor parasympathetic fibres to lacrimal, submandibular, and sublingual glands and the mucous membrane of the nose and palate.

The facial nerve divides into five terminal branches:

- Temporal
- Zygomatic
- Buccal
- Mandibular
- Cervical

These branches supply the muscles of facial expression (*vide infra*). Other motor branches provide innervation to the stylohyoid and posterior belly of the digastric muscle.

The muscles of the face (**Figure 2.23**) are arranged as follows:

- Around the eyelids (see **Table 2.3**) in addition to the occipitofrontalis.
- Around the mouth. The orbicularis oris arises from the medial aspect of the maxilla and the mandible and inserts into the skin of the upper and lower lips. It acts as a sphincter of the mouth, and is supplied by the buccal branch of the facial nerve.
  - *Levator labii superioris:* lifting the upper lip
  - *Depressor labii inferioris:* pulling the lower lip down
  - *Levator anguli oris and depressor anguli oris:* act on the corners of the mouth
  - *Zygomaticus major:* from the zygomatic bone; inserts into the modiolus, helps in smiling
  - *Zygomaticus minor:* arises from the zygomatic bone, inserts into the skin of the lateral upper lip
  - *Mentalis:* from the anterior aspect of the mandible to the skin of the chin
  - *Risorius:* arises from the parotid fascia and inserts into the modiolus; helps in smiling
- Muscles around the nostrils (see **Table 2.4**).
- *Buccinator:* from the alveolar processes of both the mandible and the maxilla and the pterygomandibular raphe; inserts into the orbicularis oris; supplied by the buccal branch of the facial nerve; compresses the cheek against the teeth and helps in mastication and whistling

The modiolus is a fibromuscular structure at the angles of the mouth, where several muscles converge. The modiolus helps in integrating the muscles around the mouth.

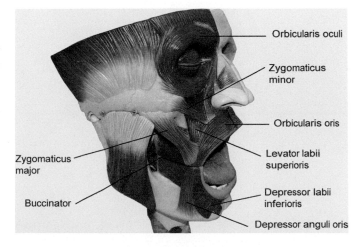

FIGURE 2.23 Muscles of facial expression. (Courtesy of Department of Anatomical Sciences, SGUL.)

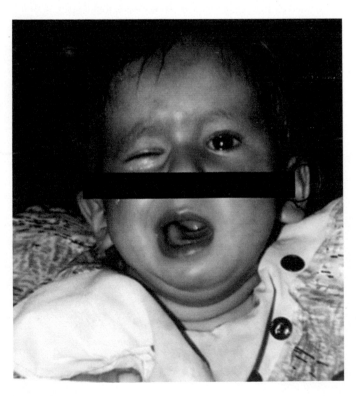

FIGURE 2.24 Child with viral encephalitis. (Courtesy of Qassim F. Baker.)

The Vestibulocochlear Nerve (CN VIII)
See "The Ear".

Glossopharyngeal Nerve (CN IX)
Exits the medulla oblongata, where it originates from four nuclei, emerges through the jugular foramen, and innervates the following:

- Motor supply to the stylopharyngeus muscle
- Parasympathetic innervation to the parotid gland
- Receives information from the baroreceptors of the carotid sinus and chemoreceptors of the carotid body in response to changes in blood pressure and blood gases (O_2 and CO_2)
- General sensory information from the external ear, inner side of the tympanic membrane, upper pharynx, and posterior third of the tongue
- Special sensory (taste sensation) from the posterior third of the tongue

Vagus Nerve (CN X)
The term vagus nerve translates to "wandering nerve" in Latin. It emerges from the anterior surface of the medulla oblongata and exits the cranial cavity through the jugular foramen. It is accompanied by the internal carotid artery (ICA) and subsequently the common carotid artery (CCA) and internal jugular vein (IJV) as it descends within the carotid sheath of the neck. In the neck, the vagus nerve and its branches supply the following:

- Soft palate muscles (except tensor veli palatini)
- Pharyngeal muscles (except stylopharyngeus), including palatoglossus
- Muscles of the larynx
- Sensation at the back of the ear, external auditory meatus, and external aspect of the temporomandibular joint
- Sensation to the larynx and laryngopharynx

The vagus nerve continues as the parasympathetic supply to the thoracic (pulmonary, cardiac, bronchi, oesophageal) and abdominal viscera (down to splenic flexure) (see **Section 5**).

Recurrent Laryngeal Nerve
The recurrent laryngeal nerve (RLN) originates from the vagus nerve in the thorax and ascends to the neck. The left RLN loops around the aortic arch at the ligamentum arteriosum, while the right loops around the right subclavian artery and therefore has a shorter course. Ascending in the neck, the RLN lies within the tracheo-oesophageal groove. The RLN supplies all the intrinsic muscles of the larynx except the cricothyroid, and supplies sensory innervation to the mucous membrane inferior to the vocal cords. The nerve should always be identified prior to thyroidectomies (*vide infra*). The final 2 cm of the nerve before entering the larynx are the most vulnerable to injury. The RLN is lateral but close to the lateral thyroid ligament (ligament of Berry).

Accessory Nerve (CN XI)
The accessory nerve is composed of two roots: the spinal root arising from the upper six cervical nerves and the cranial root emerging from the lateral side of the medulla oblongata.

The spinal root enters the posterior cranial fossa through the foramen magnum and unites with the cranial root. Both roots leave the cranial cavity through the jugular foramen, where they separate. The cranial root joins the vagus nerve to provide motor innervation to the muscles of the pharynx and larynx.

The spinal root supplies the sternocleidomastoid muscle and passes through the posterior triangle of the neck to supply the trapezius. Within the posterior triangle it lies in close proximity to cervical lymph nodes. This is of clinical importance during the removal of cervical lymph nodes for biopsy.

Hypoglossal Nerve (CN XII)

The hypoglossal nerve originates from the hypoglossal nucleus in the medulla oblongata as a series of rootlets. It subsequently exits the cranial cavity via the hypoglossal canal. It is related to the carotid arteries within the carotid triangle and can be injured during carotid endarterectomy. It swings from the carotid triangle to the submandibular triangle for its destination to supply all the intrinsic and extrinsic muscles of the tongue except for the palatoglossus. Injury results in ipsilateral tongue atrophy. The superior root of the ansa cervicalis (C1, C2) is closely related to the hypoglossal nerve, but not part of it. Remember that the nerve supply of the geniohyoid muscle (C1) courses with the hypoglossal nerve but doesn't originate from it.

The Oral Cavity

The oral cavity (mouth) is bounded by the lips anteriorly and extends to the palatoglossal folds, where it is continuous with the oropharynx.

Mucous membrane lines the oral cavity, giving it its red appearance, covered by stratified squamous epithelium.

The oral cavity is divided into two parts: the vestibule and the oral cavity proper. If you blow your cheeks out, air fills the vestibule of the mouth. This is the "slit-like" space external to the teeth and between the gums. The oral cavity proper is the space internal to the teeth.

The oral cavity is bound laterally by the left and right buccinator muscles. The parotid duct (salivary duct) pierces the buccinator muscle to open into the oral cavity opposite the upper second molar tooth.

A pocket of fat, the buccal fat pad, lies superficially on the buccinator muscle. The buccal fat pad is relatively large in babies and assists in suckling.

The **mylohyoid and the geniohyoid muscles form the floor of the mouth**. The tongue arises from the floor of the cavity and occupies most of it.

The roof of the oral cavity is formed by the palate (appreciate how the palate also forms the floor of the nasal cavity).

Tongue

The tongue is composed of a mass of skeletal muscle that is covered in mucous membrane. This organ is important for speech, mastication, swallowing, and taste. It is divided into left and right parts by a fibrous septum. It has oral (anterior two-thirds) and pharyngeal (posterior third) parts, demarcated by the V-shaped terminal sulcus (sulcus terminalis). The apex of the V-shaped sulcus marks a pit, the foramen caecum (see Development of the thyroid gland). The tongue has a rough dorsal surface containing the taste buds and papillae in the anterior two-thirds and a ventral smooth surface. The posterior one-third contains aggregates of lymphoid tissues (the lingual tonsil) (**Figure 2.25**).

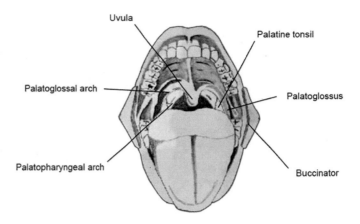

FIGURE 2.25 The tongue and the oral cavity. (Courtesy of John Ward.)

Papillae

Papillae are mucosal projections located on the dorsal surface and give the anterior two-thirds of the tongue (the pre-sulcal area) its rough texture. There are four types of papillae:

- Fungiform (mushroom-like)
- Circumvallate (means surrounded by a "vallum" or wall of mucosa), 8 to 12 in number, located at the anterior part of the terminal sulcus (supplied by the glossopharyngeal nerve)
- Foliate (leaf-like), located on the posterior lateral edge of the tongue
- Filiform (filament or thread-like), numerous and do not contain taste buds

The fungiform, circumvallate, and foliate papillae are considered gustatory papillae, as they contain taste buds. Taste buds are also present on the soft palate (supplied by the facial nerve), on the epiglottis, and on the larynx (supplied by the internal laryngeal branch of the vagus).

The muscles of the tongue arise from the occipital myotomes, which migrate ventrally, bringing their nerve supply (the hypoglossal nerves) with them.

The tongue is composed of four intrinsic and four extrinsic muscles (**Figure 2.26**). The intrinsic muscles are named for the direction of the muscle fibres and do not attach to any bones. Their function is to alter the shape of the tongue. They are classified as:

- Superior longitudinal
- Vertical
- Transverse
- Inferior longitudinal

The extrinsic muscles attach to superior or inferior bony landmarks and travel into the tongue. They function to move the tongue (**Table 2.8**).

All the extrinsic muscles are supplied by the hypoglossal nerve (CN XII), apart from the palatoglossus muscle, which is supplied by the vagus nerve (CN X).

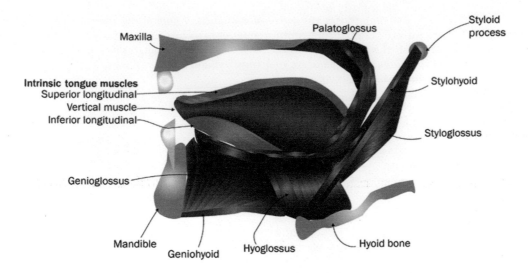

FIGURE 2.26   Sagittal view of the intrinsic and extrinsic tongue muscles. (Courtesy of John Ward.)

TABLE 2.8: Extrinsic muscles of the tongue

Muscle	Origin	Insertion	Action	Innervation
Genioglossus	Superior mental spine on the inner surface of the symphysis menti	Tongue and body of the hyoid bone	• Depress to create central furrow • Posterior part protrudes tongue, anterior part retract tongue	Hypoglossal nerve (CN XII)
Hyoglossus	Hyoid bone	Side of the tongue between styloglossus and longitudinal muscle	Depresses and retracts tongue	Hypoglossal nerve (CN XII)
Styloglossus	Styloid process of temporal bone	Tongue	Retracts tongue and helps create central furrow	Hypoglossal nerve (CN XII)
Palatoglossus	Palatine aponeurosis of the soft palate	Tongue	Elevates posterior aspect of tongue	Vagus nerve (CN X)

Sensory Supply of the Tongue

The general and special sensory innervation of the anterior two-thirds and the posterior third of the tongue is different.

Anterior two-thirds: arises from the first pharyngeal arch:

- General sensation is supplied by the **lingual nerve**, a branch of the mandibular division of trigeminal nerve (CN V3).
- Special sensory is supplied by the **chorda tympani**, a branch of the facial nerve (CN VII) which runs with the lingual nerve to enter the tongue.

Posterior third: arises from the third and the fourth pharyngeal arches.

General and special sensory fibres arise from the **glossopharyngeal nerve** (CN IX), which also supplies taste buds in the oropharynx. The glossopharyngeal nerve is responsible for the afferent pathway for the gag reflex. The motor part is mediated by the vagus nerve.

Blood Supply of the Tongue

The tongue is supplied predominantly by the lingual artery (a branch of the external carotid). It also receives contributions from the tonsillar branch of the facial artery and from the ascending pharyngeal artery. The lingual veins drain into the internal jugular veins.

Lymphatic Drainage of the Tongue

Lymph from the:

- Tip of the tongue drains to the submental lymph nodes.
- Lateral part of the anterior two-thirds of the tongue drains to submandibular lymph nodes, which drain into the inferior deep cervical lymph nodes.
- Posterior third of the tongue drains into the superior deep cervical lymph nodes.

CLINICAL NOTES

The tongue, historically, is looked at as a reflection of body health. Examination of the tongue is an integral part of the physical examination, looking for dehydration (dry tongue), blue tongue (central cyanosis), and bald tongue (nutritional deficiency).

SUBLINGUAL ABSORPTION OF DRUGS

Drugs placed under the tongue can be quickly absorbed into the bloodstream due to its rich blood supply – for example, sublingual nitroglycerin, a coronary vasodilator which is used by patients with angina.

TONGUE ULCERS

Causes can be classified as:

- *Traumatic* (injuries, sharp teeth, accidental biting).
- *Infections* (human papillomavirus 1, HIV, fungi such as candidiasis, tuberculosis [TB], syphilis). Ulcers due to aphthous stomatitis are usually multiple and very painful and improve within a short time.
- *Malignant* (squamous cell carcinoma), which may be preceded by leucoplakia (white patch on the tongue or on the oral mucosa). This is mostly related to smoking and excessive alcohol consumption and presents as an ulcer or a growth. The lateral aspect of the tongue is the most common site for malignant ulceration (see oropharyngeal cancer).

HYPOGLOSSAL NERVE PARALYSIS

The hypoglossal nerve can be injured during surgery (e.g., carotid endarterectomy), causing the tongue to deviate to the same side as the injury.

The Palate

The palate is composed of the hard palate anteriorly and the soft palate posteriorly. It forms the roof of the mouth and the floor of the nasal cavity.

Hard Palate

The hard palate is formed by two bones:

- Horizontal part of the palatine bone
- Palatine process of the maxillary bone

Soft Palate

The soft palate hangs from the posterior aspect of the hard palate as a mobile flap, which separates the nasal and oral parts of the pharynx (**Figure 2.27**). The soft palate is composed of five muscles:

- Musculus uvulae (the muscle of the uvula).
- Palatoglossus (from the palate to the side of the tongue within the palatoglossal arch).
- Palatopharyngeus (from the soft palate to the lateral wall of the oropharynx, within the palatopharyngeal arch; the palatine tonsil lies in between the palatoglossal and palatopharyngeal arches). This muscle inserts into the posterior border of the thyroid cartilage and is considered one of the longitudinal muscles of the pharynx.
- Levator veli palatini's contraction helps to shut the nasopharynx from the oropharynx.
- Tensor veli palatini's expanded tendon forms the palatine aponeurosis.

The five muscles are all supplied by the vagus nerve (pharyngeal plexus) except for the tensor veli palatini, which is supplied by the mandibular division of the trigeminal nerve.

The sensory innervation of the palate is by the maxillary division of the trigeminal nerve (CN V2) through the greater and lesser palatine nerves.

Blood supply is provided by branches from the maxillary, facial, and ascending pharyngeal arteries.

Lymphatic drainage is to the deep cervical group of lymph nodes.

CLINICAL NOTE

GAG OR PHARYNGEAL REFLEX

Stimulation of the pharynx wall is detected by the afferent glossopharyngeal nerve (CN IX), which initiates the gag reflex by stimulating the vagus nerve (CN X) to contract the pharyngeal muscles.

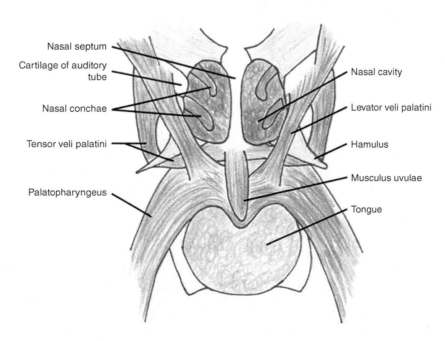

FIGURE 2.27 The muscles of the soft palate, posterior view. (Courtesy of Gabriela Barzyk.)

Cleft Palate

This is a developmental defect that results from the failure of the primary palate (intermaxillary segment) and the secondary palate (palatal shelves) to fuse, normally at the incisive foramen. There are different grades of cleft palate; some are associated with cleft lip (**Figure 2.28**) and, rarely, abnormality of the nasal septum. It can result in problems with feeding and phonation.

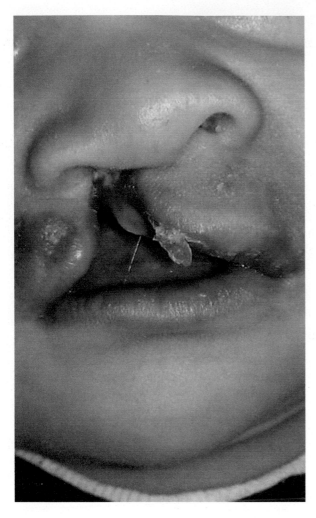

FIGURE 2.28   Cleft lip and palate. (Courtesy of Mohammed H. Aldabbagh.)

Muscles of Mastication

The muscles of mastication function to move the temporomandibular joint in order to chew and grind up food. They are **all innervated by branches of the mandibular nerve (CN V3)**.

There are four muscles of mastication on each side of the face:

- **Temporalis** arises from the temporal fossa and inserts into the coronoid process and ramus of the mandible.
- **Masseter** passes from the zygomatic arch to the ramus and angle of the mandible.
- **Medial pterygoid** originates as two heads from the lateral pterygoid plate of the sphenoid bone and from the palatine bone. It inserts into the ramus and angle of the mandible.

- **Lateral pterygoid** originates as two heads from the greater wing of the sphenoid and lateral pterygoid plate to insert into the temporomandibular joint and neck of the mandible. It divides the maxillary artery into three parts as it passes between its two heads.

Temporomandibular Joint

The temporomandibular joint is the articulation between the condylar process of the mandible and the mandibular fossa of the temporal bone. It is a bilateral hinge joint, with a biconcave fibrocartilaginous articular disc located between the condyle and the mandibular fossa. The articular disc facilitates complex movements. The capsule is reinforced laterally by the temporomandibular ligament, and there are two accessory ligaments: the sphenomandibular and stylomandibular ligaments.

Infratemporal Fossa

The infratemporal fossa is the area inferior to the zygomatic arch and deep to the masseter muscle. It contains the:

- Lateral pterygoid muscle
- Medial pterygoid muscle
- Maxillary artery (terminal branch of the external carotid artery, divided into three parts due to its relationship with the lateral pterygoid muscle)
- Pterygoid venous plexus
- Mandibular division of the trigeminal nerve (CN V3)
- Chorda tympani branch of the facial nerve
- Otic ganglion, a parasympathetic ganglion, located at the stem of the mandibular nerve, near the foramen ovale. Parasympathetic fibres, through the lesser petrosal branch of the glossopharyngeal nerve, synapse within the ganglion and supply secretomotor fibres to the parotid gland. The sympathetic fibres from the superior cervical ganglion pass without synapsing in the ganglion within the auriculotemporal nerve to supply the parotid gland

Salivary Glands

There are three paired salivary glands: the parotid, submandibular, and sublingual glands. The salivary glands produce saliva to lubricate the oral cavity, help protect the teeth from decay, and aid in digestion.

Parotid Gland

The parotid gland is the largest salivary gland and is located anterior to the external ear, enclosed in a fibrous capsule. It has two lobes (deep and superficial), which are bisected by the facial nerve. Saliva produced in the parotid gland enters the oral cavity by travelling through the parotid duct. The parotid duct is approximately 5 cm in length and emerges from the medial aspect of the gland. It passes over the masseter muscle (inferior to the zygomatic arch) and pierces the buccinator to open in the mouth opposite the upper second molar tooth. Several important anatomical structures traverse the parotid gland:

- The facial nerve branches into its terminal divisions within the gland: temporal, zygomatic, buccal, mandibular, and cervical.

- The external carotid artery travels though the gland and bifurcates posterior to the ramus of the mandible into its two terminal branches: the maxillary and superficial temporal arteries.
- The superficial temporal and maxillary veins unite within the substances of the gland to form the retromandibular vein.

Innervation of the Parotid Gland

Sensory innervation is from the great auricular nerve, a branch of cervical plexus. Autonomic innervation is secretomotor in nature (see the earlier discussion on the otic ganglion).

Sublingual Gland

The sublingual salivary gland opens into the floor of the mouth via multiple ducts. This small gland lies on top of the mylohyoid muscle.

Submandibular Gland

The submandibular salivary glands produce the most saliva. The saliva produced by the submandibular glands is mucoid in nature to facilitate lubrication of the bolus before swallowing. The gland is described as having superficial and deep parts due to its relationship to the mylohyoid muscle. The submandibular salivary gland opens to the side of the frenulum of the tongue. Parasympathetic supply runs with the chorda tympani and increases the amount of saliva secreted (vide infra, the submandibular triangle).

CLINICAL NOTES

- Mumps (a viral infection) is the most common cause of parotid swelling (parotitis). Mumps is particularly painful because the swelling is compressed by the tough capsule covering the gland.
- Pleomorphic adenoma is the most common parotid tumour (**Figures 2.29** and **2.30**).

QUIZ QUESTION

This swelling has been slowly enlarging over many years (**Figure 2.29**).

Q1. *What is the most prominent physical sign?*

Q2. *What should be examined next?*

The facial nerve should always be identified and preserved during surgical removal of the parotid gland (parotidectomy).

With salivary duct calculi (sialolithiasis), the parotid duct is blocked by stones. This is a rare condition.

Submandibular Calculi

Salivary gland calculi (stones) are most commonly located in the submandibular gland and duct. The history of a swelling under the jaw, which is intermittent and appears with food ingestion, represents blockage of the submandibular duct. Examination of the mouth includes looking for the orifice of the submandibular duct (Wharton's duct) below the tongue, to the side of the frenulum, and bimanual palpation of floor of the mouth and the submandibular region. The orifice of the duct may reveal the presence of

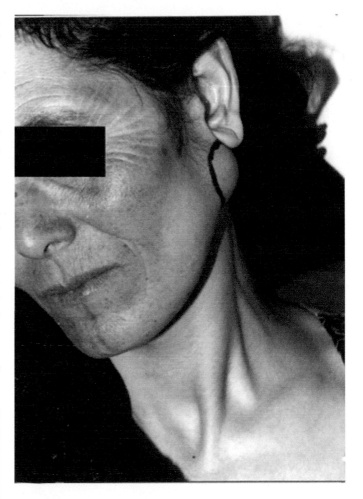

FIGURE 2.29 Mixed parotid tumour. (Courtesy of Qassim F. Baker.)

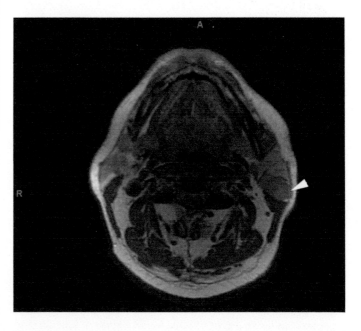

FIGURE 2.30 MRI neck: Axial T1 with contrast: Left parotid adenoma *(arrowhead)*. (Courtesy of Asha Ali.)

a stone (**Figure 2.31**). The diagnosis may be confirmed by X-ray of the floor of the mouth or by sialography (injecting a dye through the cannulation of the orifice of the submandibular duct), which may dislodge the stone as well.

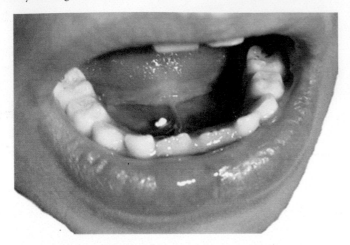

FIGURE 2.31   Stone at the orifice of the right submandibular duct. (Courtesy of Ali M. Hasan.)

Anatomy of the Neck

Cervical Vertebrae

There are seven cervical vertebrae in the neck region, of which four are typical (C3–C6) and three are atypical (C1, C2, and C7).

The Atlas (C1)

The first cervical vertebra is called the atlas (**Figures 2.32 and 2.33**). It is shaped like a ring and does not have a body. The lateral sides are expanded as two masses, which articulate with the occipital condyles of the skull at the atlanto-occipital joint. This joint allows for the nodding movement of the head.

The Axis (C2)

The second cervical vertebra is called the axis (**Figure 2.34**). The most prominent feature is the short odontoid process, or dens, that projects from the superior aspect of the body. The odontoid process articulates with the atlas at the atlantoaxial joint. This joint allows for rotation of the skull, as the dens acts as a pivot.

Vertebra Prominens (C7)

The seventh cervical vertebra has the longest spinous process, which is not bifid. It can be easily palpated at the back of the neck (**Figure 2.35**).

Important cervical landmarks:

- *C1:* base of nose and hard palate
- *C2:* teeth in closed mouth
- *C3:* mandible and hyoid
- *C4:* bifurcation of the carotid artery
- *C3–C6:* larynx
- *C4–C5:* thyroid cartilage
- *C6–C7:* cricoid cartilage
- *C6:* laryngopharynx becomes continuous with the trachea and oesophagus

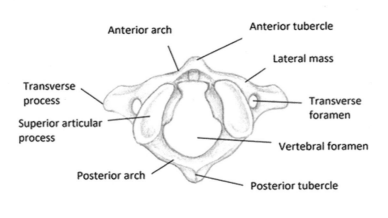

FIGURE 2.32   Superior view of C1 vertebra. (Courtesy of Callum Moffitt.)

Typical Cervical Vertebrae

The bodies of the cervical vertebrae are relatively small, as they do not have to support the weight of the trunk. The vertebral foramen is relatively large and triangular. The cervical spinous processes of C2–C6 are bifid. They each possess a foramen in their transverse processes, the foramina transversaria. The vertebral artery, which supplies the spinal cord and brain, ascends through only six transverse foramina (C6–C1), whereas the vertebral vein descends through all seven (C1–C7). Note that the C7 foramina are small and sometimes absent. Joints between superior and inferior articular processes (zygapophyseal joints) allow flexion and extension of the column.

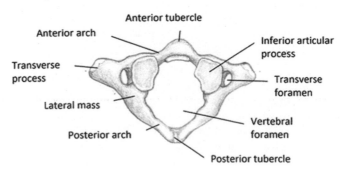

FIGURE 2.33   Inferior view of atlas (C1). (Courtesy of Callum Moffitt.)

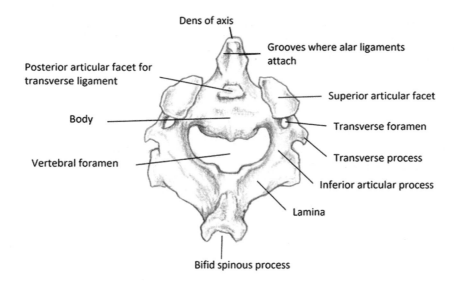

FIGURE 2.34 The axis (C2). (Courtesy of Callum Moffitt.)

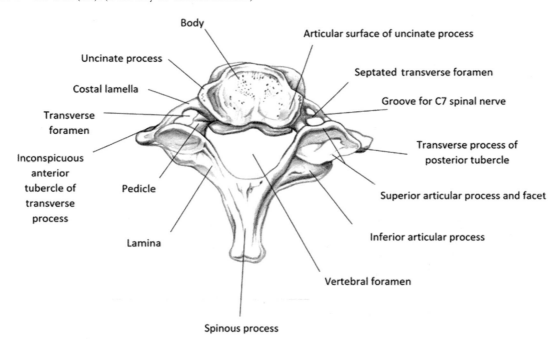

FIGURE 2.35 Superior view of C7. (Courtesy of Callum Moffitt.)

CLINICAL NOTES

CERVICAL SPINE INJURY

- The cervical spine is the most common site of spinal injury, particularly at C7.
- Common patterns of fractures include occipital condyle fractures, Jefferson's fracture (burst fracture of the anterior and posterior arches of C1), atlantoaxial dislocation, hangman's fracture (fracture of the pars interarticularis of C2), odontoid process fracture, compression fractures, and C7 facet joint dislocation.
- The most common cause of cervical spine injury is road traffic accidents (RTAs) resulting in a whiplash injury mechanism. This involves shear, tensile, and rotational forces from acute flexion, compression, extension, and distraction movement all occurring in less than a second.
- Other causes of cervical spine injury include violent assaults, shallow water diving (axial force producing vertical compression fractures), and falls (common in the elderly).
- All major trauma patients should be presumed to have a cervical spine injury until proven otherwise, due to the high risk of spinal cord injury. Initial management of a severely injured patient at the scene of the accident must include applying cervical spine immobilisation with a rigid collar, lateral head supports, and strapping across. The patient should be very carefully lifted. The cervical collar and other precautions should be kept until the CT scan of the spine reveals no evidence of injury.

(Continued)

- After initial resuscitation (ABCDE) and assessment, a CT scan should be done in accordance with Advanced Trauma Life Support (ATLS) guidelines. A lateral X-ray is only to be used if a CT scan is unavailable.

CERVICAL DEGENERATIVE DISEASES

Spondylosis is a form of osteoarthritis in the vertebral column and leads to the formation of osteophytes. Symptoms arise from osteophyte compression of the nerve root, leading to unilateral radiculopathy. Degenerative disc disease results from dehydration and alterations in the collagen composition of the nucleus pulposus and annulus fibrosus, which occur with age.

CHASSAIGNAC'S (CAROTID) TUBERCLE

The tubercle of the fourth cervical vertebrae separates the carotid and vertebral arteries. The carotid artery can be massaged against this tubercle to relieve symptoms of supraventricular tachycardia.

QUIZ QUESTION

Q. *How do you differentiate the seventh cervical vertebra from the first thoracic vertebra?*

Fascia of the Neck

The superficial fascia on the front of the neck contains the platysma (a sheet of voluntary muscle that extends from the lower jaw to the front of the upper chest, supplied by the cervical branch of the facial nerve).

Deep cervical fascia is the fibrous connective tissue which surrounds different compartments of the neck. It is composed of the following layers:

- The investing layer is the more superficial layer, which completely invests the sternocleidomastoid and trapezius muscles. Inferiorly, it attaches to the manubrium sterni, clavicles, and acromion and spine of the scapula; superiorly it attaches to the external occipital protuberance, superior

nuchal line, zygomatic arches, and mastoid processes. Posteriorly, it attaches to the ligamentum nuchae, along the spinous processes of the cervical vertebrae. It also splits to enclose the parotid and the submandibular salivary glands.

- Prevertebral fascia is located in front of the vertebral column, the deep muscles of the back, and the scalene muscles. Superiorly, it attaches to the base of the skull and is continuous inferiorly with the endothoracic fascia of the chest and the anterior longitudinal ligament of the vertebral column. Laterally, it extends as the axillary sheath to envelope the axillary vessels and brachial plexus.
- Pre-tracheal fascia is located in the front of the neck and is attached superiorly to the hyoid. It encapsulates the thyroid gland, trachea, and oesophagus, as well as the infrahyoid muscles. The pre-tracheal fascia is weak posteriorly, meaning infection can easily spread backwards in the neck (*vide infra*, the lateral thyroid ligament). Swellings related to the thyroid gland (goitre) move on swallowing, a very important clinical sign (see the later discussion on the anatomy of the thyroid gland).
- The carotid sheath is the fascia which surrounds the common and internal carotid arteries, internal jugular vein, vagus, ansa cervicalis, and deep cervical lymph nodes on each side of the neck from the base of the skull to the root of the neck. The cervical sympathetic trunk is located posterior to the carotid sheath.

Suprahyoid Muscles

The suprahyoid muscles are a group of muscles that attach to the superior part of the hyoid, and thus their contraction results in elevation of the hyoid (**Table 2.9**).

Infrahyoid Muscles

The infrahyoid muscles are a group of strap muscles that attach to the inferior surface of the hyoid, and hence their contraction depresses the bone itself, Mnemonic: TOSS (**Table 2.10**).

CLINICAL NOTE

In order to mobilise the thyroid lobes in thyroid gland surgery, the infrahyoid strap muscles must be retracted. Only in extreme operative difficulty are the muscles cut.

TABLE 2.9: Suprahyoid muscles

Muscle	Origin	Insertion	Innervation	Function
Mylohyoid (diaphragm of the mouth)	Mylohyoid line of mandible	Hyoid	Nerve to mylohyoid from mandibular branch of trigeminal (CN V3)	Elevates hyoid
Digastric (anterior belly)	Digastric fossa of mandible, close to symphysis menti	Intermediate tendon attached to the body and greater cornu of the hyoid bone through a fibrous sling	Nerve to mylohyoid (CN V3)	Elevates hyoid, depresses mandible
Digastric (posterior belly)	Intermediate tendon (between the two bellies)	Mastoid notch of the temporal bone	Facial nerve (CN VII)	Elevates hyoid, depresses mandible
Geniohyoid	Inferior mental spine of mandibular symphysis	Hyoid	C1 via hypoglossal (CN XII)	Helps in swallowing by widening pharynx
Stylohyoid	Styloid process of the temporal bone	Hyoid	Facial nerve (CN VII)	Retracts, elevates hyoid to increase length of floor of the mouth
Hyoglossus (see **Table 2.8**)				

TABLE 2.10: Infrahyoid muscles

Muscles	Origin	Insertion	Innervation	Function
Thyrohyoid	Thyroid cartilage	Hyoid	C1 via hypoglossal (CN XII)	Depresses hyoid
Sternohyoid	Manubrium sterni	Hyoid	Ansa cervicalis (C1–C3)	Depresses hyoid and larynx
Sternothyroid	Manubrium sterni	Oblique line on the lamina of thyroid cartilage	Ansa cervicalis (C1–C3)	Depresses larynx
Omohyoid (see **Table 2.11**)				

Nerves of the Neck

There are three major nervous structures which travel through the neck: the vagus nerve, phrenic nerve, and cervical sympathetic trunk. (Note: the accessory, glossopharyngeal, and hypoglossal nerves also give branches to structures in the neck.)

The Cervical Plexus

This is formed from the ventral rami of C1–C4 and supplies sensory nerves to the neck and motor branches, mainly via the ansa cervicalis, to the infrahyoid and prevertebral muscles and levator scapulae. Branches from C3 and C4 join C5 to form the phrenic nerve. The plexus lies deep to the sternocleidomastoid muscle. Each nerve, except the first (suboccipital nerve) gives rise to both descending and ascending roots in the form of loops.

The sensory branches, which arise at the punctum nervosum (Erb's point) (the middle of the posterior border of the sternocleidomastoid muscle) are:

- *Lesser occipital nerve* (C2) supplies the back of the scalp (see "Innervation of the scalp").
- *Greater auricular nerve* (C2, C3), sensory fibres from the skin over the parotid gland, back of the pinna of the external ear and mastoid process.
- *Transverse cervical nerve* (C2, C3), sensory supply of the anterior aspect of the neck.
- *Supraclavicular nerves* (C3, C4), medial, intermediate, and lateral, supply sensory fibres to part of the skin of the neck and over the shoulder and upper chest down to the second rib (see **Section 5** for gallbladder-referred pain to the tip of the right shoulder).

QUIZ QUESTION

Q. *What is the importance of the punctum nervosum to the anaesthetist?*

Phrenic Nerve (C3–C5, mainly C4)

The major branch from the cervical plexus, the phrenic nerve provides motor innervation to the diaphragm in addition to sensory branches to the pericardium, diaphragmatic pleura, and peritoneum. It runs anterior to the scalenus anterior (see **Section 4**).

Ansa Cervicalis (Latin: "Handle of the Neck")

The ansa cervicalis is a looped nerve that is composed of a superior root (C1), which is continuous with an inferior root (C2–C3). The superior root (*descendens hypoglossi*) travels with the hypoglossal nerve, then passes inferiorly to form a loop with the inferior root, which ascends anterior to the internal jugular vein in the carotid triangle. Both roots supply the infrahyoid muscles.

Cervical Sympathetic Trunk

The cervical sympathetic trunk lies on the prevertebral muscles, behind the prevertebral fascia. It is composed of three ganglia (inferior, middle, and superior). The pre-ganglionic fibres arise from the thoracic spinal nerves. The post-ganglionic fibres travel with the cervical nerves to supply blood vessels and glands, such as the lacrimal and salivary glands.

Vagus Nerve (CN X)

See above, Cranial nerves.

Triangles of the Neck

Each side of the neck can be divided into anterior and posterior triangles by the sternocleidomastoid muscle (**Table 2.11**).

CLINICAL NOTE

TORTICOLLIS

Torticollis is a condition that results in an abnormal tilting of the top of the head to one side while the chin tilts to the other side. It is caused by the shortening of the sternocleidomastoid, usually as a result of trauma to the muscle during birth.

TABLE 2.11: Key muscles of the neck triangles

Muscle	Origin	Insertion	Innervation	Function
Sternocleidomastoid	Superior surface of manubrium sterni, medial third of the clavicle (sternal and clavicular heads, respectively)	Mastoid process and lateral half of superior nuchal line	Spinal root of the accessory nerve (CN XI)	Laterally rotate the head and flex the neck
Trapezius Has three parts: descending, transverse, and ascending	The medial third of the superior nuchal line, nuchal ligament, spinous processes of the vertebra C7–T12	The lateral third of the clavicle, acromion, and spine of the scapula, respectively	Spinal root of the accessory nerve (CN XI)	Upper fibres pull the scapula upwards, middle fibres pull the scapula medially, and the lower fibres pull the scapula downwards
Omohyoid (inferior belly)	Superior aspect of scapula	Intermediate tendon, which unites the two bellies	Ansa cervicalis (C1–C3)	Depress hyoid and larynx
Omohyoid (superior belly)	Intermediate tendon	Hyoid	Ansa cervicalis (C1–C3)	Depress hyoid and larynx

TABLE 2.12: The scalene muscles

Muscle	Origin	Insertion	Innervation	Action
Scalenus anterior	Anterior tubercles of transverse processes of the third to sixth cervical vertebrae	Scalene tubercle on the inner border of the first rib	Cervical plexus (C4–C6)	Acts as an accessory muscle of respiration by elevating the first rib, also bends the cervical spine forwards and laterally
Scalenus medius (the longest of the scalene muscles)	Transverse processes of the lower five cervical vertebrae	Upper surface of the first rib	Cervical plexus	Elevates first rib
Scalenus posterior	Transverse processes of the fourth to sixth cervical vertebrae	Second rib	Ventral rami of lower three cervical spinal nerves	Elevates the second rib

Scalene Muscles

The term scalene refers to a triangle with sides of unequal lengths. There are three scalene muscles in the neck: scalenus anterior, scalenus medius, and scalenus posterior (**Table 2.12**).

The anterior scalene has important anatomical relations:

- It divides the subclavian artery into three parts (**Figure 2.36**).
- The subclavian vein lies anterior to the muscle belly, so it is readily accessible for cannulation.
- The phrenic nerve descends on its anterior surface to travel into the thorax.
- The brachial plexus emerges between the scalenus anterior and medius at the lateral border of the scalenus anterior. Anaesthetists will perform upper limb nerve blocks here.
- Brachial plexus roots lie posterior to the muscle.

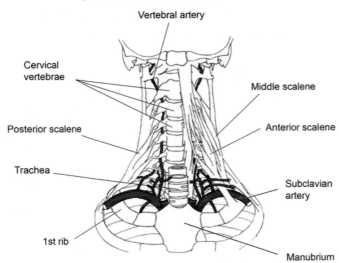

FIGURE 2.36 The anterior scalene (scalenus anterior) muscle divides the subclavian artery into three parts. (Courtesy of Calum Harrington-Vogt.)

Posterior Triangle of the Neck

The boundaries of the posterior triangle are as follows:

- *Anterior:* posterior border of sternocleidomastoid
- *Posterior:* anterior border of trapezius
- *Inferior:* clavicle

The posterior triangle of the neck can be further subdivided into the occipital triangle and the supraclavicular triangle by the inferior belly of the omohyoid (**Figure 2.37**).

The floor of the posterior triangle is covered by the following muscles:

- Inferior belly of omohyoid
- Anterior, middle, and posterior scalenes
- Levator scapulae
- Splenius capitis

A number of important structures are located within the triangle:

- Branches from the cervical plexus, including the phrenic nerve
- Spinal root of the accessory nerve (CN XI)
- Roots of the brachial plexus
- Third part of the subclavian artery lies partly within the supraclavicular triangle and may be palpable

Anterior Triangle of the Neck

The boundaries of the anterior triangle are as follows:

- *Superior:* ramus of mandible
- *Lateral:* anterior border of sternocleidomastoid
- *Medial:* midline of the neck

It can be subdivided into the following triangles:

- Submental
- Digastric
- Muscular
- Carotid

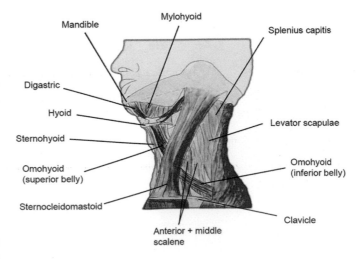

FIGURE 2.37 Triangles of the neck. (Courtesy of Xi Ming Zhu.)

Submental triangle (unpaired) boundaries are as follows:

- *Lateral:* anterior bellies of the right and left digastric muscles
- *Inferior:* body of hyoid bone
- Apex is at the lower part of the symphysis menti

The main content is the submental lymph nodes (drain the tip of the tongue) and the nerves to the mylohyoid muscles, which are united by the mylohyoid raphe and form the floor of the triangle.

Digastric (submandibular) triangle boundaries are as follows:

- *Anteroinferior:* anterior belly of digastric
- *Posteroinferior:* posterior belly of digastric
- *Superior:* mandible

The main contents are the submandibular salivary gland and lymph nodes. The mandibular and cervical branches of the facial nerve pass through the roof of the triangle (skin, superficial fascia, and platysma). The facial artery passes through the triangle deep to the submandibular gland and sometimes indents the gland. It curls towards the inferior border of the mandible. (See "Hypoglossal nerve", earlier, and information on the facial vein, later.)

CLINICAL NOTES

- Injury to the mandibular and cervical branches of the facial nerve can occur while raising the skin flaps to access the submandibular salivary gland.
- Ludwig's angina is an aggressive cellulitis of the floor of the mouth, commonly following a lower tooth abscess, which extends to the submandibular triangle. It may compromise the airway by causing laryngeal oedema.

Muscular triangle boundaries include the following:

- *Anterior:* midline of the neck, from the hyoid bone to the sternum
- *Inferoposterior:* anterior border of sternocleidomastoid
- *Posterosuperior:* superior belly of omohyoid

It also contains the infrahyoid muscles.

Carotid triangle boundaries include the following:

- *Superior:* posterior belly of digastric
- *Lateral:* anterior border of sternocleidomastoid
- *Inferior:* superior belly of omohyoid

Its contents include the common, internal, and external carotid arteries, the IJV, and CN X (within the carotid sheath), and CNs XI and XII and the ansa cervicalis (superficial to the carotid sheath).

Arterial Supply of the Head and Neck

Common Carotid Artery

The CCA originates in the thorax (see **Section 4**). It travels superiorly from the superior mediastinum to enter the neck, deep to the sternocleidomastoid muscle (lateral retraction of this muscle is of surgical importance during exposure of the artery). It bifurcates into the external and internal carotid arteries at the level of the superior border of the thyroid cartilage (C4). This is an important landmark for the palpation of the carotid pulse.

The **carotid body** is a cluster of chemoreceptors located at the bifurcation of the CCA (**Figure 2.38**). It is influenced by changes in the partial pressure of oxygen and carbon dioxide.

The **carotid sinus** is a dilatation at the proximal internal carotid artery, immediately superior to the common carotid bifurcation. The carotid sinus contains baroreceptors which influence systemic blood pressure. The glossopharyngeal nerve (CN IX) transmits information from the carotid sinus and body to the central nervous system.

For details on the internal carotid artery, see **Section 1A**.

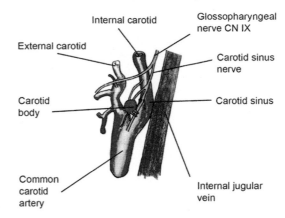

FIGURE 2.38 Carotid sinus and carotid body. (Courtesy of Aditya Mavinkurve.)

CLINICAL NOTE

Carotid endarterectomy is a surgical procedure to remove atherosclerotic plaques from the carotid artery in order to reduce the risk of stroke (**Figure 2.39**). The vagus nerve (CN X), ansa cervicalis, and hypoglossal nerve (CN XII) are at risk of damage during this procedure.

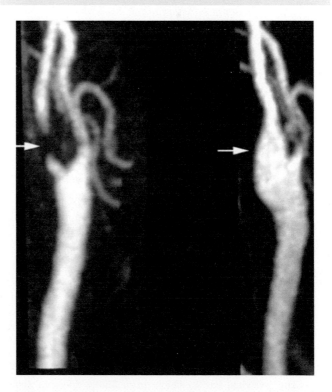

FIGURE 2.39 Carotid angiogram before (*left*) and after (*right*) carotid endarterectomy. (Courtesy of Munther Aldoori.)

Massage of the carotid sinus is a therapeutic measure used to slow down the heart rate in supraventricular tachycardia.

Carotid body tumours (carotid body paraganglioma, chemodectoma) arise from the paraganglion cells of the carotid body, at the bifurcation of the CCA. They are usually benign. They present as an asymptomatic, hard, slowly growing neck mass, which can be moved from side to side but not up and down. A small percentage can secrete catecholamines, increasing the sympathetic drive. Patients may therefore have signs such as elevated blood pressure.

External Carotid Artery

The external carotid artery lies anteromedial to the ICA within the carotid triangle. It then travels superiorly, lateral to the internal carotid, to supply structures of the head and neck. From proximal to distal it gives rise to the following branches:

- Superior thyroid artery to upper pole of the thyroid gland, close to the external laryngeal nerve (of surgical importance when clipping or ligating the artery during thyroid surgery)
- Ascending pharyngeal artery to the pharyngeal wall
- Lingual artery to the tongue
- Facial artery to the superficial face
- Occipital artery to the occipital region
- Posterior auricular to the area behind the ear

The external carotid artery passes within the parotid gland behind the neck of the mandible and terminates by bifurcating into two terminal branches:

- Maxillary artery to the deep face and jaw muscles.
- Superficial temporal artery to the side of the head. This is a common site for taking biopsy specimens for the diagnosis of temporal arteritis.

A mnemonic for remembering the branches of the external carotid (proximal to distal) is "some anatomists like freaking out poor medical students" (*s*uperior thyroid, *a*scending pharyngeal, *l*ingual, *f*acial, *o*ccipital, *p*osterior auricular, *m*axillary, *s*uperficial temporal).

Subclavian Artery

The right subclavian artery arises from the brachiocephalic trunk, while the left arises from the aortic arch.

The **scalenus anterior muscle divides the artery into three parts**. The third part continues as the axillary artery at the outer border of the first rib.

Branches of the first part (may have aberrant sites of origin) include the following:

- Vertebral artery ascends in the foramina transversaria of all the cervical vertebrae except C7 and enters the skull through the foramen magnum (see **Section 1A**). Extracranially, it gives rise to spinal branches to supply the spinal cord and the meninges.
- Internal thoracic artery (see **Section 4**).
- Thyrocervical trunk, which immediately divides into the inferior thyroid, transverse cervical, and ascending cervical branches

Branches of the second part include the costocervical trunk, which gives rise to the superior (supreme) intercostal and the deep cervical branches.

The third part of the subclavian artery gives origin to the dorsal scapular artery.

The Subclavian Vein

This is a continuation of the axillary vein at the outer border of the first rib to the medial border of the scalenus anterior, which lies posterior to it, where it joins the internal jugular vein to form the brachiocephalic vein. It receives the external jugular vein and the thoracic duct on the left side and the right lymphatic duct on the right side.

Venous Drainage of the Head and Neck

The facial vein drains the structures of the face and is formed by a union of the supratrochlear and supraorbital veins at the medial angle of the eye. It follows the same oblique course as the facial artery. When entering the submandibular triangle (deep to the platysma and the deep fascia), it lies superficial to the submandibular salivary gland.

It drains into the IJV after its union with the anterior division of the retromandibular vein.

The retromandibular vein is formed by the union of the superficial temporal and maxillary veins. It divides into an anterior division, which joins the facial vein, and a posterior division, which joins the posterior auricular vein to form the external jugular vein.

The external jugular vein descends in the neck upon the sternocleidomastoid muscle and drains into the subclavian vein in the root of the neck.

The anterior jugular vein descends in the front of the neck; it joins the opposite vein superior to the suprasternal notch and drains into the external jugular vein.

The IJV is the major vein of the head and neck, including the brain. It is the continuation of the sigmoid sinus and leaves the skull through the jugular foramen. It continues inferiorly within the carotid sheath, usually lateral to the carotid artery. The IJV unites with the subclavian vein to form the brachiocephalic vein, posterior to the sternoclavicular joint. It receives tributaries from the face, tongue, and thyroid gland through the superior and middle thyroid veins.

CLINICAL NOTE

CENTRAL IV LINES

Central lines can be inserted into the internal jugular vein for easy and quick access to the venous system, for example, in cases of shock and prior to major surgery. This procedure is performed under ultrasound guidance.

Jugular Venous Pressure

The IJV is of clinical importance in examining jugular venous pressure (JVP), which reflects venous pressure in the right side of the heart. It is measured with the patient positioned at 45 degrees and looking for the pulsation between the clavicular and the sternal heads of the sternocleidomastoid muscle. The measurement in centimetres is taken from the angle of Louis (sternal angle).

High JVP is a sign of congestive heart failure, excessive fluid overload, and constrictive pericarditis.

Hyoid Bone

The hyoid bone is the only bone in the body that does not articulate with any other bone and is therefore suspended by muscles and ligaments. It is composed of a body and two lesser and two greater horns and is located at the C3 level.

It gives attachment to the infrahyoid and suprahyoid strap muscles, in addition to ligaments including the thyrohyoid membrane, which attaches to the thyroid cartilage, and the stylohyoid ligament, which connects the lesser horn of the hyoid to the styloid process of the temporal bone.

> ### CLINICAL NOTE
>
> Hyoid bone fractures are characteristically associated with strangulation.

Larynx

The larynx is a collection of structures in the neck which function collectively to produce sound (phonation) and protect the airways from foreign bodies, especially during swallowing (**Figure 2.40**).

thyrohyoid, and thyropharyngeus (see inferior pharyngeal constrictor). The upper borders of the laminae are separated by the V-shaped superior thyroid notch.

Cricoid cartilage, a signet-ring structure of hyaline cartilage, is composed of an arch anteriorly and a lamina posteriorly. The lamina measures 2 to 3 cm from the upper to the lower border, while the arch measures 5 to 7 mm. It articulates with the bases of the arytenoid cartilages and the inferior horn of the thyroid cartilage. Inferiorly, it is attached to the trachea via the cricotracheal ligament (*vide infra*, the cricothyroid membrane).

And **four paired cartilages**:

- Arytenoids (*vide infra*).
- Cuneiform cartilages are small, club-shaped, whitish nodules within the aryepiglottic folds (because of their colour they might be mistaken for lesions).
- Corniculate cartilages are small, conical elastic structures that lie in the posterior part of the aryepiglottic fold and articulate with the apex of the arytenoid cartilage.
- Triticeal cartilages are small elastic nodules variably present within the posterior part of the thyrohyoid membrane.

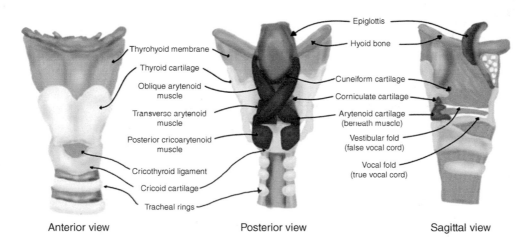

FIGURE 2.40 Anterior, posterior, and lateral views of the larynx. (Courtesy of John Ward.)

The larynx begins at the level of C2–C3 in neonates, but in adults, the level is slightly lower at C3. The adult larynx is continuous with the trachea at the level of C6.

The laryngeal skeleton is composed of **three single cartilages**:

Epiglottis, a leaf-like structure which is composed of elastic cartilage and lies behind the root of the tongue. Its stalk is attached to the posterior aspect of the upper part of the angle formed by the two laminae of the thyroid cartilage through the thyroepiglottic ligament.

- It acts as a protector of the inlet of the larynx. The aryepiglottic fold on each side runs from the side of the epiglottis to the arytenoid cartilage.

Thyroid cartilage, composed of hyaline cartilage, consists of two laminae and superior and inferior horns on each side. The two laminae unite in the midline anteriorly to form the laryngeal prominence (Adam's apple). The oblique line on the external surface of each lamina gives attachment to three muscles: sternothyroid,

Arytenoid cartilage has the following features:

- Is pyramidal in shape and has three surfaces, an apex, and a base.
- The base has a vocal process (anteriorly) for the attachment of the vocal ligament (*vide infra*) and a muscular process, which projects backwards and laterally, for the attachment of lateral and posterior arytenoid muscles. The base articulates with the lamina of the cricoid cartilage through a synovial joint.

Ligaments of the larynx include the following:

- **Thyrohyoid membrane** is between the hyoid and the thyroid cartilage. The lateral part of the thyrohyoid membrane is called the lateral thyrohyoid ligament. The thickened middle part is the median thyrohyoid ligament.

  It is pierced by the superior laryngeal artery, from the superior thyroid artery, and the superior thyroid vein and the internal laryngeal nerve, a branch of the superior laryngeal nerve from the vagus nerve.

- The **hyoepiglottic ligament and the thyroepiglottic ligament** connect the epiglottis to the hyoid bone and the thyroid cartilage, respectively.
- **Cricothyroid membrane** is the fibroelastic membrane connecting the thyroid and cricoid cartilages of the larynx. It is composed of a median part (median or anterior cricothyroid ligament) and two lateral parts (conus elasticus). The **upper free margin of the conus elasticus is the vocal ligament**, which runs from the angle of the thyroid cartilage (about midway between its upper and lower margins) in the midline anteriorly to the tip of the vocal process of the arytenoid cartilage posteriorly (see information on cricothyroidotomy later).
- The **quadrangular membrane** extends between the epiglottis and the arytenoid cartilages. Its lower end is called the vestibular ligament, which is the core of the vestibular fold (false vocal cord) and looks pink in colour and fixed (in contrast to the mobile white vocal cord). The ventricle is the space between the vestibular fold above and the vocal cord below on each side of the laryngeal cavity.

Important landmarks of the larynx include the following:

- The **superior laryngeal aperture** is composed of the epiglottis anteriorly, the apices of the arytenoid cartilages with the attached corniculate cartilages and the interarytenoid notch posteriorly, and the aryepiglottic folds laterally.
- The **vallecula** is the space between the back of the tongue and the epiglottis.
- The **rima glottidis** is the space between the true vocal cords and the arytenoid cartilages and is the narrowest part of the laryngeal cavity (**Figure 2.41**).

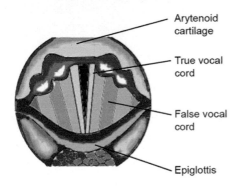

Arytenoid cartilage

True vocal cord

False vocal cord

Epiglottis

FIGURE 2.41   Vocal folds. (Courtesy of Aditya Mavinkurve.)

The **vocal cord** (the vocal ligament) is composed of elastic tissue and is covered by the mucosa. It consists of the lamina propria (three layers) and the vocalis and thyroarytenoid muscles. It appears pearly white on laryngoscopy, as it is relatively avascular. It is supplied by the recurrent laryngeal nerve.

Muscles of the Larynx
The muscles of the larynx are grouped into extrinsic and intrinsic muscles.

Extrinsic Muscles
The extrinsic muscles function to depress or elevate the larynx, depending on their relationship to the hyoid bone.

- Suprahyoid muscles (**Table 2.9**) and the three extrinsic muscles of the pharynx, *vide infra*. They all elevate the hyoid bone.
- Infrahyoid muscles (**Table 2.10**). They all depress the hyoid.

Intrinsic Muscles
The intrinsic muscles of the larynx function to tense and lengthen the vocal cords by opening (abduction) and closing (adduction) the rima glottidis, which allows for phonation.

- *Cricothyroid:* between the cricoid cartilage and the lower part of the thyroid lamina. The cricothyroid muscle is the only tensor of the vocal cords.
- *Thyroarytenoid:* runs between the inner surface of the thyroid lamina and the arytenoid cartilage. Some muscle fibres run lateral to the vocal ligament, under the name of vocalis.
- *Posterior cricoarytenoid:* from the back of the cricoid cartilage to the muscular process of the ipsilateral arytenoid cartilage. It is the only muscle that opens (abducts) the rima glottidis.
- *Lateral cricoarytenoid:* from the upper border of the cricoid arch to the ipsilateral muscular process of the arytenoid cartilage. It opposes the posterior arytenoid muscle by closing the rima glottidis.
- *Transverse (inter) arytenoid:* this is a single muscle which lies on the back of the larynx between the arytenoid cartilages and acts to approximate them.
- *Oblique arytenoid:* these two muscles cross each other. Each originates from the muscular process of the arytenoid cartilage and inserts into the apex of the contralateral arytenoid cartilage. They are superficial to the transverse arytenoid muscle. Some fibres extend to the aryepiglottic fold and are called the aryepiglottic muscle.

Innervation of the Larynx
The superior laryngeal branch of the vagus divides into the external laryngeal nerve (motor) and internal laryngeal nerve (almost wholly sensory).

All muscles of the larynx are supplied by the RLN, apart from the cricothyroid, which is supplied by the external laryngeal nerve. The RLN is also the sensory nerve supply below the vocal cords. The internal laryngeal nerve is the sensory supply to the level of the vocal cords.

Blood supply is via laryngeal branches of the superior and inferior thyroid arteries. Venous drainage is via the corresponding veins (see information on the superior and inferior thyroid veins).

Lymphatic Drainage

This is very important in regard to the spread of laryngeal cancer, in order to plan surgical or radiotherapy treatment. The part above the vocal cords (supraglottic, the second most common site for malignant tumours) drains to the upper deep cervical lymph nodes, often early and bilaterally. The lower part (subglottic) drains to the pre-tracheal and paratracheal lymph nodes and finally to the inferior deep cervical lymph nodes.

CLINICAL NOTES

Epiglottitis is an acute infection of the epiglottis. The numbers of affected children with *Haemophilus influenzae* as the cause has dramatically reduced with the introduction of Hib vaccination (*H. influenzae* B is the most common causative organism).

The clinical features include drooling, fever, odynophagia (painful swallowing), and dyspnoea.

Epiglottitis is an ear/nose/throat (ENT) emergency because of the potentially rapid and fatal airway obstruction.

A key sign to remember is stridor, which indicates significant airway narrowing.

Cricothyroidotomy is an emergency procedure to relieve upper respiratory obstruction. It entails making a small cut in the skin and underlying median cricothyroid membrane to pass a breathing tube down to the trachea. It is used as a last resort when orotracheal or nasotracheal intubation is not possible (see **Section 4**).

Laryngeal obstruction can follow the swallowing of foreign bodies, inflammation (e.g., epiglottitis), and allergic reactions like anaphylactic shock. Diphtheria is a highly dangerous bacterial infection which can cause acute upper airway obstruction.

Vocal cord nodules (singer's nodules) are benign and typically occur in the superficial mid-portion of the membranous vocal cords. They are associated with heavy voice use and are typically seen in professions such singing, acting, and teaching.

Laryngeal papillomatosis are viral warts from human papillomavirus infection (HPV 6-11) can affect the vocal cords. This condition, called recurrent papillomatosis, can cause hoarseness or stridor due to incomplete adduction of the vocal cords.

Laryngeal cancer, the majority of laryngeal cancers are squamous cell carcinoma. Risk factors include heavy smoking, alcohol misuse, and HPV infection (rare with laryngeal cancer, but more common with cancer of the oropharynx). Hoarseness of voice is an early sign in the glottic type (of the vocal cords, the most common type), and the patient usually seeks clinical opinion a earlier than in the other types, supraglottic and subglottic, above and below the vocal cords, respectively. Lymph node metastasis is rare, with the glottic type due to the minimal lymphatic drainage of the vocal cords (**Figure 2.42**).

Other clinical features include dysphagia, cough, haemoptysis, or a neck lump. The diagnosis depends on laryngoscopy and tissue biopsy.

Learning Point

All patients with a persistent change of voice for 2 to 3 weeks should be referred to the ENT clinic.

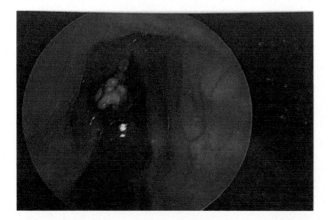

FIGURE 2.42 Intraoperative image of a suspicious left vocal cord lesion in a patient with persistent hoarseness. Note the patient is intubated. (Courtesy of Professor Dae Kim, St. George's Hospital, London.)

Trachea

The trachea, or windpipe, is about 12 cm in length and is the continuation of the larynx at the lower border of the cricoid cartilage. It is composed of multiple C-shaped hyaline cartilaginous rings which are incomplete posteriorly. The incomplete gap is bridged by the trachealis muscle. The trachea bifurcates at the carina into two principal bronchi (T4 level).

CLINICAL NOTES

Foreign bodies are more likely to get lodged in the right bronchus, as it is more vertical, shorter, and wider than the left (see **Section 4**).

Endotracheal intubation is accomplished by passing a tube, usually via the mouth, through the vocal cords down to the trachea, with the aid of a laryngoscope. This procedure is the gold standard for airway protection and preventing aspiration of gastric contents into the respiratory passages, especially in emergency settings, as the tube is cuffed. This procedure should be performed by a skilled professional.

Tracheostomy is performed by making a small opening in the trachea, at the level of the second to third tracheal rings, to allow the passage of a breathing tube. This can be performed as an open surgical procedure in the theatre or percutaneously using Seldinger's technique. Patients in the intensive care unit (ICU) will need replacement of mechanical ventilation with a tracheostomy after a certain period, usually between 1 and 2 weeks. It is more difficult than a cricothyroidotomy in emergency settings.

Stridor is a high-pitched respiratory sound mainly produced during inspiration and is caused by turbulent airflow within the larynx. Stridor is a sign of upper respiratory obstruction (due to infections like epiglottitis, laryngitis, laryngotracheobronchitis, or foreign body inhalation) and is especially important to observe in children with upper respiratory tract infections. Examination of children with stridor should be done by a senior clinician, and care taken not to distress them.

Stertor is a low-pitched, heavy, snoring-like sound heard during inspiration. Stertor is caused by a partial obstruction above the level of the larynx. This sound is often heard in sleep apnoea or as a result of hypoglossal nerve damage. Causes include infections such as epiglottitis or inhalation of a foreign body.

Thyroid Gland

Embryology

The thyroid gland is a butterfly-shaped gland located anteriorly in the neck and is composed of two lobes, which are connected by a band of thyroid tissue called the isthmus, which runs over the second to fourth tracheal rings. It is the first endocrine gland that develops, around 24 days into the gestational period. The median thyroid originates from the primitive pharynx, while the lateral thyroid originates from neural crest cells in between the first and second pharyngeal pouches. The thyroid gland originally develops on the posterior aspect of the tongue at the foramen caecum. The gland descends into the neck through the thyroglossal duct, a hollow tube that is formed as a result of the thickening of the thyroid primordium at its midline. This duct usually disappears; however, in some individuals the thyroglossal duct is retained, closely associated with the hyoid bone.

In some cases, the gland does not descend adequately and remains located in the back of the tongue, where it is known as a lingual thyroid, which may be the only functioning thyroid tissue available.

The thyroid gland is encased in pre-tracheal fascia (see the discussion on the inferior constrictor of the pharynx). The lateral thyroid ligament (ligament of Berry) is a condensation of the pre-tracheal fascia which connects the posteromedial aspect of each thyroid lobe to the trachea and the cricoid cartilage.

A third lobe, the pyramidal lobe, can be found occasionally arising from the superior border of the isthmus. The pyramidal lobe is suspected to be an embryological remnant of the thyroglossal duct.

The gland lies deep to the infrahyoid strap muscles sternothyroid (medially) and sternohyoid (more laterally) (see earlier, including information on the RLN).

Surface Anatomy of the Thyroid Gland
The thyroid isthmus can be found by palpating inferiorly from the cricoid cartilage downwards towards the second to fourth tracheal rings. The thyroid lobes can be palpated from the isthmus laterally when standing behind the seated patient.

Arterial Supply of the Thyroid Gland
The thyroid gland has a rich blood supply.

The arterial supply of the thyroid gland (**Figure 2.43**) is as follows:

- The superior thyroid artery, the first branch of the external carotid artery, gives the largest contribution.
- The inferior thyroid artery, a branch of the thyrocervical trunk, supplies the inferior and posterior portion of the thyroid gland and the parathyroid glands.
- The *thyroidea ima* is a small inconstant artery which arises from the aortic arch or brachiocephalic trunk.

Venous Drainage of the Thyroid Gland
The venous drainage of the thyroid gland is by three sets of veins:

- The superior thyroid vein runs with the superior thyroid artery to the upper pole of the gland and drains to the IJV.
- The middle thyroid vein drains to the IJV.
- The inferior thyroid vein drains to the innominate (brachiocephalic) veins.

The hormones T3 and T4 are secreted by the thyroid gland. Their secretion is controlled by thyroid-stimulating hormone (TSH) from the anterior pituitary gland through a negative feedback mechanism. The parafollicular C cells of the thyroid gland are responsible for secreting calcitonin, partly responsible for calcium balance (medullary thyroid cancer is a rare type arising in these cells).

CLINICAL NOTES

GOITRE

Goitre is the clinical term for enlargement of the thyroid gland. It can be uninodular (single nodule), multinodular (many nodules) (**Figures 2.44** and **2.45**), or diffuse (entire gland appears swollen). The swelling moves with swallowing.

THYROID CANCER

Cancer of the thyroid gland usually presents with goitre. There are four main types of thyroid cancer: papillary (the most common type, comprising around 85% of all thyroid cancers), follicular, medullary, and anaplastic.

RETROSTERNAL GOITRE

Rarely, the goitre may extend inferiorly to the superior mediastinum (retrosternal goitre) and can compress the trachea and neck veins. The goitre can usually be surgically removed through a neck incision. Rarely, a median sternotomy incision is needed when there is difficulty in delivering the goitre through the neck (**Figure 2.46**).

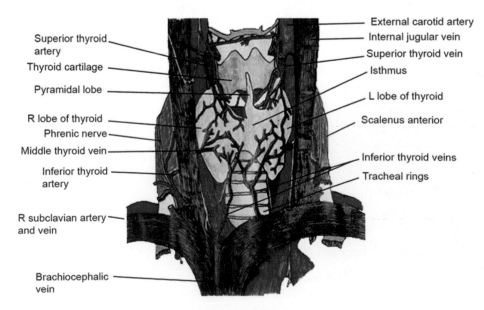

FIGURE 2.43   Blood supply of the thyroid gland. (Courtesy of Aditya Mavinkurve.)

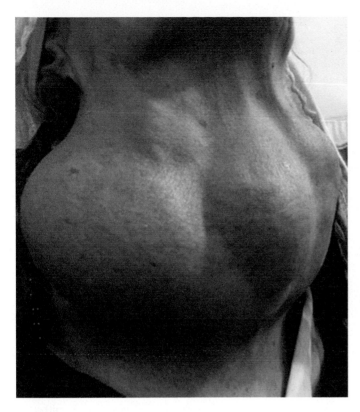

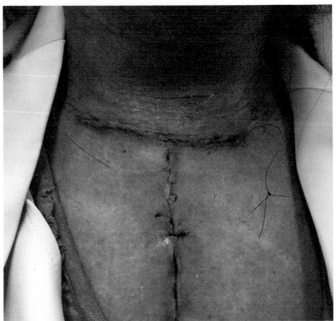

FIGURE 2.46 Postoperative wound: Large retrosternal goitre; a median sternotomy was needed for access. (Courtesy of Asha Ali.)

FIGURE 2.44 Patient with multinodular goitre. (Courtesy of Mohammed M. Habash.)

THYROTOXICOSIS

Thyrotoxicosis results from an overactive thyroid and most commonly presents as Graves' disease (primary hyperthyroidism).

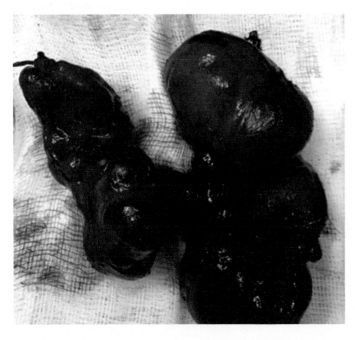

FIGURE 2.45 Specimen showing multinodular goitre following total thyroidectomy. (Courtesy of Mohammed M. Habash.)

Learning Points

- *Thyroid surgery:* total thyroidectomy, removal of the whole thyroid gland. Lobectomy is removal of one of the thyroid lobes and is not advised for localised papillary cancer, which tends to be multifocal. Thyroidectomy is indicated to treat multinodular goitre with pressure symptoms, hyperthyroidism not responding to medical treatment, cosmesis, or to treat thyroid cancer, except the most aggressive anaplastic type.
- While undertaking this surgery several key structures must be maintained, such as the thyroid arteries (bleeding from these can be severe) and the RLNs, which run posterior to the thyroid lobes. Injury to the external laryngeal branch of the superior laryngeal nerve affects the pitch and projection of the voice. This nerve can be injured while ligating the superior thyroid artery at the upper pole. The other important structures to preserve are the parathyroid glands (*vide infra*).
- The lateral thyroid ligament (ligament of Berry) should be divided to ensure removal of the whole lobe (lobectomy).
- Damage to the RLN, whether unilateral or bilateral, results in paralysis of all of the intrinsic muscles of the larynx (except the cricothyroid) on the damaged side. This would result in a hoarse voice due to the fact that the larynx cannot close properly. The patient will be unable to project their voice, reach high notes in singing, and will have a bovine cough (non-explosive cough due to an inability to close the glottis). Due to the close relation of the thyroid gland to the trachea, oesophagus, and thus the tracheoesophageal groove, it is vital to identify the

(Continued)

RLN before proceeding too far into the operation (Figure 2.47).
- Bilateral RLN injury is an anaesthetic emergency resulting in rima glottis closure, stridor, and falling oxygen saturations, as the airway cannot be maintained. This is managed by immediate intubation or emergency tracheostomy.
- Laryngoscopy immediately following thyroidectomy is a medicolegal requirement to ensure the integrity of the vocal cords and should be recorded in the patient's notes.

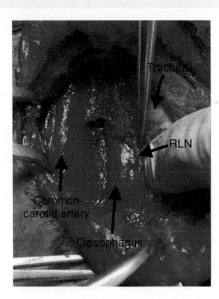

FIGURE 2.47 Perioperative identification of the right recurrent laryngeal nerve within the tracheo-oesophageal groove. (Courtesy of Mohammed M. Habash.)

Thyroglossal Cyst

If the thyroglossal duct remains in adults, it can lead to the appearance of a midline neck swelling, which moves with both swallowing and tongue protrusion (**Figure 2.48a**). Sistrunk's operation can be performed to treat thyroglossal cysts. Surgeons remove the cyst and duct, in addition to the mid-portion of the hyoid to prevent recurrence (**Figures 2.48b** and **2.48c**).

Parathyroid Glands

The parathyroid glands are four small, yellowish-brown endocrine glands located on the posterior aspect of the thyroid gland. The parathyroid glands originate from the pharyngeal pouches, which arise from the endoderm. The inferior parathyroid glands originate from the third pharyngeal pouch, while the superior parathyroid glands originate from the fourth pharyngeal pouch. The superior parathyroids have a more constant location than the inferior, which may even migrate to the superior mediastinum.

Arterial Supply of the Parathyroid Glands

The parathyroid glands are mainly supplied by branches from the inferior thyroid arteries.

Function of the Parathyroid Glands

The parathyroid glands secrete parathyroid hormone (parathormone), which regulates calcium metabolism.

CLINICAL NOTE

HYPERPARATHYROIDISM

Hyperparathyroidism is a condition of increased parathyroid hormone in the bloodstream. It can lead to hypercalcaemia (increased calcium level in the blood). Primary hyperparathyroidism is caused by parathyroid tumours, commonly adenomas (benign tumour), and rarely, due to parathyroid cancer. When medical management fails, these patients undergo surgical excision (parathyroidectomy).

Surgical Damage to the Parathyroid Glands

Iatrogenic damage to the parathyroid glands can follow total thyroidectomy and cause postoperative hypocalcaemia (low level of serum calcium).

Postoperative calcium levels are therefore monitored in these patients. Signs and symptoms of hypocalcaemia include perioral and digital paraesthesia, tetany, and less commonly, abnormal heart rhythm (arrhythmia). Tetany involving laryngeal muscles and arrhythmias can be life-threatening.

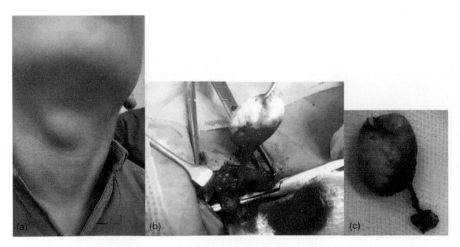

FIGURE 2.48 (a) Thyroglossal cyst; (b) excision of the thyroglossal cyst with dissection of the central portion of the hyoid bone; (c) excised thyroglossal cyst with the central part of the hyoid bone (Sistrunk's operation). (Courtesy of Mohammed M. Habash.)

Lymphatic Drainage of the Neck

Lymphatic drainage of the head and neck can be divided as follows (**Figure 2.49**).

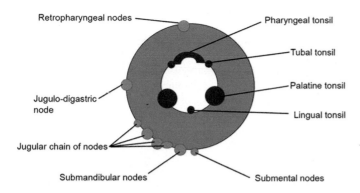

FIGURE 2.49 Lymphatic drainage of neck. (Courtesy of Aditya Mavinkurve.)

Outer ring comprises:

- Submental triangle
- Submandibular triangle
- Pre-auricular
- Occipital

Inner ring of mucosa-associated lymphoid tissue (MALT) or Waldeyer's ring. Waldeyer's ring refers to lymphatic tissue that surrounds the nasopharynx and oropharynx. It consists of the lingual tonsil (at the back of the tongue), the palatine tonsils (between the palatoglossal arch anteriorly and palato-pharyngeal arch posteriorly), the tubal tonsils (located near the opening of the auditory tube in the nasopharynx), and the pha-ryngeal/adenoid tonsil (on the posterior aspect of the roof of the nasopharynx).

The **deep cervical lymph nodes** are arranged longitudinally along the IJV in the carotid sheath. They can be divided into upper, middle, and inferior jugular nodes.

The level of cervical lymph nodes is important when treating metastatic cancers, commonly from the thyroid, tongue, larynx, etc. The levels of lymph nodes can be classified according to the American Academy of Otolaryngology as:

- *Level I:* the submental and submandibular groups
- *Level II:* upper jugular lymph nodes, e.g., the jugulodigastric node
- *Level III:* middle jugular lymph nodes
- *Level IV:* lower jugular lymph nodes
- *Level V:* lymph nodes in the posterior triangle, including the supraclavicular nodes
- *Level VI:* the anterior neck, between the hyoid and the suprasternal notch (infrahyoid, pre-tracheal, paratracheal, pre-laryngeal), jugulodigastric.

The deep cervical lymph nodes on the right side finally drain into the right jugular trunk (for the right upper limb, right side of the head and neck, and right side of the thorax), which drains into the venous system at the subclavian-jugular junction (the right venous angle). The left jugular trunk enters the thoracic duct.

The Clinical Approach to the Diagnosis of Neck Swellings

A proper clinical approach starts with good history taking and thorough physical examination.

Midline swellings:

- Thyroglossal cyst (see earlier)
- Enlarged pyramidal lobe of the thyroid gland
- Submental lymphadenopathy
- Dermoid cyst

Lateral swellings (anterior triangle):

- Goitre, localised (thyroid adenoma, thyroid cancer) (**Figure 2.50**) or generalised swelling (multinodular goitre, Graves' disease)
- Submandibular triangle swellings (salivary gland inflam-mation and tumours, obstruction of the submandibular duct, enlarged lymph nodes)
- Cervical lymphadenopathy (see earlier), can be in any of the triangles that contain lymph nodes

- Branchial cyst (**Figure 2.51**), a remnant of the second and third branchial arches, lies deep to the sternocleidomastoid, at the junction of the upper third and lower two-thirds
- Chemodectoma (see earlier)
- Cystic hygroma (lymphangioma) usually appears at birth but may appear later

Characteristics of a neck lump (the criteria you are expected to mention in clinical exams or clinical briefings, for example, a ward round with your consultant) can also be applied, with some modification, to examination of lumps elsewhere in the body:

- *Site:* anterior or posterior triangles, and their subdivisions
- *Size:* usually measured in centimetres, for example, a 3 X 2 cm mass in the anterior aspect of the neck
- *Shape:* rounded, irregular margin
- *Consistency:* soft, hard, or cystic (positive fluctuation test)

Mobile or fixed to the skin or the underlying structures. Attachment to skin, e.g., sebaceous cyst is attached to the skin; subcutaneous lipoma is separate from the skin.

- Tender or not, e.g., inflammatory swelling is prone to be painful (always ask the patient if it hurts before doing the palpation)
- Watching the movement of the swelling with deglutition while the patient drinks a sip of water is a very important part of the clinical examination (thyroid-related masses)
- *Overlying skin:* temperature (warm skin associated with abscess formation), redness (erythema), presence of sinus/sinuses, e.g., TB lymphadenitis (**Figure 2.52**)

- Transillumination by shining a light torch through the lump, if indicated, for example, cystic hygroma (see examination of hydrocele, Section 6)
- Pulsatile mass suggests the presence of a carotid body tumour or aneurysm
- Examination of the regional lymph nodes; for example, when finding an ulcer on the tongue, the submandibular and submental lymph nodes should be examined next

Common skin and subcutaneous conditions such as sebaceous cysts (**Figure 2.52**) and lipomas can occur anywhere on the neck.

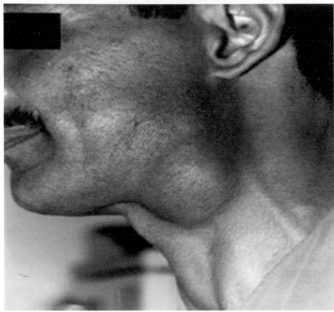

FIGURE 2.51   Large left branchial cyst. (Courtesy of Qassim F. Baker.)

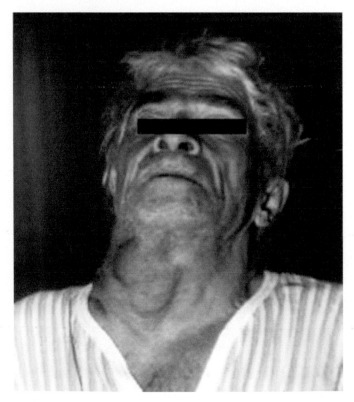

FIGURE 2.50   Right thyroid mass due to papillary thyroid carcinoma. (Courtesy of Qassim F. Baker.)

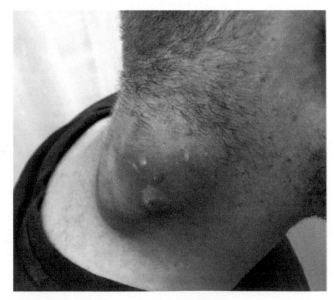

FIGURE 2.52   A 20-year-old male presenting with a large infected sebaceous cyst in the posterior triangle. Note the overlying erythema and punctum. (Courtesy of Asha Ali.)

The Pharynx and the Cervical Oesophagus

The pharynx (Greek, "throat") is a fibromuscular tube approximately 12 cm in length that extends from the base of the skull to the inferior border of the cricoid cartilage (C6), where it becomes continuous with the oesophagus (**Figure 2.53**). It is located directly anterior to the bodies of the cervical vertebrae (C1–C6). The pharynx is responsible for the passage of both air (to the larynx, trachea, and lungs) and food (to the oesophagus and then stomach). It can be described as funnel-shaped and sits behind the nasal cavity, mouth, and larynx; it is therefore divided into three sections: nasopharynx, oropharynx, and laryngopharynx, respectively.

There are three layers to the wall of the pharynx: mucosal, muscular layer, and fibrous (median raphe, which extends posteriorly from the pharyngeal tubercle on the occipital bone down to the oesophagus):

- The mucosal layer is continuous with that of the nasal cavities, mouth, larynx, and tympanic cavity by means of the auditory (pharyngotympanic or eustachian) tubes.
- The upper part of the pharynx (nasopharynx) is lined with ciliated columnar epithelium, and the lower part (oropharynx and laryngopharynx) is lined with stratified squamous epithelium. There is a transitional epithelial zone (cuboid epithelium) where the two layers come together.

Muscles of the Pharynx

There are two layers of muscles in the pharynx: the circular muscles (constrictor muscles) and the longitudinal muscles (**Figure 2.54**).

Circular muscles

- The three pharyngeal constrictor muscles overlap each other in a vertical arrangement, similar to stacked plant pots.
- The superior, middle, and inferior constrictor muscles are supplied by the pharyngeal plexus, which is in turn supplied by the vagus nerve (CN X).
- They function to propel the bolus of food into the oesophagus through their successive contractions.

Superior Constrictor Muscle

- *Origin:* lower posterior border of the medial pterygoid plate, pterygoid hamulus, pterygomandibular ligament, posterior end of mylohyoid line on the mandible, and the side of the tongue
- *Insertion:* upper fibres curve superiorly and medially and attach to the pharyngeal tubercle of the occipital bone, middle fibres insert into the median fibrous raphe on the posterior wall, and lower fibres curve medially and inferiorly and join the fibrous raphe
- *Function:* upper fibres have a specific function; when they contract, they pull the posterior pharyngeal wall forward, aiding the soft palate in closing off the upper part of the pharynx

Middle Constrictor Muscle

- *Origin:* lower part of the stylohyoid ligament and from the greater and lesser cornua of the hyoid
- *Insertion:* fibres radiate out medially and join the median fibrous raphe attached to the posterior wall of the pharynx.

Inferior Constrictor Muscle

- *Origin:* has two parts, the thyropharyngeus and cricopharyngeus, originating from the oblique line on the outer surface of the lamina of the thyroid cartilage and the cricoid cartilage, respectively.
- *Insertion:* all fibres insert into the median fibrous raphe on the posterior wall of the pharynx. The lower fibres also run inferiorly and are continuous with the circular muscle of the oesophagus below
- *Specific function:* lowest fibres (the cricopharyngeus muscle) act as a sphincter on the lower end of the pharynx (upper oesophageal sphincter).

Longitudinal Muscles

Stylopharyngeus

- *Origin:* styloid process of the temporal bone
- *Insertion:* enters the pharyngeal wall by passing between the superior and middle constrictor muscles and inserts into the posterior border of the thyroid cartilage, along with the palatopharyngeus
- *Action:* elevates the larynx and pharynx when swallowing

Palatopharyngeus

- *Origin:* posterior aspect of hard palate and palatine aponeurosis
- *Insertion:* passes inferiorly and posteriorly to form the palatopharyngeal arch and then inserts into the posterior aspect of the thyroid cartilage
- *Action:* pulls the pharynx superiorly and pulls the palatopharyngeal arch towards the midline

Salpingopharyngeus

- *Origin:* lower part of the cartilage of the auditory tube (pharyngotympanic tube)
- *Insertion:* passes downwards and joins the palatopharyngeus
- *Action:* aids in elevation of the pharynx

The muscles of the pharynx are supplied by the vagus nerve (CN X), except for the stylopharyngeus, which is supplied by the glossopharyngeal nerve.

Blood Supply of the Pharynx

From the branches of the external carotid artery (ascending pharyngeal, facial, maxillary, and lingual arteries).

Venous drainage is via the venous plexus around the pharynx, which drains into the IJV.

Lymphatic drainage is to the deep cervical lymph nodes.

Learning Point

The anatomical basis of deglutition (the action of swallowing). As the two parts of the inferior constrictor muscle are attached to the thyroid cartilage and cricoid cartilage, when the patient swallows, the muscle contracts, and the respective parts of the larynx, thyroid, and cricoid cartilages elevate. The thyroid gland is attached to the larynx by the suspensory ligament of Berry (see earlier), part of the pre-tracheal fascia, which envelops the gland. With this close relationship and attachment of the thyroid gland to the larynx, the gland will move up and down with deglutition (see "Thyroid Gland" earlier).

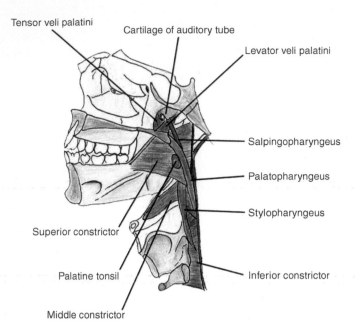

FIGURE 2.53 The inner and outer muscles of the pharynx. (Courtesy of Gabriela Barzyk.)

Parts of the Pharynx (Figure 2.54)

Nasopharynx – Sensory innervation (CN V2)

- The anterior part is the posterior borders of the nasal apertures (choanae) and the posterior edge of the nasal septum.
- The floor is formed by the soft palate.
- The posterior wall and roof contain the pharyngeal tonsils (adenoids).
- The auditory tube (eustachian or pharyngotympanic tube) communicates with the middle ear and opens in the lateral wall of the nasopharynx at the tubal elevation.
- The pharyngeal recess is located behind the tubal elevation.
- The function of the nasopharynx is to purify the inhaled air, in addition to the nasal cavity.

Oropharynx – Sensory innervation (CN IX)

- The oropharynx extends from the inferior border of the soft palate to the superior border of the epiglottis and lies posterior to the mouth.
- The roof is formed by the inferior surface of the soft palate.
- The floor consists of the epiglottis, which closes the larynx to prevent food aspiration.
- The posterior wall is supported by the bodies of the second vertebra and upper part of the third cervical vertebra.
- The anterior aspect contains the opening of the mouth into the oropharynx, known as the isthmus of the fauces (oropharyngeal isthmus), and is formed by the palatoglossal arches laterally, the soft palate superiorly, and the dorsum of the tongue inferiorly.
- The lateral walls contain the palatopharyngeal and palatoglossal arches and the palatine tonsil, which is located between them.

Laryngopharynx (hypopharynx) – Sensory innervation (CN X):

- Extending from the pharyngoepiglottic folds superiorly to the upper oesophageal sphincter inferiorly (level of C3–C6). Posterior to the laryngopharynx lie the bodies of the cervical vertebrae (C3–C6).
- The larynx lies anterior to the laryngopharynx.
- The inferior edge of the cricoid cartilage marks the inferior border.
- The piriform sinus (smuggler's fossa) is a depression posterolaterally on each side of the laryngeal opening lateral to the aryepiglottic fold; swallowed foreign bodies such as fish bones are likely to lodge here.

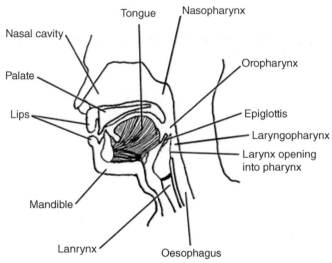

FIGURE 2.54 Parts of the pharynx. (Courtesy of Aditya Mavinkurve.)

CLINICAL NOTE

PHARYNGEAL CANCER
Pharyngeal cancer has a strong association with smoking and alcohol consumption. Other factors include infections with Epstein-Barr virus and HPV, which can be linked to sexual contact.

Killian's Triangle
The inferior constrictor muscle can be subdivided into the thyropharyngeus and cricopharyngeus muscles. Killian's triangle (or Killian's dehiscence) is a potential triangular gap between these two parts of the muscle (**Figure 2.55**). It represents an area of weakness, through which the pharyngeal mucosa can herniate, known as Zenker's diverticulum, or pharyngeal pouch. The pouch most commonly herniates on the left-hand side, and symptoms include dysphagia, cough, and regurgitation. Imaging in the form of a barium swallow is needed for diagnosis (**Figure 2.56**).

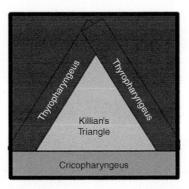

FIGURE 2.55 Simplified diagram of Killian's triangle.

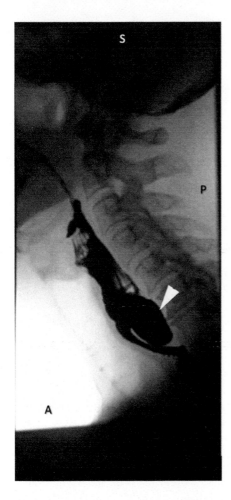

FIGURE 2.56 Lateral view of a barium swallow showing large pharyngeal pouch *(arrowhead)* with posterior outpouching from the hypopharynx (laryngopharynx) at level of C6 vertebral body. (Courtesy of Asha Ali.)

Cervical Oesophagus

The oesophagus is a fibromuscular tube approximately 25 cm in length. It extends from the cricoid cartilage (C6) to the stomach. The mucosa is lined by non-keratinised squamous epithelium. The muscular layer consists of two types of muscles: longitudinal (outermost) and circular (innermost). The function of the oesophagus is to transport food to the stomach for digestion. The upper third has striated (voluntary) muscle for both the outer longitudinal and the inner circular muscle layers. The middle third has both striated and smooth (involuntary) muscle for both the outer and inner muscle layers, whereas the lower third has smooth muscle in both of its layers. The oesophagus has three anatomical constrictions: one in the neck (see cricopharyngeus muscle), and two in the thorax and the abdomen (see **Section 4**).

Anatomical Relations of the Cervical Oesophagus

- The trachea lies anterior to the oesophagus. There is a narrow groove between the trachea and the oesophagus, known as the tracheo-oesophageal groove. This is where the RLN runs.
- Posterior to the cervical oesophagus is the longus coli muscle and the bodies of the C6 and C7 vertebrae.
- Lateral to the oesophagus in the neck lie the respective left and right lobes of the thyroid gland and the carotid sheath. On the left-hand side, the thoracic duct runs for a short distance.

Blood Supply

The blood supply to the upper third of the oesophagus stems from the inferior thyroid arteries and veins.

Lymphatic Drainage

Lymph from the upper third of the oesophagus drains to the deep cervical lymph nodes. Cancer of the cervical oesophagus may spread to these nodes.

Nerve Supply

The cervical oesophagus is innervated by the recurrent laryngeal nerve and post-ganglionic fibres from the sympathetic cervical ganglia.

CLINICAL NOTES

DYSPHAGIA

Dysphagia is defined as difficulty in swallowing (sensation of obstruction) and can be a very serious presenting symptom that may warrant urgent investigation to rule out a sinister cause, such as malignancy. It must be distinguished from other oesophageal symptoms such as odynophagia (pain on swallowing, for example, due to acute tonsillitis and peritonsillar abscess) and regurgitation (reflux of oesophageal contents). The possible causes are categorised in **Table 2.13**.

Notes:

- Dysphagia may also be a result of neurological pathologies, such as cerebral vascular accidents, brainstem tumours, motor neuron disease (MND), and MS.
- Pharyngeal pathologies like cancer can clinically present as dysphagia.

(Continued)

OESOPHAGEAL CANCER

The majority of cervical oesophageal cancers are squamous cell carcinoma (compare with lower oesophageal cancer, see **Section 5**). It is related to heavy smoking, alcohol intake, and infection with HPV. The UK mortality rate is the highest in Europe for both men and women.

SYSTEMIC SCLEROSIS (SYSTEMIC SCLERODERMA)

This is an autoimmune multiorgan connective tissue disease affecting the skin and internal organs (such as the GIT), including the joints and blood vessels (**Figure 2.58**).

PLUMMER-VINSON SYNDROME (SIDEROPAENIC DYSPHAGIA)

Characterised by glossitis, angular stomatitis, and oesophageal webs, due to iron-deficiency anaemia.

TABLE 2.13: The categorical causes of dysphagia

Intraluminal	Intramural	Extraluminal
Foreign body such as food bolus, swallowed denture (**Figure 2.57**)	*Stricture:* • Malignant (mainly carcinoma) or benign tumour (e.g., leiomyoma) • Oesophagitis (reflux oesophagitis due to sliding hiatus hernia), ingestion of chemical solution like caustic soda and bleaches • Scleroderma • Pharyngeal pouch • Plummer-Vinson syndrome (oesophageal web) • Achalasia	• Hiatus hernia (rolling type) • Retrosternal goitre • Bronchial carcinoma • Thoracic aortic aneurysm

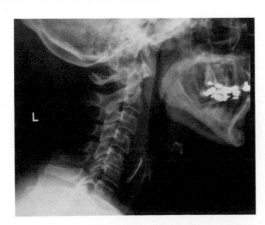

FIGURE 2.57 Lateral neck X-ray of a 30-year-old male with foreign body (shellfish) in the proximal oesophagus, causing absolute dysphagia. The patient required endoscopy and urgent removal of the foreign body to prevent complications such as upper airway swelling and oesophageal perforation. (Courtesy of Asha Ali.)

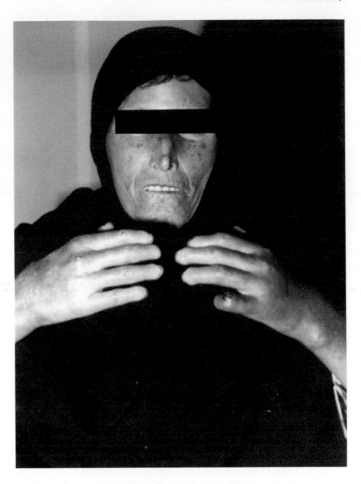

FIGURE 2.58 Systemic sclerosis in a 35-year-old female who presented with dysphagia and Raynaud's phenomenon; note the ulceration on left little finger. (Courtesy of Qassim F. Baker.)

Answers to Quiz Questions on the Eye

1.
   - *Fibrous layer:* contains the sclera and cornea which provide support for the eyeball.
   - *Vascular layer:* contains the choroid, iris, and ciliary body. Supplies blood and manipulates the lens and pupil to aid in accommodation.
   - *Inner layer:* contains the retina with photoreceptors and is responsible for vision.
2. The ophthalmic artery is the main blood supply to the eyeball of which a prominent branch is the central artery of the retina, which supplies the inner surface of the retina. The ophthalmic artery is a branch of the internal carotid artery.
3. Open angle glaucoma occurs when the trabecular meshwork is partially occluded and leads to a slow loss of peripheral vision, whereas closed angle glaucoma is when the iris fully occludes the trabecular meshwork, and the rapid build-up of aqueous humour can lead to blindness if not treated swiftly.

Answer to Quiz Question on the Ear

A1. d. Facial nerve

Revision Questions

Q1.

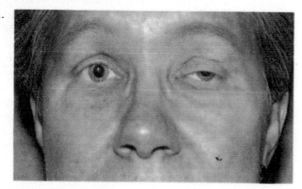

Q1A. Which of the following best describes the muscle that is affected, causing the patient's ptosis?
   a. Lateral rectus
   b. Levator palpebrae superioris
   c. Orbicularis oculi
   d. Superior oblique
   e. Superior rectus

Q1B. Which of the following nerves supplies the patient's affected muscle?
   a. Abducens
   b. Facial
   c. Maxillary
   d. Oculomotor
   e. Ophthalmic

Q2.

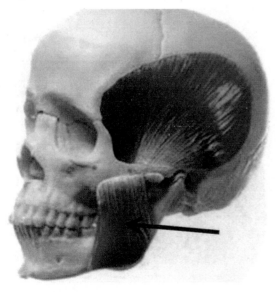

Q2A. The arrow is pointing to:
   a. Buccinator
   b. Lateral pterygoid
   c. Medial pterygoid
   d. Masseter
   e. Temporalis

Q2B. The nerve supply of this muscle is:
   a. Facial nerve
   b. Lingual nerve
   c. Maxillary nerve V2
   d. Mandibular nerve V3
   e. Ophthalmic division of trigeminal V1

Q3.

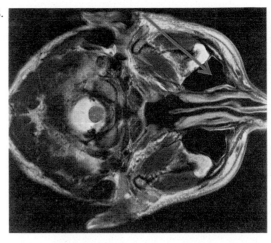

Q3A. Identify the feature indicated by the arrow.
   a. Clinoid process
   b. Maxillary sinus
   c. Orbit
   d. Pituitary fossa
   e. Sphenoid sinus

Q3B. Which of the following best describes the type of image shown?
   a. Contrast radiograph
   b. CT scan
   c. MRI scan
   d. Plain film radiograph
   e. Ultrasound scan

Q4.

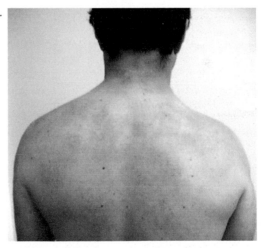

Q4A. Which of the following muscles is likely to have been paralysed in the patient illustrated in the image, who sustained injury to his right posterior triangle?
   a. Deltoid
   b. Levator scapulae
   c. Rhomboid minor
   d. Supraspinatus
   e. Trapezius

Q4B. Which nerve supplies the muscle that appears to be paralysed?
   a. Accessory
   b. Ansa cervicalis
   c. Phrenic
   d. Sympathetic chain
   e. Vagus

Q5.

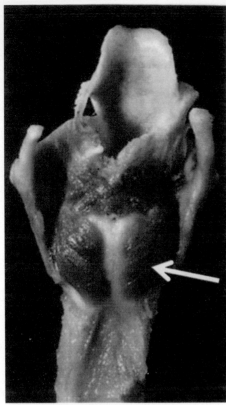

Q6A. Which of the following best describes the structure indicated by the arrow?
   a. Lingual tonsil
   b. Palatine tonsil
   c. Pharyngeal tonsil
   d. Tubal tonsil
   e. Waldeyer's ring

Q6B. Which of the following best describes sensory nerve supply
to the region indicated by the arrow?
   a. Glossopharyngeal
   b. Lingual
   c. Mandibular branch of the trigeminal
   d. Recurrent laryngeal
   e. Superior laryngeal

Q7.

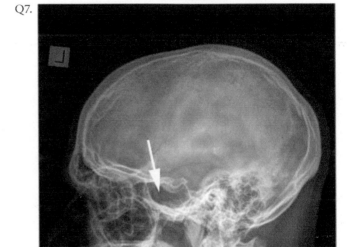

Q5A. Identify the muscle indicated by the arrow.
   a. Cricothyroid
   b. Omohyoid
   c. Posterior cricoarytenoid
   d. Sternothyroid
   e. Thyrohyoid

Q5B. Which statement best describes the effects of paralysis of
the muscle indicated by the arrow?
   a. Difficulty in swallowing
   b. Inability to abduct the vocal cords
   c. Inability to relax the vocal cords
   d. Inability to tense the vocal cords
   e. Spasm of the vocal cords

Q6.

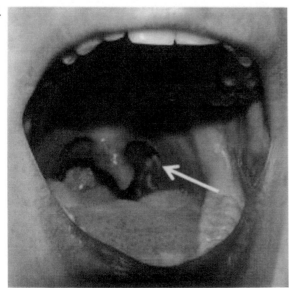

Q7A. What is the structure indicated by the arrow?
   a. Anterior ethmoidal air cells
   b. Maxillary sinus
   c. Middle ethmoidal air cells
   d. Posterior ethmoidal air cells
   e. Sphenoid sinus

Q7B. What does this structure drain into?
   a. Ethmoidal bulla
   b. Inferior meatus
   c. Semilunaris hiatus
   d. Sphenoethmoidal recess
   e. Superior meatus

Additional Questions on the Anatomy of the Neck

Q8. What are the branches of the external carotid artery?
Q9. What are the motor and sensory nerves that supply the
larynx?
Q10. What are the borders of the posterior triangle?
Q11. What nerve can get injured in a lymph node biopsy of that
triangle?
Q12. What is the carotid sheath? Enumerate its contents.
Q13. What is the blood supply of the thyroid gland?
Q14. What type of epithelium is found lining the vestibule of the
nose?

Q15. What is the blood supply of the nasal septum?

Q16. What arteries anastomose to form the Kiesselbach's plexus?

Q17. Where does the maxillary sinus drain into?
- a. Middle meatus
- b. Superior meatus
- c. Inferior meatus
- d. Sphenoethmoidal recess

Further Reading

Corbridge R, Steventon, N. Oxford Handbook of ENT and Head and Neck Surgery. (2020) Oxford: Oxford University Press.

McLatchie G, et al. Oxford Clinical Handbook of Clinical Surgery (2013) Oxford: Oxford Press. 4e. Pages: 554–555.

Mehta R, Chinthapalli K. Glasgow Coma Scale explained. *BMJ* (2019) 365 doi: https://doi.org/10.1136/bmj.l1296

Raine T, et al. Oxford Handbook for the Foundation Programme (2018) Oxford: Oxford Press. 5e. Page 440.

Answers

A1A.	b	A4B.	a
A1B.	d	A5A.	c
A2A.	d	A5B.	b
A2B.	d	A6A.	b
A3A.	b	A6B.	a
A3B.	c	A7A.	e
A4A.	e	A7B.	d

A8–16. see text

A17. a

3

ANATOMY OF THE UPPER LIMB

Reviewed by Philip J. Adds and Joanna Tomlinson

Learning Objectives

- Osteology of the bones of the pectoral girdle and common pathology
- Anatomy of the shoulder, elbow, and wrist joints
- Anatomy of the brachial plexus, cubital fossa and carpal tunnel, and clinical applications
- Anatomy of the muscles of the upper limb, their compartments and pathology
- Functional anatomy of the upper limb, including movements and types of grips
- Boundaries, contents, and surgical importance of the axilla
- Revision questions

Bones of the Pectoral Girdle

The pectoral girdle comprises the clavicle and scapula (**Figure 3.1**). Together, they form a strut to keep the upper limb positioned lateral to the thoracic cage and allow for rotation, abduction, adduction, flexion, and extension of the glenohumeral joint.

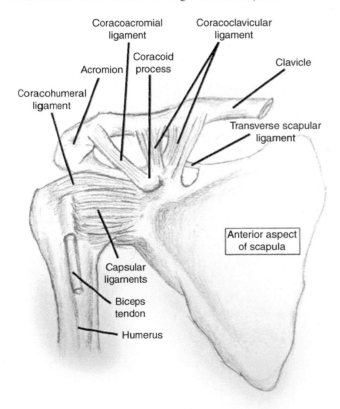

FIGURE 3.1 The pectoral girdle and the ligaments of the shoulder. (Courtesy of Jordan Bethel.)

Clavicle

The clavicle (collar bone) is an S-shaped bone. It is the first bone to ossify in fetal life and the last bone to fuse. The lateral one-third is flattened and wider (**Figure 3.2**). The weakest part is the junction of its medial two-thirds (convex) and lateral one-third (concave), which is therefore a common site for fractures. The medial end articulates with the manubrium sterni at the sternoclavicular joint (a synovial joint divided into two cavities by a fibrocartilage disc) and the lateral end with the acromion at the acromioclavicular joint, a plane-type synovial joint, stabilised by ligaments.

The conoid tubercle is a projection located inferiorly on the acromial end and gives attachment to the conoid ligament (*vide infra*).

The clavicle has several important roles:

- Shock absorption of the upper limb by transferring forces to the thoracic cage
- Suspension of the scapula to maintain the upper limb lateral to the trunk
- Protection of the subclavian vessels and brachial plexus (despite its role in protection, the clavicle is the most common bone to fracture)
- Attachment site for many important muscles; these are the:
    - Sternocleidomastoid (clavicular head) and sternohyoid (see **Section 2**)
    - Pectoralis major (sternoclavicular head)
    - Trapezius
    - Deltoid
    - Subclavius

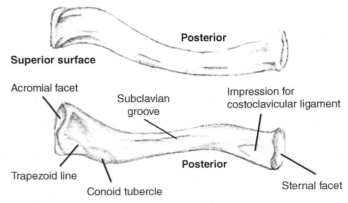

FIGURE 3.2 Diagram of the superior and inferior surfaces of the right clavicle. (Courtesy of Jordan Bethel.)

DOI: 10.1201/9781003312895-4

Scapula

The scapula (shoulder blade) is a flat triangular bone that connects the clavicle to the humerus (**Figure 3.3**). It extends from the second to the seventh ribs posteriorly. Fractures to the scapula are rare because the scapula is well protected by muscles and usually follow severe trauma to the back.

- Deltoid
- Trapezius (see **Section 2**)
- Long head of biceps (from the supraglenoid tubercle)
- Long head of triceps (from the infraglenoid tubercle)
- Muscles of the posterior axillary wall (teres major and latissimus dorsi)

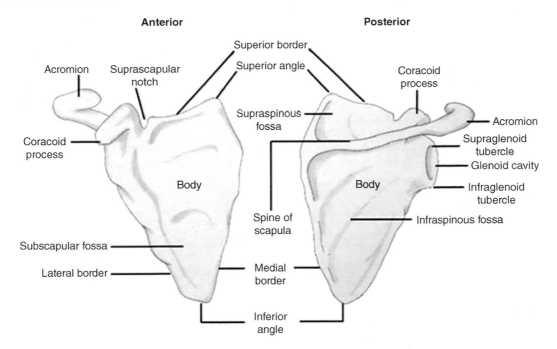

FIGURE 3.3 The anterior and the posterior surfaces of the scapula. (Courtesy of Calum Harrington-Vogt.)

The scapula is composed of several important bony parts:

- Ventral/anterior/costal surface for the origin of the subscapularis muscle.
- Dorsal or posterior surface, which is divided into the supraspinous and infraspinous fossae by the spine of the scapula, for the origin of the supraspinatus and infraspinatus muscles, respectively.
- Coracoid process (Greek: *korakos*, "crow"), a beak-like projection from the superior border of the scapula.
- Acromion (Greek: *akros*, "outermost"; *omos*, "shoulder"), a bony projection from the spine of the scapula laterally.
- Glenoid fossa (Greek: *glene*, "socket"; *eidos*, "shape" or "form"), which is located laterally and accommodates the head of the humerus to form the glenohumeral joint.
- The scapula has three angles (inferior, lateral, and superior) and three borders (superior, lateral, and medial). The suprascapular notch is located medial to the base of the coracoid process, and the transverse scapular ligament converts the notch to the foramen, where the suprascapular nerve passes to innervate the supraspinatus and infraspinatus muscles.

Several muscles are attached to the scapula and play a role in the stabilisation of the scapula:

- Four rotator cuff muscles (supraspinatus, infraspinatus, teres minor, and subscapularis; you can use the acronym SITS to help you remember these)

- Muscles attached to the coracoid process (short head of biceps brachii, pectoralis minor, and coracobrachialis)
- Serratus anterior
- Omohyoid
- Rhomboid major and minor
- Levator scapulae

For ligaments attached to the scapula, see **Figure 3.1**.

The scapular anastomosis is formed by major three arteries which supply the scapula and the attached muscles and help support the blood supply of the upper limb. These arteries are the suprascapular, dorsal scapular, and branches from the subscapular arteries.

Humerus

The humerus (**Figure 3.4**) is the bone of the arm ("arm" is the correct anatomical term for the upper arm). Proximally, it articulates with the scapula to form the glenohumeral joint, and distally, it articulates with the ulna and radius to form the elbow joint.

The humerus has several important bony landmarks (**Table 3.1**).

The articulation of the scapula, clavicle, and humerus (**Figure 3.1**) is maintained by several strong ligaments:

- *Coracoacromial ligament*, between the coracoid process and acromion. This protects the head of the humerus.
- *Coracoclavicular ligament*, between the coracoid process and clavicle; this is split into a trapezoid and conoid portion, which prevent movement at the acromioclavicular joint and aid in transmission of weight of the upper limb to the skeleton.

TABLE 3.1: Summary of the anatomical features of the humerus

Bony Feature	Description
Head	• Located at the superior aspect of the humerus • It is spherical and articulates with the glenoid cavity to form the glenohumeral joint
Anatomical neck	• Acts as a bridge between the head and the greater and lesser tubercles of the humerus
Surgical neck	• This is the part distal to the head, anatomical neck, and tubercles of the humerus • The surgical neck forms a bridge between the tubercles and the shaft of the humerus
Greater tubercle	• Forms the lateral aspect of the proximal humerus • Acts as a site of attachment for three muscles of the *rotator cuff*: supraspinatus, infraspinatus, and teres minor
Lesser tubercle	• Forms the medial aspect of the proximal humerus and acts as a site of attachment for the subscapularis muscle
Bicipital groove (intertubercular groove)	• A deep depression on the proximal shaft of the humerus between the greater and lesser tubercles • This contains the tendon of the long head of the biceps brachii • The borders (lips) and floor of the bicipital groove also form a site of attachment for *three muscles*: pectoralis major (lateral lip), teres major (medial lip), and latissimus dorsi muscles (floor)
Shaft of the humerus	• Distal to the surgical neck • The shaft is the longest part of the bone and contains the deltoid tuberosity and radial (or spiral) groove
Deltoid tuberosity	• Small ridge on the lateral aspect of the shaft of the humerus. It forms a site of attachment for the deltoid muscle
Radial (spiral) groove	• Located along the posterior aspect of the humeral shaft • The radial groove contains the radial nerve and the deep artery of the arm (profunda brachii)
Medial and lateral supracondylar ridges	• Formed towards the distal end of the shaft, as it begins to widen • The lateral supracondylar ridge gives origin to the brachioradialis and the extensor carpi radialis longus
Medial and lateral epicondyles (Greek: *epi*, "upon")	• Pointed projections that lead to bony projections on either side of the supracondylar ridges
Medial epicondyle	• The **common flexor origin** • Forms a site of attachment for some flexor muscles of the anterior compartment of the forearm • It also protects the ulnar nerve, which runs posteriorly to it
Lateral epicondyle	• The common extensor origin • Forms a site of attachment for some extensor muscles in the forearm • Inflammation of the common extensor tendon is referred to as lateral epicondylitis, or **tennis elbow** • Patients with this condition will present with pain around the elbow region and a reduction in grip strength
Trochlea	• Meaning pulley, this is the only structure which extends to the posterior aspect of the humerus • The trochlea forms the medial aspect of the articular surface of the elbow joint • It articulates with the trochlear notch of the ulna • The olecranon fossa can also be found on the posterior aspect of the distal humerus
Capitulum	• Meaning "little head", this forms the lateral aspect of distal articular surface of the humerus • It articulates with the head of the radius • The coronoid and olecranon fossae are involved in receiving the respective processes on the ulna during full flexion and full extension of the forearm, respectively • The radial fossa is involved in receiving the head of the radius during full flexion

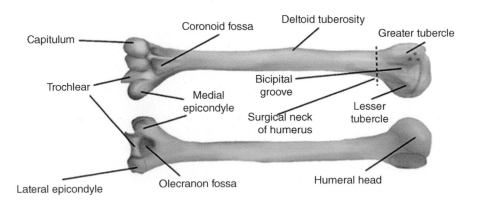

FIGURE 3.4 The bony landmarks of the humerus. (Courtesy of Katie Michaels.)

- *Acromioclavicular ligament*, between the acromion and clavicle; this reinforces the capsule of the joint.
- *Costoclavicular ligament*, between the clavicle and first rib; this provides additional protection for the subclavian artery and vein and acts as an axis of movement for the clavicle.
- *Ligaments of the shoulder capsule* (these are explained in more detail in the "Glenohumeral Joint" section).

Glenohumeral Joint (Shoulder Joint)

A synovial ball-and-socket joint between the head of the humerus and the shallow glenoid fossa of the scapula. The glenoid fossa is deepened by a fibrocartilaginous rim, called the glenoid labrum. This increases the congruency of the joint. Both the head of the humerus and the glenoid fossa are covered by hyaline cartilage. The joint articulation is maintained by the ligamentous capsule, which holds the two bones together and is strengthened by the rotator cuff muscles. The inner aspect of the joint is lined by synovial membrane, which produces synovial fluid to lubricate the joint and communicates with the bursa of the subscapularis.

Stability of the joint is also derived from the ligaments, which are under tension during movement of the shoulder, and muscles acting on the glenohumeral joint. The muscles are included in **Table 3.2** and are explained in more detail in the Muscles of the Upper Limb section.

The ligaments include:

- *Superior glenohumeral ligament*, which is under tension in adduction.
- *Middle glenohumeral ligament*, which is under tension in external rotation.
- *Inferior glenohumeral ligament*, which is under tension in abduction and internal or external rotation.
- *Coracohumeral ligament*, which is under tension in extreme flexion, extension, or external rotation.

TABLE 3.2: Muscles acting on the glenohumeral joint

Muscle	Action
Anterior fibres of the deltoid, pectoralis major, biceps	Flexion
Posterior fibres of the deltoid and muscles of the posterior axillary wall, teres major, and latissimus dorsi	Extension
Subscapularis, teres major, and latissimus dorsi	Internal rotation
Infraspinatus, teres minor, and posterior fibres of the deltoid	External rotation
Supraspinatus and the middle fibres of the deltoid	Abduction
Pectoralis major, latissimus dorsi, and teres major	Adduction

Blood supply is provided by the anterior and posterior circumflex humeral and subscapular arteries (branches of the third part of the axillary artery).

Nerve supply is provided by the articular branches from axillary, suprascapular, and musculocutaneous nerves.

FRACTURES AND DISLOCATION OF THE HUMERUS

Three nerves are closely related to the humerus: the axillary, radial, and ulnar nerves. Fractures of associated anatomical landmarks can lead to damage of these structures:

- *Surgical neck of the humerus:* this is narrow in nature and therefore is a common site for fracture (**Figure 3.5**). Fractures of the proximal humerus can lead to damage of the axillary nerve (*vide infra*).
- *Shaft of the humerus:* as the radial nerve and profunda brachii artery run in the spiral groove, these structures may be damaged during fracture of the shaft of the humerus. This can result in wrist drop, as the radial nerve supplies the muscles of the posterior compartment of the forearm.
- *Medial epicondyle:* the ulnar nerve runs posteriorly to this structure, and therefore is at risk of damage during compression or fracture of this bony landmark.

ANTERIOR DISLOCATION OF THE SHOULDER

The glenohumeral joint is commonly the most dislocated joint in the human body in view of its wide ranges of movement. This is due to its poor congruency, as it has a shallow glenoid fossa in relation to the relatively large humeral head.

- Anterior dislocation of the shoulder forms the majority of all shoulder dislocations, as the head of the humerus slips down into the least protected part of the capsule and lies below the coracoid process (subcoracoid position) (**Figure 3.6**).
- This may be caused by a fall on an outstretched hand or during sports.
- Typically, a sign of anterior dislocation is that there is loss of the normal contour of the deltoid (flat shoulder deformity). This is due to the loss of the bulge of the greater tubercle, as it is displaced medially (**Figure 3.7**).
- Axillary nerve function should be assessed, as the displaced humeral head can damage the nerve in the quadrangular space. Rotator cuff muscles may also be affected. However, injury to the axillary artery or the brachial plexus is rare.

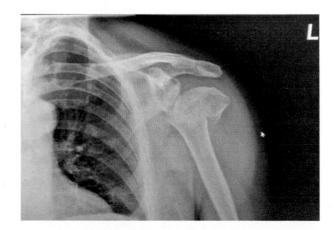

FIGURE 3.5 Fracture of the surgical neck of the left humerus in an 85-year-old patient. (Courtesy of Muthana Alqassab.)

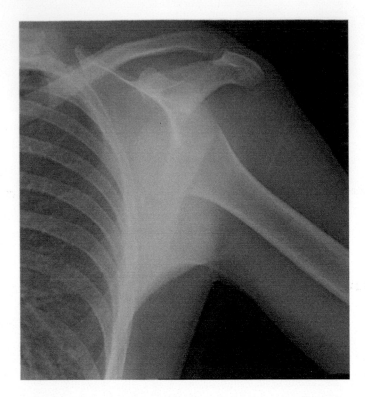

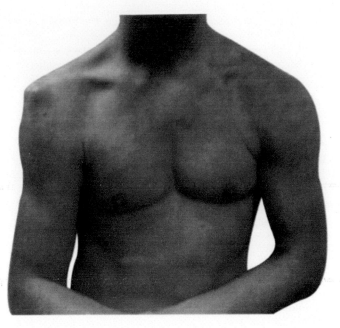

FIGURE 3.7 Image of an anterior dislocation of the right shoulder; note the flat shoulder appearance. (Courtesy of Department of Anatomical Sciences, SGUL.)

FIGURE 3.6 Anterior dislocation of the left shoulder of a 29-year-old patient after a skiing injury. There is anterior displacement of the humeral head on the glenoid fossa. (Courtesy of Salam Ismael.)

Brachial Plexus

The brachial plexus is formed from the union of the ventral rami of spinal nerves of C5–C8 and T1. This forms the roots, trunks, divisions, cords, and terminal branches (**Figure 3.8**).

The axillary sheath is a prolongation of the prevertebral fascia, which encloses the axillary artery and the cords of the brachial plexus. T1 divides into a large nerve, which contributes to the brachial plexus, and a small branch, which runs as the first intercostal nerve (see **Section 4**).

In the neck, the roots pass between the anterior and middle scalene muscles to emerge on the lateral border of the scalenus anterior.

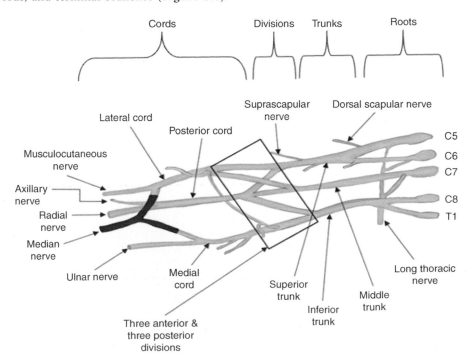

FIGURE 3.8 Diagram of the brachial plexus showing the roots, trunks, divisions, cords, and branches. (Courtesy of Katie Michaels.)

Several nerves originate from the roots:

- C5–C7 roots give the **long thoracic nerve** (nerve of Bell), which supplies the serratus anterior
- C5 **contributes to the phrenic nerve** (C3–C5), which innervates the diaphragm
- **Dorsal scapular nerve** (C5) innervates the rhomboid muscles and levator scapulae

The roots converge to form the trunks, which are present in the lower part of the posterior triangle of the neck behind the middle one-third of the clavicle:

- *Superior trunk:* C5 and C6; forms branches for the **nerve to the subclavius** (which may give rise to the accessory phrenic nerve)
- *Suprascapular nerve:* supplies the supraspinatus and infraspinatus muscles and articular branches to the acromioclavicular and shoulder joints
- *Middle trunk:* C7
- *Lower trunk:* C8 and T1

Each trunk divides into anterior and posterior divisions in the axilla (six divisions in total).

Cords are named in their relation to the axillary artery:

- *Medial cord:* anterior division of lower trunk
- *Posterior cord:* all posterior divisions
- *Lateral cord:* anterior divisions of upper and middle trunks

Branches of the medial cord:

- Ulnar nerve (C8, T1, and occasionally C7)
- Part of the median nerve
- Medial pectoral nerve, to both the pectoralis major (sternocostal part) and minor muscles, with a communicating branch from the lateral pectoral nerve (ansa pectoralis)
- Medial cutaneous nerve of the arm
- Medial cutaneous nerve of the forearm

Branches of the lateral cord:

- Musculocutaneous nerve (C5–C7), supplies the biceps brachii, brachialis, and coracobrachialis
- Part of median nerve
- Lateral cutaneous nerve of the forearm
- Lateral pectoral nerve to the clavicular part of the pectoralis major muscle

The branches of the posterior cord:

- Axillary nerve (C5–C6) to deltoid and teres minor
- Radial nerve (C5–C8, T1) to all arm and forearm extensors (in addition to supinator, anconeus, and brachioradialis) and skin on the dorsal arm, forearm, and hand
- Upper subscapular nerve to subscapularis and lower subscapular nerve to subscapularis and teres major
- Thoracodorsal nerve to latissimus dorsi, which may become injured during the operation of axillary node clearance

Terminal Branches of the Brachial Plexus

The Axillary Nerve

This arises from the posterior cord of the brachial plexus (ventral rami of C5 and C6).

The axillary nerve exits the axilla with the posterior circumflex artery via the quadrangular space. It then divides into three terminal branches: anterior, articular branches to the shoulder joint, and posterior branches. It supplies the deltoid, teres minor and the long head of the triceps, and a patch of skin covering the inferior region of the deltoid muscle (the "regimental badge" area).

The nerve may be injured during trauma to the shoulder joint and surgical neck fractures and can follow iatrogenic injuries, such as shoulder arthroscopy, intra-articular steroid injections, and intramuscular injections into the deltoid muscle. Patients will experience a loss of ability in abducting their shoulder (paralysis of the deltoid muscle) and a loss of sensation in the regimental badge area. To check the integrity of the axillary nerve in patients with fractures of the surgical neck by examining the function of the deltoid in its three parts, see later in the text.

Musculocutaneous Nerve (C5–C7)

The musculocutaneous nerve has both sensory and motor functions. It begins at the axilla at the level of the lower border of the pectoralis minor muscle. It gives rise to motor branches to the coracobrachialis muscle, which it pierces; runs between the biceps brachii and the brachialis muscle; and gives rise to branches to both respective muscles (the acronym BBC can be used to help you remember this). These muscles are flexors of the anterior compartment of the arm. The biceps brachii is also a strong supinator.

After descending the length of the arm, the musculocutaneous nerve emerges lateral to the biceps tendon and continues into the forearm as the lateral cutaneous nerve of the forearm, which provides sensory innervation to the lateral aspect of the forearm.

The musculocutaneous nerve supplies articular branches to the shoulder and elbow joints.

Ulnar Nerve (C8, T1)

The ulnar nerve courses inferiorly to the elbow, on the medial aspect of the brachial artery, until it pierces the medial intermuscular septum to enter the posterior compartment of the arm.

It then loops behind the medial epicondyle of the humerus. Here, the ulnar nerve runs between the medial epicondyle and skin, leaving it vulnerable to irritation upon impact at this point. Hence, this nerve can cause an electric shock-like sensation when striking the medial epicondyle with the elbow flexed, colloquially referred to as the "funny bone". **It supplies no branches in the upper arm**.

Median Nerve (C5–C8, T1)

This is formed from both lateral and medial cords of the brachial plexus in the axilla. It makes up the middle nerve of the characteristic "M-shaped" part of the brachial plexus.

- The median nerve runs superficial to the brachial artery, just lateral to the closely related ulnar nerve.
- Midway down the arm, the median and ulnar nerves diverge. The median nerve continues lateral to the brachial artery.
- As the median nerve approaches the elbow, it crosses over the brachial artery and thus enters the cubital fossa medial to the brachial artery.
- **It does not supply branches above the elbow.**

Radial Nerve (C5–T1)

The radial nerve exits the axilla and descends into the arm, running posterior to the axillary artery and then the brachial artery.

The course of the radial nerve is as follows:

- It enters the anterior compartment of the arm through the intermuscular septum, where it becomes surrounded by both brachialis and brachioradialis.
- It firstly gives rise to branches which provide **motor innervation to the medial and long heads of the triceps brachii**.
- It also gives rise to a sensory branch called the **posterior cutaneous nerve of the arm**, which provides sensory innervation for the majority of the skin on the posterior aspect of the arm.
- It then accompanies the profunda brachii artery along the radial (spiral) groove (see above, anatomy of the humerus). Here it supplies the **lateral head of the triceps in addition to brachialis, brachioradialis, and extensor carpi radialis longus**, after leaving the radial groove.
- At the lower aspect of the arm, the radial nerve gives rise to two more sensory branches:
  - The **lateral cutaneous nerve of the arm** (which supplies the lower half of the lateral aspect of the arm)
  - The **posterior cutaneous nerve of the forearm**, which innervates a small area of skin along the middle section of the dorsal aspect of the forearm

- The nerve then divides into its two terminal branches (superficial and deep radial branches) anterior to the lateral epicondyle.

The **deep radial branch continues into the forearm as the posterior interosseous nerve** (which can get injured in proximal injuries to the radius) to provide motor innervation for the posterior compartment of the forearm (extensor muscles).

The superficial radial branch runs distally and anterolaterally, deep to the brachioradialis, along with the radial artery. When near the distal end of the forearm, the superficial radial branch courses laterally to enter the anatomical snuff box. Once it passes the anatomical snuff box, it helps to provide sensory innervation to the lateral surface of the palm and the dorsal surface of the lateral three and a half digits of the hand.

Quadrangular Space

The axillary nerve and the posterior circumflex humeral vessels pass through this space (**Figure 3.10**) which is bound by the:

- Teres minor superiorly
- Teres major inferiorly
- Surgical neck of the humerus laterally
- Long head of the triceps medially
- Subscapularis muscle, which covers the space anteriorly

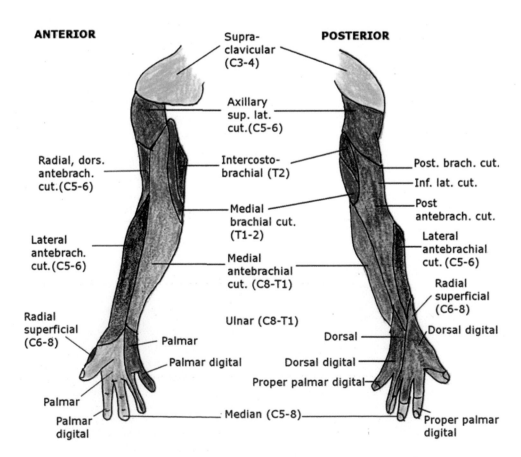

FIGURE 3.9 Sensory innervation of the upper limb. (Antebrach: Antebrachial, Cut: Cutaneous, Dors: dorsal, Inf: Inferior, Lat: Lateral, Sup: Superior.) (Courtesy of Gabriela Barzyk, adapted from Dermatome Maps of Foerster [1933] and Fender [1939].)

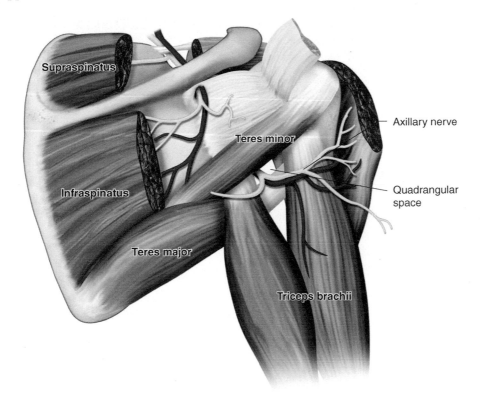

FIGURE 3.10 The anatomy of the quadrangular space. (Courtesy of Kathryn DeMarre.)

CLINICAL NOTES

BRACHIAL PLEXUS

Injury at the superior aspect of the shoulder

Musculocutaneous nerve injury is relatively uncommon because the nerve is well protected at the axilla. However, injury to the nerve can occur during heavy backpacking by injuring the superior trunk (C5–C6) of the brachial plexus.

Radial nerve injury at the axilla

If the injury occurs at the axilla, e.g., during dislocation of the shoulder, stabbing, "Saturday night palsy" (compression of the radial nerve typically follows deep sleep with the arm hanging over the arm rest of a chair, usually following heavy alcohol consumption), or "crutch palsy", the patient will present with the following motor deficits:

- Inability to extend their forearm, wrist, and fingers; as a result, patients present with wrist drop.

They will also present with the following sensory deficits:

- Loss of sensation in the upper lateral aspect of the arm, posterior surface of the arm, posterior forearm, lateral aspect of the palm, and dorsal aspect of the lateral three and half digits

Injury at the middle part of the upper arm

If the injury occurred at the middle part of the arm, e.g., when there is damage to the radial groove due to fracture of the humeral shaft, patients will present with the following motor deficits:

- Inability to extend the wrist and fingers; therefore, patients present with a **wrist drop** (note that at this level, the radial nerve would have provided motor innervation to the triceps, and therefore patients retain their ability to extend the forearm)
- Weakness in supination due to paralysis of the supinator

They will also present with the following sensory deficits:

- Loss of sensation at the posterior forearm, lateral aspect of the palm, and dorsal aspect of the proximal part of the lateral three and a half digits except the nailbeds. Note that at this level, the radial nerve would have already given rise to the lower lateral cutaneous nerve of the arm and posterior cutaneous nerve of the arm.
- This is why there is no loss of sensation in the upper lateral and posterior aspect of the arm. Therefore, only the superficial radial branch and the posterior cutaneous nerve of the forearm become affected if the injury occurs at this level.

(Continued)

Injury inferior to the elbow

If the injury to the radial nerve occurred just below the elbow (e.g., elbow dislocation), patients will present with the following motor deficits:

- Inability to extend fingers (paralysis of extensors of the digits)
- Weakness in extending hand (partial wrist drop; there is partial wrist drop because the extensor carpi radialis longus is not affected, as it is already innervated)

They will also present with the same sensory deficit as injuries at the middle part of the upper arm.

Injury at the distal aspect of the forearm

- **Wartenberg's syndrome** results from compression of the superficial radial branch of the radial nerve at the wrist, e.g., due to wearing tight jewellery.
- Patients will only present with a loss of sensation in the lateral aspect of the palm and the dorsal aspect of the lateral three and a half digits of the hand. This happens as the superficial branch would be affected. **Note that the nailbeds would be spared because they are supplied by the median and ulnar nerves.**

Learning Point

Remember the radial nerve supplies the BEST muscles (brachioradialis, extensors, supinator, and triceps).

Other injuries of the brachial plexus include:

- *Birth injuries* during difficult vaginal delivery, due to traction on the upper limb.
- *Blunt and penetrating injuries* to the shoulder and axillary regions.
- *Postoperative injuries* (following injuries during operations such as the removal of axillary lymph nodes, i.e., axillary clearance and diagnostic lymph node biopsy). Examples include injury to the thoracodorsal and long thoracic nerves.

The Shoulder

Muscles of the Shoulder

Deltoid

A triangle-shaped muscle that spans superficially over the glenohumeral joint, forming the rounded appearance of the shoulder. The anterior and posterior parts are unipennate, with the muscle fibres inserted into the tendon on one side. The central part is multipennate – muscle fibres are inserted on both sides of the tendon (**Table 3.3**).

The Rotator Cuff Muscles

Four muscles form the rotator cuff; their tendons converge to blend with the capsule of the glenohumeral joint. They help to maintain the stability of the shoulder by keeping the head of the humerus within the shallow glenoid fossa (**Table 3.4**). Additional functions include medial and lateral rotation of the arm and initiation of abduction by the supraspinatus.

TABLE 3.3: Details on the origin, insertion, innervation, and action of the deltoid muscle

Muscle	Origin	Insertion	Innervation	Action
Deltoid, consists of three parts: • Anterior • Central • Posterior	Lateral third of the clavicle, acromion, and spine of scapula	Inserts onto the deltoid tuberosity of the humerus	Axillary nerve	*Anterior:* flexion and medial rotation of arm *Central:* abductor of shoulder *Posterior:* extensor and lateral rotator of shoulder

TABLE 3.4: Rotator cuff muscles

Muscle	Origin	Insertion	Innervation	Action
Supraspinatus	Supraspinous fossa of the scapula	Greater tubercle of the humerus	Suprascapular nerve (C4–C6)	Abductor of the arm
Infraspinatus	Infraspinous fossa	Greater tubercle of the humerus	Suprascapular nerve (C5 and C6)	Lateral rotator of the arm
Teres minor	Middle of the lateral border of the scapula	Greater tubercle of the humerus	Axillary nerve (C5 and C6)	External arm rotator
Subscapularis	Subscapular fossa (ventral surface of the scapula)	Lesser tubercle	Upper and lower subscapular nerves (C5–C7)	Internal rotator of the arm

CLINICAL NOTES

- **Painful arc syndrome** is the impingement of the supraspinatus tendon below the acromion, usually due to wear and tear with age. A sign of this is that the patient may feel pain on abduction of the arm between 60 and 120 degrees. This is diagnosed by history taking and physical examination.
- **Jobe's test** (also known as the empty can test) is used to diagnose painful arc syndrome. The patient's arm is elevated to 90 degrees of abduction with internal rotation (arm up and out with the thumb turned inward toward the floor). A downward pressure is then applied against the arm. A positive test is the provocation of pain.
- The function of the deltoid muscles (and the axillary nerve which supplies the deltoid) can be tested as the patient abducts their arm 15 degrees from the body against resistance, and simultaneously the examiner should feel the contraction of the deltoid muscle. The deltoid muscle is assisted by the supraspinatus muscle in the initial 10 to 15 degrees.

The Upper Arm

Muscles of the Upper Arm
(Figures 3.11–3.13 and Tables 3.5–3.6)

Flexors: anterior compartment (biceps brachii, coracobrachialis, and brachialis)
Extensor: posterior compartment (triceps muscle)

Posterior Compartment of the Upper Arm
The triceps is the only muscle in the posterior compartment of the arm (**Figure 3.13**).

TABLE 3.5: Origin, insertion, innervation, and action of the muscles of the upper arm flexor compartment

Muscle	Origin	Insertion	Innervation	Action
Biceps brachii	Originates from two heads The long head of the biceps is intra-articular and arises from the supraglenoid tubercle of the scapula The short head of the biceps arises from the coracoid process of the scapula	Radial tuberosity of the proximal radius Bicipital aponeurosis of the cubital fossa	Musculocutaneous nerve	Flexor of the elbow and supinator of the forearm, e.g., opening a bottle with corkscrew
Brachialis	Anterior surface of the shaft of the humerus, below the deltoid tuberosity; it lies under the biceps	Coronoid process and tuberosity of ulna	Musculocutaneous nerve (with additional innervation from the radial nerve in 70%–80% of people)	Flexor of the elbow joint
Coracobrachialis	Coracoid process of the scapula	Medial surface of the shaft of the humerus	Musculocutaneous nerve	Flexor and adductor of the arm in addition to stabilisation of the humeral head within the shoulder joint

TABLE 3.6: Origin, insertion, innervation, and action of the triceps brachii muscle

Muscle	Origin	Insertion	Innervation	Action
Triceps muscle	Long head originates from the infra-glenoid tubercle of the scapula Lateral and medial heads from the posterior aspect of the shaft of the humerus	The olecranon process of the ulna	Radial nerve, (although some anatomy books mention the axillary nerve as the nerve supply of the long head)	Helps to stabilise the shoulder joint inferiorly Extensor of the elbow joint

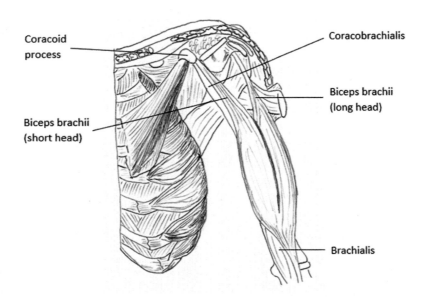

FIGURE 3.11   The anterior upper arm muscles. (Courtesy of Alina Humdani.)

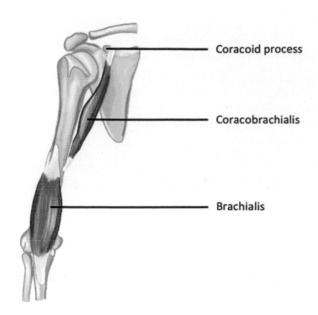

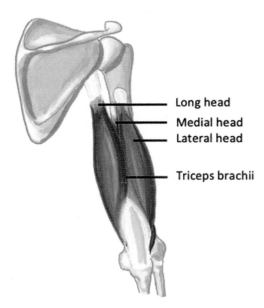

- Muscular branches to flexor compartment of the arm
- Superior and inferior ulnar collateral arteries (form an anastomosis around the elbow)

Venous drainage is by the venae comitantes accompanying the brachial artery, which will form the axillary vein.

Cubital Fossa

This is the triangular space at the ventral aspect of the elbow, which is bounded on the ulnar side by the pronator teres, on the radial side by the brachioradialis, and proximally by an imaginary line between the medial and lateral epicondyles.

The floor of the cubital fossa is formed by the brachialis and supinator muscles. The roof is composed of skin and deep fascia, reinforced by the bicipital aponeurosis. The median cubital vein (a common site for venepuncture) runs in the roof of the fossa, alongside the medial and lateral cutaneous nerves of the forearm.

Bicipital Aponeurosis

This is an important band of tissue formed from thickened deep fascia, and represents an extension of the tendon of the biceps brachii muscle. It separates the contents from the superficial structures found within the roof of the fossa. The aponeurosis helps to prevent damage to the brachial artery during venepuncture (the "*grace à Dieu* fascia").

Contents (Figure 3.14):

- *Biceps tendon (most lateral):* the tendon inserts into the radial tuberosity.
- *Brachial artery (medial to the biceps tendon):* often the brachial artery divides into the radial and ulnar arteries at the apex of the cubital fossa.
- The median nerve is the most medial structure.

FIGURE 3.12 The anterior upper arm muscles with the biceps brachii removed. (Courtesy of Avni Kant.)

FIGURE 3.13 Posterior view showing the heads of the triceps brachii. (Courtesy of Avni Kant.)

Arterial Supply and Venous Drainage of the Arm

The main artery of the upper arm is the **brachial artery**, which terminates at the level of the neck of the radius by dividing into the radial and ulnar arteries.

The main branches are:

- Profunda brachii follows the radial nerve in the spiral groove and supplies the triceps muscle

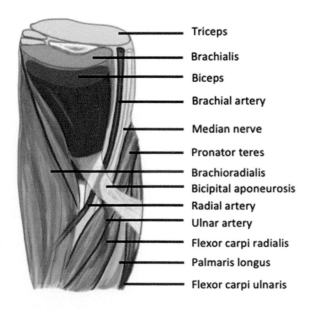

FIGURE 3.14 The contents of the cubital fossa. Note the relationship of the median nerve, brachial artery, and biceps brachii aponeurosis. (Courtesy of Avni Kant.)

BRACHIAL ARTERY

The brachial artery is an important landmark when taking blood pressure and is where the bell of the stethoscope is positioned.

It may become damaged following a **supracondylar fracture** (a break in the bone superior to the lateral and medial condyles) of the lower humerus (**Figure 3.15**). It is the most common elbow fracture in children, and commonly follows a fall on the outstretched hand. Neurovascular injury might be associated, so the distal radial and ulnar pulses should always be checked (as the brachial artery may get compromised by the anteriorly displaced bone segment) in addition to median and ulnar nerve examination. Improperly treated fractures can end up with ischaemia of the forearm muscles and fibrosis (fibrous tissue formation replacing the damaged muscles); this is called **Volkmann's ischaemic contracture**.

Anatomy of the Forearm and Wrist

The forearm begins distal to the elbow joint and continues to the wrist joint. The forearm has anterior and posterior compartments, which contain muscles that mainly act to produce movements at the wrist joint and fingers.

Bones

The bones of the forearm consist of the radius and ulna; these articulate with the trochlea and capitulum of the humerus at the elbow joint (**Figure 3.16**). These bones are united by the interosseous membrane, which is a strong sheet of fibrous tissue that runs between the interosseous borders. This forms a syndesmosis (fibrous joint) and provides attachment to some of the muscles of the forearm.

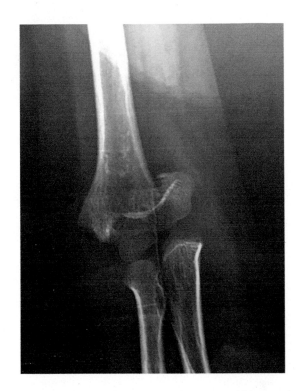

FIGURE 3.15   X-ray of the elbow of a 5-year-old boy with displaced supracondylar fracture. (Courtesy of Qassim F. Baker.)

- Posterior
- *Interosseous:* the sharp attachment ridge for the interosseous membrane, on the medial aspect of the shaft

The radius has three surfaces:

- Anterior
- *Posterior:* identified due to the large dorsal tubercle (Lister's tubercle, **Figure 3.17**), which acts as a pulley for the tendon of the extensor pollicis longus

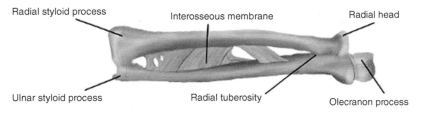

Radial styloid process   Interosseous membrane   Radial head

Ulnar styloid process   Radial tuberosity   Olecranon process

FIGURE 3.16   Radius and ulna. (Courtesy of Katie Michaels.)

The Radius

The radius has a circular proximal head, which allows it to rotate about its axis during pronation and supination. The radius forms a major component of the forearm's articulation at the wrist distally. Unlike the ulna, the head of the radius is found proximally. It is concave and articulates with the capitulum.

Moving just distal to the head, the radius narrows. This is the neck of the radius.

Just distal to the neck is a raised rough area – the **radial tuberosity**. This is the site of insertion of the biceps brachii.

The **shaft** of the radius is narrow proximally but expands distally. The shaft is triangular on cross-section. This triangular shape gives the shaft three borders:

- *Anterior:* starts as a continuation of the radial tuberosity in the proximal end of the shaft

- *Lateral:* contains a small roughening for insertion of the pronator teres

At the distal end of the radius the lateral surface extends out as the **radial styloid process**, which can be felt on the lateral side of the wrist in the anatomical position. Medially there is an impression on the radius, the **ulnar notch**, for the articulation with the head of the ulna at the distal radio-ulnar joint.

The Articulations of the Radius

The radius has four articulations:

- *Elbow joint: vide infra.*
- *Proximal radio-ulnar joint:* between the radial head and the radial notch of the ulna; the radius rotates against the ulna during pronation and supination.

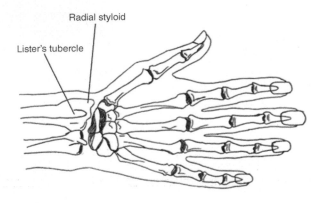

Radial styloid

Lister's tubercle

FIGURE 3.17 Posterior aspect of the wrist, showing Lister's tubercle on the distal radius. (Courtesy of Alina Humdani.)

- *Wrist (radiocarpal) joint:* distally, the radius articulates with two of the carpal bones, laterally with the scaphoid, and medially with the lunate.
- *Distal radio-ulnar joint:* see later.

The Ulna

The **olecranon** (from Greek *"olene"*, meaning elbow and *"kranon"*, meaning head) is a bony prominence projecting proximally from the ulna, forming the posterior part of the trochlear notch, with the **coronoid process** forming the anterior. The olecranon gives the elbow its hinge-like properties. On extension, the olecranon will fit into the **olecranon fossa** of the humerus.

Moving distally, the diameter of the **ulnar shaft** narrows from its maximum width at the elbow joint. Similar to the radius, the ulna cross-section is triangular and has three borders:

- *Anterior*
- *Posterior:* can be palpated in its entirety along the posterior forearm
- *Interosseous:* on the lateral aspect for the attachment of the interosseous membrane

The ulna also has three surfaces:

- *Medial:* in contrast to the radius
- *Anterior:* for the attachment of the pronator quadratus
- *Posterior:* for muscle attachments (*vide infra*)

The **ulnar tuberosity** is distal to the coronoid process on the anterior surface and, with the coronoid process, is the site for the **brachialis** muscle insertion.

Distally, the lateral aspect is roughened to allow for the attachment of the pronator quadratus.

The distally located **ulnar head** has a bony protrusion called the **styloid process** (shaped like a *stilus*, Latin for early writing instrument) arising from the posteromedial aspect. The styloid process is linked to the **pisiform** and **triquetrum** via the **ulnar collateral ligament**.

Articulations of the Ulna

The ulna has three articulation points and doesn't contribute to the wrist joint:

- Elbow joint
- Proximal radio-ulnar joint
- Distal radio-ulnar joint

CLINICAL NOTES

FOREARM

A common fracture found in the forearm is that of the **distal radius** seen following a fall on an outstretched arm, known as **Colles' fracture**. The distal fragment of the radius is forced posteriorly producing a **"dinner fork" deformity** and impacted. Although this fracture can happen in young age groups, it is most frequently seen in elderly ladies, due to the common association with osteoporosis. Fracture of the ulnar styloid process may co-exist as well (**Figure 3.18**).

Smith's fracture is a rare fracture of the distal end of the radius with volar displacement (also known as a reverse Colles').

Other fractures:

- **Monteggia's fracture**: fracture of the proximal shaft of the ulna, with associated anterior dislocation of the radius and rupture of the annular ligament; mostly seen in children, but can also occur in adults (**Figure 3.19**).
- **Galeazzi's fracture**: fracture at the junction between the middle and distal thirds of the radius and dislocation at the distal radio-ulnar joint.

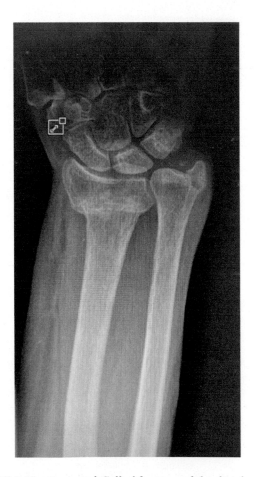

FIGURE 3.18 Impacted Colles' fracture of the distal radius in a 63-year-old female after a fall onto an outstretched hand. Also note the ulnar styloid fracture. (Courtesy of Salam Ismael.)

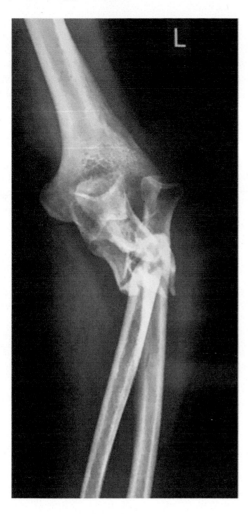

FIGURE 3.19 Monteggia's fracture (fracture of proximal ulnar diaphysis, plus dislocation of the radial head). (Courtesy of Ahmed A. Shakir.)

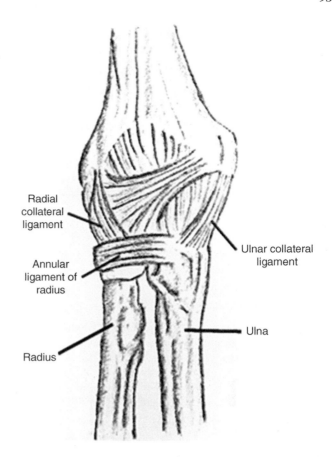

FIGURE 3.20 Diagram of the ligaments of the elbow and upper radio-ulnar joints. (Courtesy of Jordan Bethel.)

Elbow Joint

The elbow joint is a synovial hinge joint between the distal humerus and the radius and ulna. The elbow joint is surrounded by a capsule and lined by synovial membrane. The collateral radial and ulnar ligaments span over the joint along the lateral and medial aspects. These support the elbow joint during flexion and extension (**Figure 3.20**).

- The **trochlea articulates with the trochlear notch of the ulna** (consists of the olecranon posteriorly and the coronoid process anteriorly).
- The **capitulum articulates with the head of the radius** (the head and neck of the radius are encircled by the annular ligament).
- The only movements possible at the elbow joint are flexion (by flexors: biceps brachii, brachialis, and brachioradialis) and extension (by triceps and anconeus).

The **proximal radio-ulnar joint** is a synovial pivot joint between the head of the radius and the radial notch of the ulna. Rotation of the radial head within this joint **allows pronation and supination** of the forearm and wrist to occur. This is enabled by the annular ligament, which holds the radius in

place in the radial notch of the ulna and is responsible for the main integrity of this joint. Its capsule is continuous with that of the elbow joint, and the same applies to the synovial membrane (some anatomists consider the elbow and the proximal radio-ulnar joints as one joint).

CLINICAL NOTE

DISLOCATION OF THE ELBOW

Elbow dislocation is one of the most common injuries affecting the elbow, especially in children. The most common type is posterolateral, which commonly occurs in association with a fracture of the elbow. As for supracondylar fractures, it is important to always check the integrity of the neurovascular structures (brachial artery, ulnar and median nerves).

Distal Radio-Ulnar Joint

This is a synovial pivot joint between the head of the ulna and ulnar notch of the radius. A triangular disc of fibrocartilage separates the joint from the wrist joint and holds the two bones together during pronation.

The rotary movements of pronation and supination occur at the upper and lower radio-ulnar joints around a vertical axis that extends from the head of the radius above to the triangular disc below.

TABLE 3.7: Superficial forearm flexor muscles

Muscle	Origin	Insertion	Innervation	Action
Flexor carpi ulnaris	*Two heads:* • Humeral head arises from medial epicondyle • Ulnar head from olecranon of the ulna	Base of the fifth metacarpal, the pisiform bone, and hook of hamate	Ulnar nerve	Flexes and adducts the wrist
Flexor carpi radialis	Medial epicondyle of humerus	Base of the second (mainly) and third metacarpals	Median nerve	Flexes and abducts the wrist
Pronator teres	*Two heads:* • Humeral head from the medial epicondyle • Ulnar head from the coronoid process of the ulna	Lateral surface of the radius	Median nerve	Pronator of the forearm
Palmaris longus	Medial epicondyle of humerus	Flexor retinaculum and palmar aponeurosis	Median nerve	Flexion of the hand

The muscles responsible for pronation are the pronators (pronator teres and pronator quadratus) and for supination, the biceps brachii and supinator. Supination is much stronger than pronation.

Muscles of the Anterior Compartment of the Forearm

The muscles of the anterior compartment of the forearm act predominately to flex the wrist and digits. The anatomy of the hand and wrist is organised to support this motion of flexion. The anterior compartment of the wrist contains three layers of muscles: a superficial, intermediate, and deep layer (**Tables 3.7–3.9**).

Superficial Layer

The muscles of the superficial layer **all originate from the medial epicondyle** of the humerus (**Figure 3.21**).

The palmaris longus may be absent unilaterally or bilaterally, depending on the ethnicity of the individuals studied. In other mammals, this muscle is used to retract the claws. You can test for the presence of the palmaris longus by opposing the thumb to the little finger and flexing the wrist, which results in prominence of the palmaris longus tendon if it is present; this is called Schaeffer's test. The tendon of the palmaris longus may be used in tendon grafting.

The muscles of the superficial anterior compartment are innervated by the **median nerve, except for the flexor carpi ulnaris, which is innervated by the ulnar nerve**.

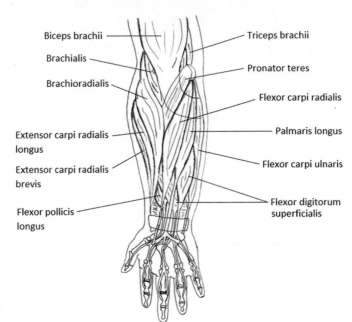

FIGURE 3.21 Muscles of the anterior compartment of the forearm showing the superficial and intermediate flexors and some extensors. (Courtesy of Alina Humdani.)

TABLE 3.8: Intermediate layer of forearm flexors

Muscle	Origin	Insertion	Innervation	Action
Flexor digitorum superficialis (FDS)	• Humero-ulnar head (from the medial epicondyle and coronoid process of the ulna) • Radial head (from anterior surface of the radius)	Middle phalanges of the second to fifth digits after forming Camper's chiasm (described later) around the flexor digitorum profundus	Median nerve	Flexes the proximal interphalangeal (PIP) joints and the metacarpophalangeal (MCP) joint of the same finger and the wrist

TABLE 3.9: Deep forearm flexor muscles

Muscle	Origin	Insertion	Innervation	Action
Flexor digitorum profundus (FDP)	Anterior surface of the ulna and medial aspect of interosseous membrane	Distal phalanges of the second to fifth digits	Median nerve, lateral half Ulnar nerve, medial half	Flexes the distal interphalangeal (DIP) joint, the MCP, and the wrist
Flexor pollicis longus (FPL)	Anterior surface of the radius	Distal phalanx of the thumb	Median nerve	Flexes the interphalangeal joint of the thumb, as well as the MCP joint
Pronator quadratus	Anterior surface of the ulnar shaft	Anterior surface of the shaft of the radius	Median nerve	Pronates the forearm

The **intermediate layer** contains one muscle (flexor digitorum superficialis [FDS]) (**Figure 3.21**).

Deep Layer
(**Figure 3.22**)

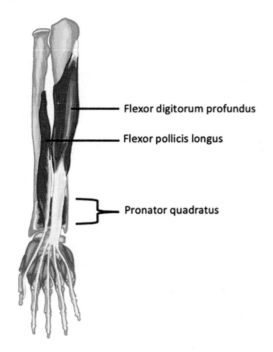

FIGURE 3.22 Muscles of the deep layer of the anterior compartment. (Courtesy of Avni Kant.)

The tendons of the flexor digitorum profundus (FDP) are deep to those of the FDS; however, the tendon of the FDP passes through the tendon of the FDS at the middle phalanx, where the FDS tendon splits into two to form Camper's chiasm (**Figure 3.23**). The FDP can be tested clinically by fixing the proximal interphalangeal joint (PIP) joint and asking the patient to flex the distal interphalangeal joint (DIP) joint.

Neurovascular Structures of the Anterior Forearm and Wrist

Arteries

The **radial** and **ulnar arteries** are the two main arteries of the anterior forearm. These arteries give rise to vessels that also supply the posterior compartment of the forearm. They are formed from the bifurcation of the brachial artery at the level of the neck of the radius.

The **radial artery** (smaller than the ulnar artery) passes laterally through the forearm, superficial to the FDS and can be located in the distal forearm, proximal to the wrist joint, immediately lateral to the flexor carpi radialis tendon.

The radial artery passes posterolaterally around the wrist to supply the thumb and lateral side of the index finger by passing obliquely through an area on the lateral aspect on the dorsum of the hand called the "**anatomical snuffbox**" (described in more detail later).

The **ulnar artery** passes medially through the forearm, deep to the FDS, and is not easily palpable in the distal forearm; hence a patient's pulse tends to be taken with the radial artery.

It gives origin to the common interosseous artery which divides into the anterior and posterior interosseous arteries, which supply the deep forearm flexors and deep and superficial forearm extensors respectively.

The ulnar artery enters the hand by passing lateral to the pisiform bone, via **Guyon's canal**, superficial to the flexor retinaculum of the carpal tunnel (described in detail later). The ulnar artery provides the major blood supply to the medial three and a half digits of the hand.

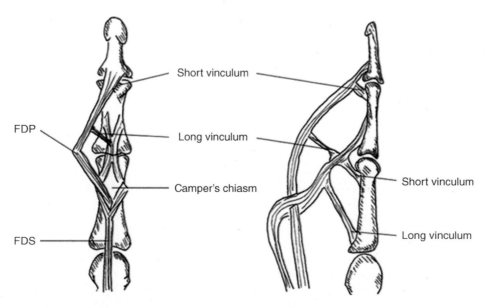

FIGURE 3.23 Camper's chiasm. (Courtesy of Alina Humdani.)

Both the radial and ulnar arteries anastomose to form the **deep and superficial palmar arches**.

CLINICAL NOTES

RADIAL ARTERY

- *Radial pulse:* as the artery lies superficially under the skin, it is a common place to measure the pulse to get an understanding of the heart rate (bradycardia, tachycardia, or normal rate), cardiac rhythm (regular, irregular, and presence of ectopic beat), and pulse volume (for example, low volume in patients with shock).
- Taking the radial pulse can be applied on both arms simultaneously to identify radioradial delay, or to the femoral and radial arteries to detect radiofemoral delays, which may indicate aortic coarctation; see **Section 4**.
- Taking an arterial blood sample for arterial blood gas (ABG) is an important clinical skill learnt by junior doctors.
- A radiocephalic fistula (between the cephalic vein and the radial artery) may be formed using the radial artery to gain vascular access in patients on chronic haemodialysis.

MODIFIED ALLEN'S TEST

- Since both radial and ulnar arteries anastomose to form the superficial and deep palmar arches, these arteries can be compressed at the wrist to produce pallor of the clenched fist. The patient then extends their fingers, and the pressure overlying the ulnar artery is released. A positive Allen's test, as shown by a return of colour to the hand within 10 seconds, signifies that the ulnar artery is sufficient to maintain arterial blood to the hand.
- This test assesses circulation in the hand and can be used to initially assess whether the radial artery can be used for coronary artery bypass graft (CABG) surgery and radial forearm flap and before taking a blood sample for ABG analysis, as thrombosis of the radial artery is a possible complication following cannulation for an arterial line or catheterisation (cardiac angiography). There is conflicting evidence to support the use of this test, although adding other tools like pulse oximetry and duplex ultrasound may help to improve the results.

Veins of the Hand and Forearm

The dorsal venous arch (or network) lies on the dorsum of the hand and continues as the **cephalic vein** laterally and the **basilic vein** medially. The cephalic vein ascends to the cubital fossa, then ascends the upper arm lateral to the biceps, and joins the axillary vein after passing through the deltopectoral groove. This vein is a common site for setting up an intravenous (IV) line (**Figure 3.24**).

The basilic vein ascends to the medial side of the biceps and joins the venae comitantes of the brachial artery to form the axillary vein.

The **median cubital vein** connects the cephalic and the basilic veins in the cubital fossa (see the notes on the bicipital aponeurosis). This vein is commonly used by phlebotomists when retrieving blood. This vein should be avoided if an IV line is set up, as flexion of the elbow kinks the IV cannula, and even risks cutting a piece of the cannula.

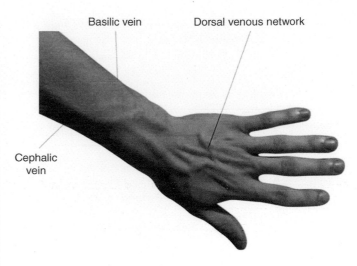

FIGURE 3.24   Dorsal venous arch and superficial veins of the forearm. (Courtesy of Jordan Bethel.)

Nerves

The main nerves of the anterior compartment are the **ulnar**, **median**, and **superficial radial nerves**.

Median Nerve

The course of the median nerve is as follows:

- It courses deep between the two heads of the **pronator teres** to enter the anterior forearm.
- In the forearm, the nerve runs between the FDP and FDS muscles.
- It passes **deep to the flexor retinaculum, through the carpal tunnel**, to enter the hand, where it divides into two terminal branches: the **recurrent branch** and the **palmar digital branch**.

Motor Innervation

Supplies **all** the **flexor muscles** of the anterior forearm **except the medial part of the FDP and flexor carpi ulnaris**.

The anterior interosseous branch of the median nerve passes over the interosseous membrane and innervates the muscles of the deep layer of the anterior compartment, except the ulnar part of the FDP. The skin of the base and central aspect of the palm is innervated by a small palmar branch of the anterior interosseous nerve (**palmar cutaneous branch**), which originates in the forearm and passes superiorly over the flexor retinaculum of the carpal tunnel, so this area is spared in carpal tunnel syndrome.

In the hand, the median nerve supplies the lateral two lumbricals and the muscles of the thenar eminence.

The acronym **LOAF** can be used to remember the muscles that are supplied by the median nerve in the hand:

- **L**umbricals 1 and 2 (by the palmar digital branch)
- **O**pponens pollicis, **A**bductor pollicis brevis, and **F**lexor pollicis brevis (the muscles of the thenar eminence), all supplied by the recurrent branch

The recurrent branch of the median nerve is sometimes referred to as the "million-dollar nerve", due to its vital importance in the opposition of the thumb to the other four fingers and litigation-related compensation when this branch is accidentally injured during hand surgery.

> Note: *pollicis* in Latin means "of the thumb"; thus, the thenar muscles act on the thumb.

Sensory Innervation

The **median nerve** carries sensory innervation from the following regions:

- The lateral aspect of the palm, including the palmar aspect and distal dorsal region of the thumb
- The palmar surface and distal dorsal aspect (including the nailbeds) of the index, middle, and lateral half of the ring finger (the second, third, and fourth digits) via the palmar digital branch

Ulnar Nerve (C8–T1)

The ulnar nerve enters the forearm by passing between the two heads (humeral and ulnar) of the flexor carpi ulnaris. At this point, muscular and cutaneous branches are given off. It courses along the medial side of the forearm, towards the lateral edge of the flexor carpi ulnaris tendon and **runs superficial to the flexor retinaculum** and the carpal tunnel. It then runs with the ulnar artery and vein in Guyon's canal into the hand, which is a fibro-osseous passage between the pisiform and the hook of hamate; the transverse carpal ligament and volar carpal ligament proximally; and the hook of hamate, abductor digiti minimi, pisohamate ligament, and fibrous arch of the hypothenar muscles distally.

The ulnar nerve runs medial to the ulnar artery and gives rise to the following cutaneous branches:

- A **palmar branch** innervates the skin on the medial side of the palm.
- A **dorsal branch** innervates the skin on the posteromedial side of the hand and the posterior surfaces of the medial one and a half digits.

Function of the Ulnar Nerve

The ulnar nerve provides motor supply to numerous muscles:

- Flexor carpi ulnaris
- Ulnar half of FDP
- All the intrinsic muscles of the hand, *except* the three muscles of the thenar eminence and two lateral lumbrical muscles, which are supplied by the median nerve. Note that the adductor pollicis is supplied by the ulnar nerve (*vide infra*, Froment's test)

The ulnar nerve provides sensory innervation to the fifth digit (little finger) and medial half of the fourth digit (ring finger) **on both palmar and dorsal aspects**.

The skin of the anterior thumb, index, middle finger, and lateral half of the fourth digit is supplied by the median nerve, while the proximal posterior skin across the same four digits is innervated by the radial nerve.

CLINICAL NOTES

ULNAR NERVE INJURY

- The ulnar nerve runs almost unprotected in its whole course and so is liable to injury.
- Ulnar nerve damage gives a **"claw hand appearance"**. Here, the fourth and fifth digits are flexed at the interphalangeal (IP) joints while hyperextended at the metacarpophalangeal joints (**Figure 3.25**). This is different from Dupuytren's contracture (due to fibrosis of the palmar fascia of the hand, forming nodules in the palm and finger contracture), which presents as flexion of the metacarpophalangeal joint, PIP, and DIP.
- More proximal ulnar lesions (at the elbow) result in the loss of function of the flexor carpi ulnaris and FDP to the medial two digits.
- Distal lesions produce a worse "clawing" of the hand, as the innervation to the FDP is intact, and so flexion still occurs at the DIP joint (this is known as the "ulnar paradox"). There is impaired sensation over areas of skin innervated by the ulnar nerve.

CUBITAL TUNNEL SYNDROME

- The ulnar nerve is pinched in the cubital tunnel, which is formed by the medial epicondyle, olecranon, and Osborne's band (an elastic tissue between the two bony landmarks).
- Usually, this syndrome follows a repetitive strain injury, e.g., continually sleeping with the arm bent behind the neck. However, often the syndrome spontaneously resolves.
- It results in altered sensation of the volar and dorsal aspects of the little and ring fingers and pain along the course of the ulnar nerve from the elbow to the ulnar side of the hand.

FROMENT'S TEST

- Used to test for ulnar nerve palsy/weakness in the adductor pollicis.
- The patient is asked to pinch a paper between the thumb and the index finger. The examining clinician tries to pull the paper away, whilst the patient applies more pressure to retain the paper by contracting the adductor pollicis.

In ulnar nerve lesions, patients start to pinch the paper by flexing the IP joints more by using the flexor pollicis longus (supplied by the median nerve) to maintain a grip.

Posterior Aspect of the Forearm Muscles

The muscles of the posterior compartment predominantly extend the wrist and digits. All muscles of the posterior forearm are innervated by the radial nerve. The posterior forearm has superficial and deep layers of muscles.

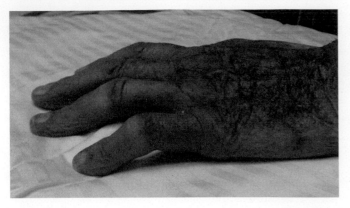

FIGURE 3.25 "Claw hand" due to ulnar nerve damage. Note hyperextension of the fourth and fifth metacarpophalangeal (MCP) joints due to paralysis of the lumbricals. (Photograph courtesy of Philip J. Adds.)

Superficial Layer

All muscles in the superficial layer originate from the **lateral epicondyle of the humerus** (the common extensor origin), except the brachioradialis and the extensor carpi radialis longus, which originate from the lateral supracondylar ridge of the humerus (**Table 3.10**).

> *Note:* The extensor carpi radialis longus and brevis and the extensor carpi ulnaris act synergistically with finger flexors, as they keep the wrist in an extended position to provide additional strength when grasping objects. This is essential for the proper formation of a **power grip**.

Deep Layer

All muscles of the deep posterior compartment originate from the posterior surface of the radius, ulna, and interosseous membrane and are innervated by the **posterior interosseous nerve**, a branch of the deep radial nerve (**Table 3.11**).

TABLE 3.10: Superficial layer of forearm extensors

Muscle	Origin	Insertion	Innervation	Action
Brachioradialis	Proximal aspect of the lateral supracondylar ridge of humerus	Radial styloid process	Radial nerve	Elbow flexion when the forearm is in pronation
Extensor carpi radialis longus	Lateral supracondylar ridge	Base of the second metacarpal	Radial nerve	Extends and abducts the wrist
Extensor carpi radialis brevis	Lateral epicondyle	Base of the third metacarpal	Radial nerve	Extends and abducts the wrist
Extensor carpi ulnaris	Lateral epicondyle of the humerus	Medial side of the fifth metacarpal	Radial nerve (deep branch)	Extends and adducts the wrist
Anconeus	Lateral epicondyle	Posterior and lateral part of the olecranon	Radial nerve	Extends and stabilises the elbow joint. Abducts the ulna during pronation of the forearm
Extensor digitorum	Lateral epicondyle	Middle and distal phalanges of the second to fifth digits	Radial nerve (deep branch)	Extension of fingers and wrist
Extensor digiti minimi	Lateral epicondyle of the humerus	Extensor hood of the fifth digit (little finger)	Radial nerve (deep branch)	Extension of little finger

TABLE 3.11: Muscles of the deep layer of the forearm

Muscle	Origin	Insertion	Innervation	Action
Abductor pollicis longus	Posterior surface of the ulna and radius	Base of the first metacarpal bone	Radial nerve (posterior interosseous branch)	Abduction of the carpometacarpal joint of the thumb and thumb extension (see information on the boundaries of the anatomical snuff box)
Extensor pollicis brevis	Posterior surface of the radius and interosseous membrane	Dorsal surface of proximal phalanx of the thumb	Radial nerve (posterior interosseous branch)	Extends the proximal phalanx of the thumb
Extensor pollicis longus	Middle third of posterior ulna and interosseous membrane	Dorsal surface of the distal phalanx of the thumb	Radial nerve (posterior interosseous branch)	Extends the interphalangeal joint of the thumb
Extensor indicis	Posterior ulna and interosseous membrane	Extensor expansion of the index finger	Radial nerve (posterior interosseous branch)	Extends the index finger
Supinator	*Two heads:* • Lateral epicondyle of the humerus • Posterior surface of the ulna and annular ligament	Lateral surface of the shaft of the radius	Radial nerve (deep branch)	Supination of the forearm, acting by rotating the radius at the proximal radio-ulnar joint

The radial nerve passes through the supinator muscle in the upper forearm. It then divides into deep (posterior interosseous nerve) and superficial (sensory) branches.

The **extensor retinaculum** is a strong thickened band of deep fascia that keeps the extensor tendons in position at the wrist. There are six tunnels for the passage of the extensor tendons lined by synovial sheaths. The retinaculum attaches laterally to the distal part of the radius and medially to the pisiform and hamate carpal bones.

The Wrist and Hand

Bones

Eight carpal bones make up the bones of the wrist. They are arranged in proximal and distal rows (**Figure 3.26**).

Proximal row (medial to lateral):

- *Pisiform* (*Latin:* "pea-shaped"): a sesamoid bone (a bone within a tendon, like the patella) within the tendon of flexor carpi ulnaris
- Triquetrum (*Latin: triquetrus*, "three-cornered")
- Lunate (*Latin: luna*, "moon-shaped/crescentic")
- Scaphoid (*Greek:* "keel-shaped")

Distal row (medial to lateral):

- The hamate has a hook (or hamulus), called "the hook of the hamate".
- The capitate is the largest carpal bone and articulates with the third metacarpal bone.
- The trapezoid articulates with the metacarpal of the index finger.
- The trapezium articulates with the thumb.
- The scaphoid, lunate, and triquetrum articulate with the radius and form the radiocarpal wrist joint.

Remember: "trapez**ium** supports the **thumb**; trapez**oid** lies in**soid**".

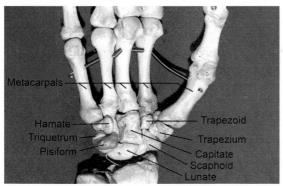

FIGURE 3.26 Carpal bones. (Photograph courtesy of Philip J. Adds.)

Anatomical Snuffbox

The "**anatomical snuffbox**" (so called because it was used in the past when taking snuff) is an anatomical landmark located on the posterolateral aspect of the hand (**Figure 3.27**).

The borders of the snuffbox consist of the:

- *Lateral border:* formed by the tendons of the **abductor pollicis longus** and **extensor pollicis brevis**
- *Medial border:* formed by the tendon of the **extensor pollicis longus**
- *Floor of the snuffbox:* formed by the **scaphoid** and **trapezium**

The **radial artery** runs obliquely through the snuffbox; the cephalic vein crosses it superficially, in addition to the terminal branches of the superficial radial nerve.

The **scaphoid** is the most commonly fractured carpal bone and commonly presents with swelling and tenderness over the area of the anatomical snuffbox (**Figure 3.28**). In around 10% of the population, blood supply comes from the distal to the proximal portion of the scaphoid bone, and so a fracture can lead to **avascular necrosis** of the scaphoid in these individuals due to interruption of the blood supply. Missed diagnosis of scaphoid fractures is a common cause of litigation.

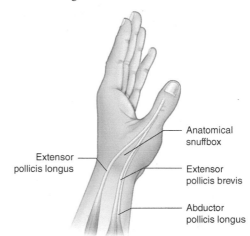

FIGURE 3.27 The anatomical snuffbox. (Courtesy of Jordan Bethel.)

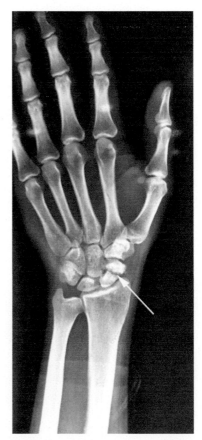

FIGURE 3.28 X-ray of the hand showing fracture of the waist of the scaphoid bone *(arrow)*. (Courtesy of Mohammed M. Altalal.)

QUIZ QUESTION

Q. *What other bones are susceptible to avascular necrosis?*

The Carpal Tunnel

This osteofascial tunnel is formed by the **flexor retinaculum** (thickened deep fascia across the flexor aspect of the wrist). Posteriorly, medially, and laterally the tunnel is formed by the **carpal arch**, which consists of the pisiform and hamate medially and the scaphoid and trapezium laterally.

Several important structures pass through the carpal tunnel from the forearm to the hand:

- FDP tendons (four)
- FDS tendons (four)
- Flexor pollicis longus tendon
- Median nerve

Note: One function of the flexor retinaculum is to prevent bowing of the FDP and FDS tendons to preserve their optimal function during flexion of the digits.

CLINICAL NOTE

CARPAL TUNNEL SYNDROME

- This is a common clinical condition, often idiopathic, due to compression of the median nerve as it travels deep to the flexor retinaculum (**Figure 3.29**). Other causes include osteoarthritis of the wrist joint, acromegaly, rheumatoid arthritis, and following injuries such as Colles' fracture.
- Compression of the median nerve interrupts its motor supply to the thenar muscles, which may lead to their atrophy, which is a late sign.
- May also lead to pain (mainly nocturnal), numbness, and paraesthesia (pins and needles) in the cutaneous distribution of the median nerve.
- More common in women than in men, especially in pregnant women, although it may disappear after labour.

If this is presented as a clinical scenario during an objective structured clinical examination (OSCE), the examiner will expect you to check for tenderness by tapping the retinaculum (Tinel's test) and for paraesthesia on flexion of the wrist (Phalen's test) and to test the function of the thenar muscles and sensation within the territory of the median nerve. Scanning by ultrasound (US) and magnetic resonance imaging (MRI) helps in reaching a clinical diagnosis.

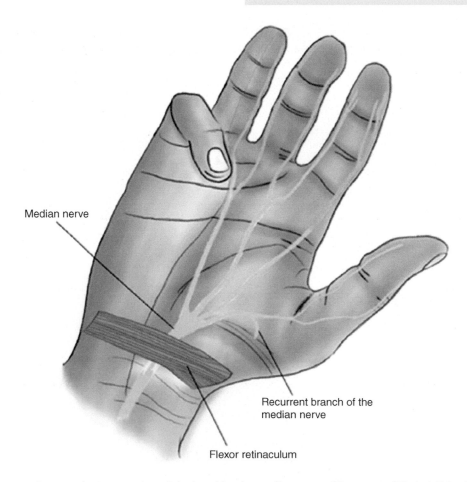

Median nerve

Recurrent branch of the median nerve

Flexor retinaculum

FIGURE 3.29 Diagram showing the innervation of the hand by the median nerve. (Courtesy of Katie Michaels.)

Skin of the Hand

The skin of the hand differs on its palmar and dorsal surfaces. The palmar skin is thicker and anchored to the deep structures and contains plenty of sweat glands but no hair follicles or sebaceous glands. The skin of the dorsum of the hand is loose, and consequently oedema is more liable to collect there.

Bones of the Hand

Distal to the carpal bones are the five **metacarpal bones**, which articulate distally with the proximal phalanges of each digit (**Figure 3.26**).

The second to fifth digits have three phalangeal bones: proximal, middle, and distal.

The thumb has only a **proximal and distal phalanx**.

The second to the fifth digits have two IP joints: PIP and DIP.

Joints of the Hand

Wrist (radiocarpal) joint

- Synovial joint between distal radius and the scaphoid, lunate, and triquetral
- *Movements:* flexion/extension, adduction, and abduction
- Wrist capsule lined by synovial membrane and reinforced by ligaments of the wrist (palmar radiocarpal, dorsal radiocarpal, ulnar collateral, and radial collateral)

Intercarpal joints

- Synovial joints between the adjacent bones of the proximal and distal rows of the carpus; each joint is surrounded by a capsule.
- There is limited intercarpal movement, which contributes to the general hand position.
- Midcarpal joints are between the bones of the proximal and distal carpal bones.

Carpometacarpal joints

- The joint between the base of the first metacarpal (i.e., of the thumb) and trapezium is a synovial saddle joint and allows for a wide range of movements (flexion/extension, adduction/abduction, and circumduction but not rotation).
- Joints of the second through fifth metacarpals allow less movement.

Metacarpophalangeal joints

- Synovial condylar joints between the head of the metacarpal and the base of the proximal phalanx.
- Allows for flexion/extension and abduction/adduction.
- Capsule reinforced by the palmar ligament and medial and lateral collateral ligaments.
- Dislocation of the metacarpophalangeal joint (MPJ) is an uncommon injury, which may be easy to reduce (**Figure 3.30**) unless major damage has occurred to the collateral ligaments.

IP joints

- Hinge joints
- Allow flexion/extension
- Reinforced by ligaments

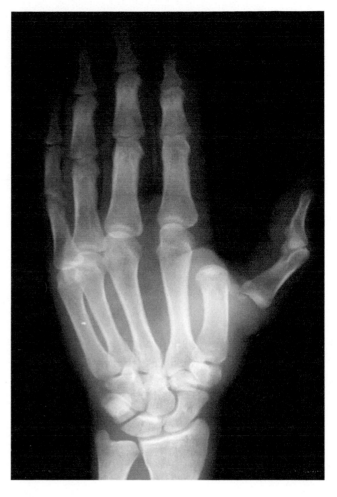

FIGURE 3.30 X-ray of the hand showing dislocation of the metacarpophalangeal joint of the thumb. (Courtesy of Mohammed M. Altalal.)

Flexion and Extension Mechanisms of the Wrist and Digits

Flexors of the Wrist and Digits

FDP

- Inserts onto distal phalanx
- Flexes digit at DIP
- Flexes the wrist

FDS

- Each tendon inserts onto the middle phalanx by splitting into two insertions, medial and lateral, forming Camper's chiasm
- Flexes digit at PIP

The FDS and FDP tendons exist in a synovial sheath as they pass through the carpal tunnel and progress distally along the palm and palmar aspect of the digits.

Pulley System of the Digits

A pulley system exists on the palmar surface of the digits. This maximises the motion of flexion by maintaining the tendon sheaths of the **FDS** and **FDP** as close to the axis of flexion as possible, thereby **preventing bowstringing**. This means that the motion of digit flexion brought about by contraction of the FDS and FDP muscles is smooth and efficient.

The pulley system contains **five annular (A) pulleys** and **three cruciate (C) pulleys (Figure 3.31)**.

The integrity of the pulley system is of the utmost importance in **flexor tendon repair surgery**, as damage to the pulleys can lead to bowstringing and adhesion formation. This means the tendon becomes stuck, or catches on the tendon sheath, and so cannot glide properly during digit flexion.

The **A2** and **A4** pulleys are the most important pulleys to preserve to maintain a suitable fulcrum through which to flex the digits and prevent bowstringing. The A2 pulley plays an important role in flexion of the proximal phalanx, and the A4 pulley is largely responsible for flexion of the distal phalanx.

The **A1** pulley is commonly involved with trigger finger, where the tendons of the digit catch on the sheath and so the finger flexes or extends in a sharp sudden motion, as if one is pulling a trigger.

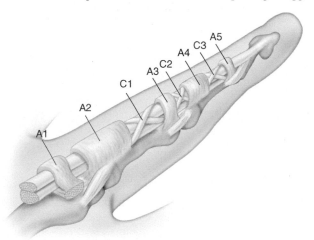

FIGURE 3.31 Pulley system of the digits, including the annular and circumferential pulleys. (Courtesy of Jordan Bethel.)

Extensors of the Wrist and Digits

The extensors of the digits form **extensor expansions (hoods)** on the **dorsal aspect** of the digits. Each expansion consists of three parts: central and two laterals.

The central is inserted into the base of the middle phalanx, second to fifth (proximal phalanx for the thumb), and the two laterals are inserted into the base of the distal phalanx.

To the corners of the extensor expansions attach the tendons of the corresponding interosseous and lumbrical muscles, allowing for complex digital movements and grips.

The extensor muscles forming the extensor hood include:

- **Extensor digitorum** (second to fifth digits)
- **Extensor pollicis longus** and **extensor pollicis brevis** (thumb)
- **Extensor digiti minimi**
- **Extensor indicis**

Intrinsic Muscles of the Hand

The intrinsic muscles of the hand can be split into the **thenar** and **hypothenar eminences, adductor pollicis, palmaris brevis, lumbricals**, and **interossei**. The eminences make up the muscle bulk on the medial and lateral sides of the palmar aspect of the hand.

Lumbricals are four "worm-like" muscles, each associated with a finger (Latin: *Lumbricus terrestris*, the common earthworm).

Each muscle originates from the tendons of the FDP and inserts onto the dorsal side of each of the medial four fingers into the extensor expansion. These act to:

- Link flexor and extensor tendons
- Flex MCP joints and extend the IP joint of the fingers (except the thumb)
- Medial two lumbricals innervated by ulnar nerve
- Lateral two lumbricals innervated by median nerve

There are four **dorsal interossei** and four **palmar interossei**. These extend between the metacarpal bones, and each has a different role.

Dorsal interossei

- Arise from the adjacent sides of the metacarpal bones and insert onto extensor expansions of the index, middle, and ring fingers and the proximal phalanges of these fingers.
- **Abduct the fingers** ("DAB"). Also have a role in flexion and extension of the fingers.

Palmar interossei

- From the first, second, fourth, and fifth metacarpals and insert into the proximal phalanges of the thumb, index, ring, and little fingers and dorsal extensor expansion of each finger (excluding the middle finger).
- **Adduct the fingers** ("PAD") towards the middle finger.

Adductor Pollicis

A fan-shaped muscle which consists of two heads (oblique and transverse). The radial artery enters the palm between its heads and continues as the deep palmar arch. It is supplied by the ulnar nerve (see discussion on Froment's test earlier). This muscle adducts and aids in flexion of the thumb.

The **palmaris brevis** arises from the flexor retinaculum and palmar aponeurosis to insert into the skin of the palm. Supplied by the superficial branch of the ulnar nerve. It helps to improve the grip of the hand.

The thenar and hypothenar eminences are both composed of three muscles, discussed next.

Thenar Eminence

Muscles of the thenar eminence arise from the carpal bones and flexor retinaculum. They are supplied by the recurrent branch of the median nerve.

- *Abductor pollicis brevis*
  - Most superficial muscle of the thenar eminence, it inserts into the base of the proximal phalanx of the thumb. It abducts the first metacarpal and the thumb.
- *Flexor pollicis brevis*
  - Has two heads, superficial and deep (the deep head may be supplied by the ulnar nerve); inserts into the base of the proximal phalanx of the thumb. It flexes the metacarpophalangeal (MCP) joint of the thumb.
- *Opponens pollicis*
  - Lies deep to abductor pollicis brevis, inserts into the first metacarpal.
  - Responsible for opposition of the thumb to touch the anterior surface of the other digits.
  - Flexes and abducts first metacarpal.

Hypothenar Eminence

All the hypothenar muscles are supplied by the ulnar nerve.

- *Abductor digiti minimi*
  - Inserts into the proximal phalanx of the little finger
  - Abducts the little finger
- *Flexor digit minimi*
  - Inserts into the proximal phalanx of the little finger
  - Flexes and adducts the little finger at the MPJ
- *Opponens digiti minimi*
  - Inserts into the fifth metacarpal
  - Deep muscle which flexes and slightly rotates the fifth metacarpal
  - Helps in cupping of the palm by pulling the fifth metacarpal forward

Palmar Aponeurosis (Palmar Fascia)

A triangular sheet of fibrous tissue. Its apex is attached to the flexor retinaculum and receives the tendon of the palmaris longus muscle. The base of the aponeurosis is divided into four slips at the bases of the fingers (except the thumb).

The palmar aponeurosis is separated from the hypothenar eminence by a fibrous septum, which is attached to the fifth metacarpal. Laterally, there is another septum which is attached to the third metacarpal and divides the palm into the **thenar** and the **midpalmar spaces**.

The thenar space is not related to the fascial compartment of the thenar muscles. It contains the first lumbrical and lies anterior to the adductor pollicis muscle. The midpalmar space is related on the dorsal aspect to the third, fourth, and fifth metacarpals. On the palmar side it is related to the long flexors and their tendon sheaths.

Note that the **radial bursa** is the sheath of the flexor pollicis longus that proximally extends into the wrist area.

The **ulnar bursa** (**Figure 3.32**) contains the common synovial sheath of the flexors of the fingers, apart from the thumb, passing through the flexor retinaculum. In the palm, it is continuous with

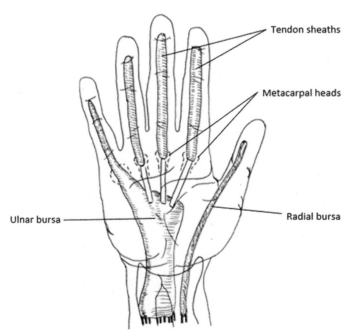

FIGURE 3.32 Ulnar bursa. (Courtesy of Alina Humdani.)

the synovial sheath of the little finger. Infection can extend to the space of Parona in the lower forearm (potential space between the tendons of the FDS and FDP and the pronator quadratus).

CLINICAL NOTES

HAND INFECTIONS

- **Felon** is pulp space infection in the tip of the finger, following needle stick injuries, for example. The distal pulp space is a confined area, and infection within this space can interrupt the blood supply to the diaphysis of the terminal phalanx, which leads to osteomyelitis, bone crumbling, and necrosis. Early treatment is imperative to avoid this serious complication.
- Distally, the thenar and midpalmar spaces are continuous into the lumbrical canals. These spaces are important, as sometimes infection can collect there and can form an abscess. Signs include severe tenderness and loss of palmar concavity.
- Inflammation of the tendon sheaths is called **tenosynovitis**.

Neurovasculature of the Hand

Arteries

- The **ulnar artery** supplies mainly the medial three and a half digits of the hand.
- The **radial artery** supplies mainly the thumb and lateral half of the index finger (*arteria princeps pollicis* and *arteria radialis indicis*, respectively).

The two arteries anastomose in the hand via the **superficial and deep palmar arches**.

Deep palmar arch: a continuation of the **radial artery** after entering the palm (see earlier). It is completed medially by the deep branch of the ulnar artery.

Superficial palmar arch: the direct continuation of the **ulnar artery**, completed laterally by a branch from the radial artery. The curve of the superficial palmar arch lies at the level of the distal border of the fully extended thumb, while the curve of the deep palmar arch lies at the level of the proximal border of the extended thumb.

The deep palmar arch is located deep to the tendons of the long finger flexors, while the superficial palmar arch is deep to the palmar aponeurosis, but anterior to the long finger flexors. Both arches give rise to the digital arteries, which pass to the fingers.

One can test clinically for a dual blood supply to the hand and an adequate radial/ulnar arterial anastomosis by using the **modified Allen's test**, which is described in the context of the clinical relevance of the radial artery (see earlier).

Nerves

Median nerve

- Innervates three thenar muscles (recurrent branch) and lateral two lumbricals (palmar digital branch).
- Innervates skin and nailbeds (palmar digital branch) on the thumb, index, and middle fingers and lateral side of ring (fourth) finger. Tactile sensation is very important to the function of the hand, so median nerve injury would be more harmful than ulnar nerve injury.

Ulnar nerve

- Divides as it leaves Guyon's canal into superficial and deep branches.
- Innervates all other intrinsic muscles of the hand, **including adductor pollicis** (*Remember:* **HILA:** H: **H**ypothenar eminence, I: **I**nterossei, L: medial two **L**umbricals, A: **A**dductor pollicis).
- The superficial branch innervates the palmaris brevis and skin on the palmar surface of the little finger and medial half of ring finger, including nailbeds.

Radial nerve

- Superficial branch innervates the skin over the dorsolateral aspect of the palm and dorsal aspect of the lateral three and a half digits proximal to the DIP joints

Arches of the Hand

There are two transverse arches and a longitudinal arch. The intrinsic hand muscles maintain the arches of the hand.

- *Proximal transverse arch*
  - The capitate carpal bone is its keystone.
  - This arch is relatively flexed and runs along the immobile distal carpal row.
- *Distal transverse arch*
  - **The head of the third metacarpal** is the keystone, and it passes through all metacarpal heads.
  - It is more mobile than the proximal transverse arch.
- *Longitudinal arch*
  - Connects the transvers arches. Central pillar consists of the **second and third metacarpals.** Thumb, third, fourth, and fifth **finger flexion** allows the palm to **flatten** or **cup.**

Functional Anatomy of the Hand

Grips

Successful grip requirements:

- Mobility of the first carpometacarpal (CMC) joint, as well as the fourth and fifth MCP joints.
- Rigidity of second and third CMC joints.
- Stability of the longitudinal and transverse arches of the hand.
- Adequate sensory input to the hand (the pulps of the fingers have a rich sensory supply, which can replace vision in the visually impaired, especially in the Braille writing system).

There are several types of grips (**Figure 3.33**):

1. *Precision grip (tip to tip):*
   - Manipulates small objects between the thumb and flexor aspect of fingers by using thumb flexion and opposition and finger flexion, like in sewing

2. *Power grip*
   - Fingers flexed at all three joints
   - Usually performed with ulnar deviation and extension of wrist, which maximise the strength of the grip
3. *Coal hammer grip*
   - Thumb wholly occupied in reinforcing the grasping action of the fully flexed digits
   - Contraction of hypothenar eminence forms a groove within which objects, such as a coal hammer, are held
4. *Dynamic tripod*
   - Involves the thumb and index finger to catch the object – a pencil, for example – and the middle finger tucks behind the object
   - One of the important skills in handwriting
   - The fourth and fifth digits are squeezed in towards the palm
   - Used for support and static control
5. *Hook grip (the thumb is not involved with this type of grip)*
   - Requires the flexion of the MPJ and IP joints
   - Used for power over a long period of time, not precision
   - Still possible even if intrinsic muscles of hand are weakened or unable to function because grip requires the use of FDS and FDP muscles

Other types of hand grips:

- *Cylindrical:* holding a glass
- *Spherical:* opening a jar
- Key grip using the flexed thumb and the middle phalanx of the index fingers

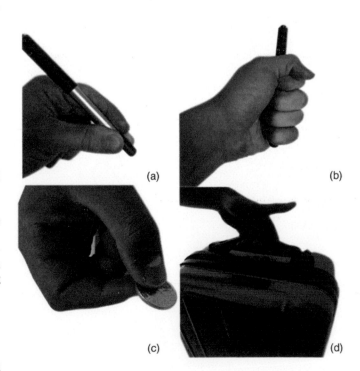

FIGURE 3.33 Photographs of types of grip. (a) Dynamic tripod, (b) coal hammer grip, (c) precision grip, (d) hook grip.

THE HAND

The hands are often used to aid in the diagnosis of systemic disorders. Some examples are given here in addition to the changes following injuries of the ulnar, median, and radial nerves (see earlier):

- Power of the grip of the hand when shaking hands with the patient
- *Warm and sweaty hand:* nervousness and thyrotoxicosis
- Tremor of the hand is an important sign in the diagnosis of Parkinson's disease, anxiety, and thyrotoxicosis (see **Section 2**)
- *Koilonychia:* spoon-shaped nails due to iron deficiency anaemia
- **Clubbing** of the fingers due to many causes, including congenital heart disease, lung cancer, bronchiectasis, right-to-left heart shunts, and endocarditis
- **Dupuytren's contracture** (fibrosis of the palmar aponeurosis), which can be associated with liver cirrhosis
- Deformities, such as the swan neck deformity of rheumatoid arthritis (**Figure 3.34**)

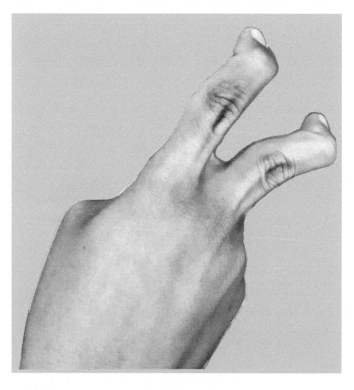

FIGURE 3.34 Swan neck deformity due to rheumatoid arthritis. (Courtesy of Sami Salman.)

The Axilla

The axilla is a region between the thorax and the upper limb, inferior to the glenohumeral joint. It is colloquially known as the armpit. The axilla is bound by several structures; the boundaries are described in **Table 3.12**.

TABLE 3.12: Boundaries of the axilla

Border	Anatomical Structure Defining the Border
Apex	Lateral border of first rib, superior border of scapula, and posterior border of clavicle
Anterior	Pectoralis major, pectoralis minor, subclavius, and clavipectoral fascia
Posterior	Subscapularis, teres major, and latissimus dorsi
Medial	Serratus anterior and thoracic wall
Lateral	Intertubercular (bicipital) sulcus of the humerus

Muscles of the Axilla

Several muscles are associated with the axilla (**Table 3.13**).

Contents of the Axilla

Several important components are found in the axilla:

1. Axillary artery
2. Axillary vein
3. Lymph nodes and axillary fat
4. Brachial plexus

The Axillary Artery

This is a continuation of the subclavian artery at the lateral border of the first rib. Alongside the brachial plexus, the axillary artery is enveloped by the axillary fascia, which is continuous with the prevertebral fascia. It is divided by the pectoralis minor into three anatomical parts:

- *First part:* one branch. Medial to the medial border of the pectoralis minor, gives rise to the superior (highest) thoracic artery.
- *Second part:* two branches. Behind the pectoralis minor, gives rise to the thoracoacromial and lateral thoracic arteries. The thoracoacromial artery divides into four branches: pectoral, clavicular, acromial, and deltoid. Each of these branches supplies the area corresponding to their name. The lateral thoracic artery follows the lateral margin of the pectoralis minor muscle.
- *Third part:* three branches. Continues as the brachial artery at the lower border of the teres major. Prior to this it gives rise to the subscapular artery, posterior circumflex, and anterior circumflex humeral arteries. The circumflex arteries are important for the anastomosis around the upper humerus.

The Axillary Vein

This is formed at the lower border of the teres major, the same location where the axillary artery ends, from the union of the venae comitantes of the brachial artery, in addition to the basilic vein. The cephalic vein joins the axillary vein after passing through the deltopectoral groove (between the deltoid and pectoralis major) towards the axilla.

The axillary vein continues as the subclavian vein at the outer border of first rib. It forms an important surgical landmark while removing axillary lymph nodes, i.e., during axillary node dissection.

TABLE 3.13: Muscles of the axilla

Muscle	Origin	Insertion	Innervation	Action
Pectoralis major A large, fan-shaped (convergent) muscle situated deep to the breast	• Sternoclavicular head (medial half of clavicle and lateral aspect of sternum) • Costal head (upper six costal cartilages)	Lateral lip of the bicipital groove of humerus (broad insertion)	Medial pectoral (C8–T1) and lateral pectoral (C5–C7) nerves	• Adduction + medial rotation of arm at glenohumeral joint • Accessory muscle of respiration with arm fixed
Pectoralis minor* A small, fan-shaped muscle deep to the pectoralis major	Third to fifth ribs	Coracoid process of scapula	Medial pectoral nerve	• Depresses scapula • Aids in raising third, fourth, and fifth ribs, with scapula fixed
Serratus anterior Slips of muscle situated laterally over the ribs, spanning posteriorly	• Upper eight ribs • Interdigitates with origin of external oblique muscle	Medial border of scapula	Long thoracic nerve (C5–C7)	• Upward rotation of scapula, enabling elevation of the arm • Protraction (as in throwing a punch) and stabilisation of scapula
Latissimus dorsi The broadest muscle of the back**	• Pelvis – iliac crest • Thoracolumbar fascia • Spinous processes of seventh thoracic to fifth lumbar vertebrae	Floor of bicipital groove of humerus	Thoracodorsal nerve From the posterior cord of brachial plexus, C6–C8	Extend arm Adduct arm

*   Regarded as the key muscle of the axilla. Lies anterior to the axillary artery and vein.

** To help you remember the insertion site of the latissimus dorsi, you can use the mnemonic "lady between the two majors" (tendons of teres major and pectoralis major).

Axillary Lymph Nodes

These receive lymph from the upper limb, the breast, and the walls of the thorax and upper abdomen, from the level of the umbilicus.

From the surgical point of view, the axillary lymph nodes are divided into three levels by the pectoralis minor muscle (**Table 3.14** and **Figure 3.35**). The bulk of lymph nodes are located within level 1. Classical clinical teaching defines these as the anterior (pectoral), posterior (subscapular), lateral (humeral), central, and apical lymph nodes (see **Section 4**).

TABLE 3.14: Surgical classification of the levels of axillary lymph nodes

Level	Location of Nodes at Each Level
Level I	Nodes are inferior and lateral to the pectoralis minor
Level II	Nodes are below the axillary vein and behind the pectoralis minor
Level III	Nodes are medial to the muscle against the chest wall towards the root of the neck

Brachial Plexus

This is described in detail in the anatomy of the nerves of the upper limb (see earlier). This structure passes through the axilla and is closely related to the axillary artery (**Figure 3.36**).

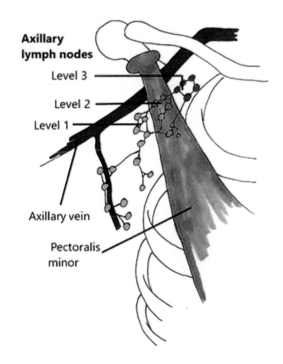

FIGURE 3.35 Levels of axillary lymph nodes in relation to the pectoralis minor muscle. (Courtesy of Calum Harrington-Vogt.)

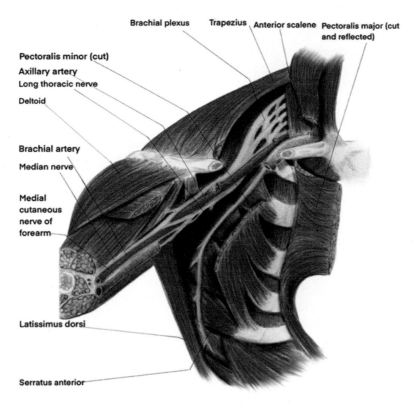

Brachial plexus   Trapezius   Anterior scalene   Pectoralis major (cut and reflected)

Pectoralis minor (cut)
Axillary artery
Long thoracic nerve
Deltoid

Brachial artery
Median nerve

Medial cutaneous nerve of forearm

Latissimus dorsi

Serratus anterior

FIGURE 3.36   The brachial plexus coursing through the axilla and its related structures. (Courtesy of Kathryn DeMarre.)

CLINICAL NOTES

AXILLA

The axilla is of surgical importance and is used as an access point during several procedures (**Table 3.15**).

Further to this, the axilla is also used as a location of reference for several procedures:

- Subpectoral space is the space deep to the pectoralis major is now commonly used to insert synthetic prostheses to augment the breast.
- Latissimus dorsi flap (LD flap) reconstruction is one of the options offered to women following mastectomy. The muscle can be mobilised and positioned on the anterior chest wall without interference to either nerve or blood supply, which come from the axilla.
- Poland syndrome is the congenital unilateral absence or underdevelopment of the muscles of the chest, shoulder, arm, or hand. Typically, individuals with Poland syndrome lack a pectoralis major, resulting in a concave appearance of the chest.
- The long thoracic nerve has the nerve roots C5–C7. Injury to this nerve, which may occur during axillary node clearance for metastatic breast cancer, can result in a winged scapula (**Figure 3.37**). This is the reason why this nerve, and the thoracodorsal nerve (which supplies the latissimus dorsi), should be identified and safeguarded during surgery.

TABLE 3.15: Surgical importance of the axilla

Procedure	Description
Sentinel node biopsy (SNB)	• This is a relatively new modality in treating conditions such as breast cancer and melanoma • It is based on the theory of the first lymph node to where the cancer spreads (see **Section 4**)
Axillary node dissection	• Removal of lymph nodes in levels I and II • The main long-term complication is the development of lymphoedema of the upper limb due to interruption of lymphatic drainage
Excisional biopsy of a suspicious axillary lymph node	• This may be used to prove the diagnosis of malignant conditions like lymphoma

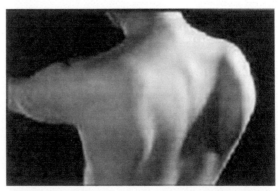

FIGURE 3.37   Image of a patient with a winged right scapula due to injury to the long thoracic nerve. The serratus anterior muscle, which receives its nerve supply from the long thoracic nerve, is clinically examined by asking the patient to push up against a wall. (Courtesy of the Department of Anatomical Sciences, SGUL.)

Revision Questions

Q1.

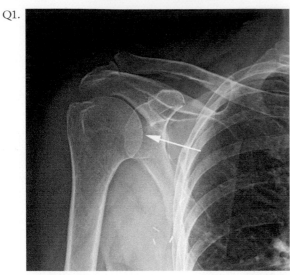

(Courtesy of Department of Anatomical Sciences, SGUL.)

Q1A. Which of the following best describes the type of joint indicated by the arrow?
   a. Ball and socket
   b. Hinge
   c. Plane
   d. Saddle
   e. Symphysis

Q1B. Which of the following nerves is commonly damaged when this joint is dislocated?
   a. Axillary
   b. Musculocutaneous
   c. Radial
   d. Subscapular
   e. Ulnar

Q2.

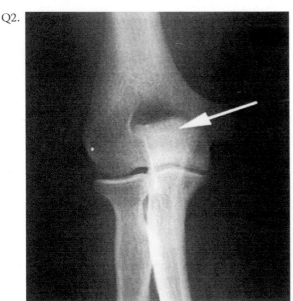

(Courtesy of Department of Anatomical Sciences, SGUL.)

Q2A. What is the name of the structure indicated by the arrow?
Q2B. Which important muscle is inserted at this structure, and what is its nerve supply?

Q3.

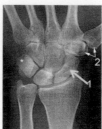

(Courtesy of Department of Anatomical Sciences, SGUL.)

Q3A. What is the structure indicated by arrow 1?
Q3B. What is the main clinical condition that can affect this structure?
Q4A. Identify the bones indicated by arrow 2.
Q4B. What type of joint do they form?
Q5. Identify the bone indicated by the asterisk.
Q4A. What type of bone is it?
Q5B. Which tendon attaches here?
Q6. What are the most common upper limb injuries following a fall onto an outstretched hand (FOOSH)?
Q7. What are the terminal branches of the brachial plexus?
Q8. What are the causes for a missed diagnosis of scaphoid fracture?
Q9. What are the muscles involved in a precision hand grip?

Answers

A1A. a
A1B. a
A2. (A) Olecranon, (B) Triceps muscle supplied by the radial nerve
A3. (A) Scaphoid, (B) Fracture scaphoid
A4. (A) Trapezium, (B) First metacarpal; synovial saddle-joint (first carpometacarpal joint)
A5. (A) Pisiform, (B) Sesamoid bone, flexor carpi ulnaris
A6. Fractured clavicle, anterior shoulder dislocation, supracondylar fracture of the humerus, fracture of the head of the radius, Colles' and Smith's fracture, Galeazzi's and Monteggia's fracture dislocation.
A7. Median, ulnar, radial, axillary, and musculocutaneous nerves.
A8. Ignoring the tenderness in the snuff box, an early X-ray may not show the fracture (if in doubt, recheck the patient in the fracture clinic).
A9. Flexors of the thumb and fingers, opponens pollicis.

Further Reading

Bumbasirevic M, et al. Radial nerve palsy. EFORT Open Rev (2016) 1(8):286–294.

Fender F. Foerster's scheme of the dermatomes. Arch Neurol Psychiatry (1939) 41:688–693.

Foerster O. The dermatomes in man. Brain (1933) 56:1–39.

Fuhrman TM, et al. Evaluation of collateral circulation of the hand. J Clin Monitor (1992) 8(1):28–32.

Ioannis D et al. Palmaris longus muscle's prevalence in different nations and interesting anatomical variations: review of the literature. J Clin Med Res (2015) 7(11):825–830.

Lu X, et al. Epidemiologic features and management of elbow dislocation with associated fracture in pediatric population. Medicine (Baltimore) (2017) 96(48):e8595.

Maroukis BL, et al. Guyon canal: the evolution of clinical anatomy. J Hand Surg Am (2015) 40(3):560–565.

Mousa AY, et al. Radiocephalic fistula: review and update. Ann Vasc Surg (2013) 27(3):370–378.

Rehim SA, et al. Monteggia fracture dislocations: a historical review. J Hand Surg Am (2014) 39(7):1384–1394.

Staples JR, Calfee R. Cubital tunnel syndrome: current concepts. J Am Acad Orthop Surg (2017) 25(10):e215–e224.

4

ANATOMY OF THE THORAX

Reviewed by Qassim F. Baker and Mohammed Al Janabi

Learning Objectives

- The thoracic wall and the diaphragm and their clinical applications
- The thoracic cavity and the mediastinum
- The lungs and the pleura
- The heart and the great vessels
- The anatomy of the breast and its clinical notes

Introduction

The thorax is defined as the region between the neck and the abdomen, which includes the cavity enclosed by the ribs, sternum, and thoracic vertebrae. It is normally described as an irregularly shaped cylinder with a relatively small opening at the top (**superior thoracic aperture**) compared to a larger opening at the base (**inferior thoracic aperture**).

Note that the superior thoracic aperture may also be referred to as the thoracic inlet in other texts. Confusion often arises with regard to thoracic outlet syndrome, where the superior thoracic aperture is referred to as the thoracic outlet. Thoracic outlet syndrome refers to compression of the subclavian artery and lower trunk of the brachial plexus.

The constituents of the thorax can be separated into the thoracic wall and three cavities.

Thoracic Wall

The main components of the thoracic wall are the musculoskeletal elements:

- Anteriorly, the wall comprises the sternum and costal cartilages. The sternum is made up of the manubrium, sternal body, and xiphisternum (also known as the xiphoid process). The pectoralis major and minor muscles form an important part of the anterior chest wall.
- Laterally, the 12 ribs on either side make up the wall along with the three-layered intercostal muscles, which enclose the intercostal spaces formed between neighbouring ribs. The serratus anterior is an important muscle on the lateral aspect of the chest wall (medial wall of the axilla).
- Posteriorly, the bony structure is composed of the 12 thoracic vertebrae and the intervertebral discs that hold them together, in addition to the scapulae. Important muscles of the back include the erector spinae, latissimus dorsi, and trapezius.

The superior thoracic aperture is bounded as follows:

- *Anteriorly:* by the suprasternal notch
- *Laterally:* by the first ribs and their costal cartilages
- *Posteriorly:* by the body of the first thoracic vertebra

The suprapleural membrane, which is a dense fascia originating from the endothoracic fascia, closes the thoracic outlet on each side of the structures passing through the aperture, including the trachea, oesophagus, and great vessels, and attaches laterally to the inner border of the first ribs and their costal cartilages. The cervical pleura underlies the suprapleural membrane.

The inferior thoracic aperture is bounded by the T12 vertebra posteriorly, xiphisternal joint anteriorly, and costal margin on both sides laterally. This aperture is closed by the diaphragm.

Functions of the Thoracic Wall

The thoracic wall has **two main functions**: to enable the lungs to expand and hence facilitate breathing, in which the actions of the ribs and the sternum are likened to the bucket handle and pump handle movements (**Figure 4.1**), and to provide protection to the internal cavities which house the heart, lungs, and other important internal organs such as the upper abdominal organs.

Thoracic Skeleton and Joints

The skeleton in the thorax comprises the sternum, ribs, costal cartilages, and thoracic vertebrae (T1–T12). The scapulae lie posteriorly and are attached by muscles to the thoracic cage. The clavicles articulate with the manubrium sterni at the sternoclavicular joint, which is a synovial joint.

Joints of the Thoracic Wall

The skeletal system of the chest wall involves many joints to hold the bones together. The main joints are summarised here:

- *Interchondral:* synovial joints formed between the costal cartilages of the ribs (e.g., fusion of eighth costal cartilage with the seventh).
- *Sternocostal:* synovial joints between the costal cartilage and sternum (except for the first rib, where it is a primary cartilaginous joint.)

Sternum

The sternum is a combination of three bones which are held together by two joints: the **manubriosternal** (between the manubrium and sternal body) and **xiphisternal** (between the sternal body and xiphoid process) (**Figure 4.2**). Both these joints are symphysis joints, which is a type of cartilaginous joint that allows for some minimal movement. The first costal cartilage is connected to the sternum by a primary cartilaginous joint (to fix the first rib on inspiration), while second to the seventh costal cartilages are connected to the sternum by synovial joints. The suprasternal or jugular notch is a depression on the upper part of the manubrium. The trachea is felt in the centre of this notch. It lies opposite the lower border of T2.

DOI: 10.1201/9781003312895-5

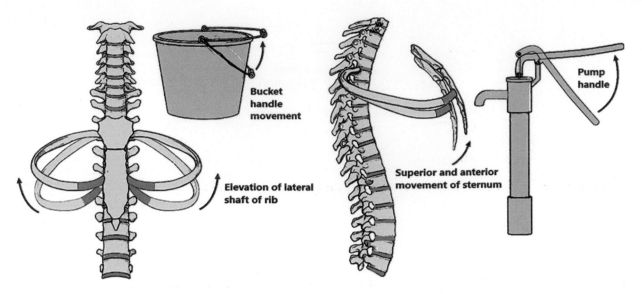

FIGURE 4.1 The bucket handle and pump handle movement represents the actions of the ribs and sternum during inspiration. (Courtesy of Kathryn DeMarre.)

The manubriosternal joint is at an angle (also referred to as the **angle of Louis** or **sternal angle**), which is felt as a transverse ridge on the anterior aspect, where the second costal cartilage articulates. This junction forms an important landmark which is used in identifying the ribs and intercostal spaces during physical examinations of the chest and electrocardiogram (ECG) lead placement, as the first rib is not clinically palpable. The angle of Louis lies opposite the intervertebral disc between T4 and T5.

The xiphisternal joint lies at the level of the body of the T9 vertebra. The xiphoid process can become calcified or ossified in adult life and be mistaken for a hard lump in the epigastric region, and even referred to surgical clinics on that assumption.

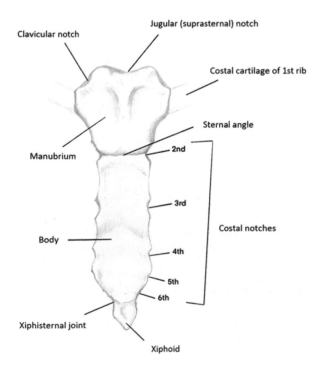

FIGURE 4.2 Bony anatomy of the sternum. (Courtesy of Kathryn DeMarre.)

Ribs

There are **12 pairs** of ribs in the thorax, each associated with their corresponding vertebrae. The ribs are subdivided according to their attachments to the sternum (**Figure 4.3**):

- *True ribs (ribs 1 to 7):* the costal cartilages of these ribs are directly connected to the sternum individually via the synovial sternocostal joints. The joint formed between the ribs and costal cartilage is known as the costochondral joint. The costochondral joints (and the joint between the first costal cartilage and the sternum) are primary cartilaginous joints, or synchondroses. Synchondrosis joints are immovable, so the manubrium of the sternum and the two first ribs move up and down as a unit.
- *False ribs (ribs 8 to 10):* the costal cartilages of each rib do **NOT** attach directly to the sternum, but rather to the **costal margin**. The cartilage fuses with the cartilage of the next higher rib. Hence, the costal cartilage of rib 8 fuses with the cartilage of rib 7 and so on down to rib 10.
- *Floating ribs (ribs 11 and 12):* these ribs are free and do not attach anteriorly to anything, as their costal cartilages end within the muscles of the abdominal wall.

Most of the ribs have the same basic anatomy, with a few exceptions.

The posterior end of a typical rib is called the **head of the rib**. The head has two facets to articulate with the costal demifacets of the respective thoracic vertebra and the vertebra immediately above it. The tubercle of the rib articulates with the facet on the transverse process of the vertebrae. The **neck of the rib** is a small narrowing between the head and the **body**. The tubercle is a protuberance on the outer aspect at the junction between the neck and the body. The neck follows on to join the body of the rib (shaft). The body of the rib is curved, with a groove on the inferior interior aspect (the **costal groove**) in which the neurovascular bundle of veins, arteries, and nerves runs to supply the chest wall.

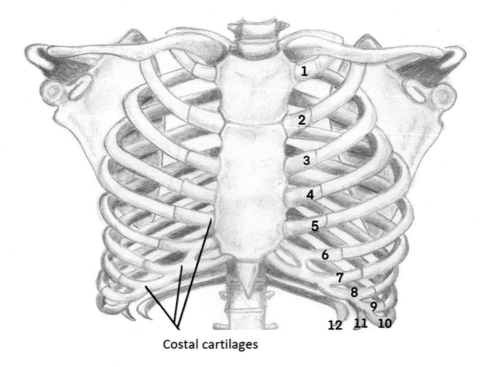

Costal cartilages

FIGURE 4.3 Skeletal anatomy of the thorax. (Courtesy of Kathryn DeMarre.)

The **angle** is where the shaft bends sharply forward and is the most common site for rib fractures (**Figure 4.4**).

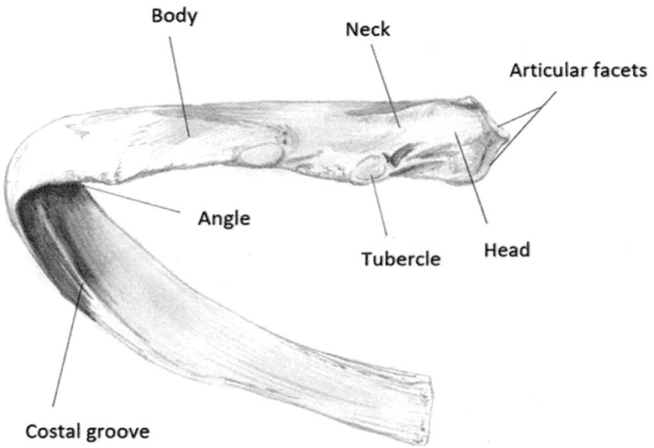

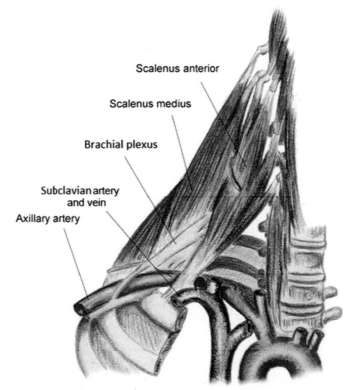

FIGURE 4.4 True rib anatomy. (Courtesy of Kathryn DeMarre.)

The exceptions are the "atypical" ribs 1, 11, and 12.

The first rib is the strongest, shortest, broadest, and flattest of the 12 ribs. It has no costal groove and is the only rib to have a protuberance on the superior surface, the scalene tubercle, where the scalenus anterior muscle is attached. Anterior to the tubercle, the subclavian vein crosses over the rib and passes through the superior thoracic aperture.

Posterior to the tubercle, the subclavian artery and lower trunk of the brachial plexus run in between the scalenus anterior and scalenus medius. The superior surface is marked by grooves for the subclavian vein and artery. This rib is rarely fractured due to its protected position below the clavicle. In this position, the rib cannot be palpated, and hence it shows how well the subclavian vessels and brachial plexus are protected by the first rib and the clavicle (**Figure 4.5**).

FIGURE 4.5 Relationship of subclavian vessels and brachial plexus with scalene muscles on the clavicle. (Courtesy of Kathryn DeMarre.)

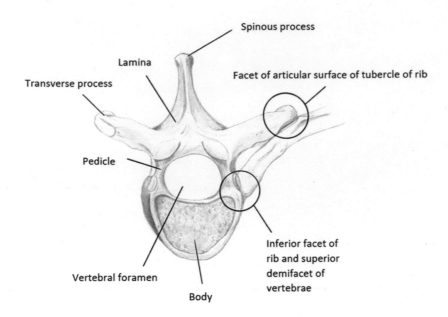

FIGURE 4.6   Thoracic vertebra and articulation of a rib with both the body (**costovertebral**) and transverse process (**costotransverse**) of the vertebra. (Courtesy of Kathryn DeMarre.)

The **1st, 11th, and 12th ribs are considered atypical** as they have only one facet on their head for articulation to the corresponding vertebra. The 11th and 12th ribs have no neck or tubercles, and the 12th rib has no costal groove.

Thoracic Vertebrae

There are 12 thoracic vertebrae.
   How to recognise thoracic vertebrae:

- The vertebral body of thoracic vertebrae is heart shaped.
- Thoracic vertebrae are easily identified by their spinous processes, which project inferiorly.

Thoracic vertebrae also have **costal demifacets** on the vertebral bodies and transverse processes which **articulate with the head and tubercle of the rib, respectively** (**Figure 4.6**). There is very little movement of the vertebral column in the thoracic region due to the presence of the sternum and ribs. It is the most stable region of the column.

Musculature of the Thoracic Wall

The muscles play an important role in the thoracic wall's main functions. They may assist during breathing and allow the thorax to be more mobile. The most important set of muscles on the chest wall are the intercostal muscles. These muscles are involved in ventilation by changing the position of the ribs (**Table 4.1**).

There are also **accessory muscles of respiration** which aid in forced respiration during exercise. These include the sternocleidomastoid, pectoralis major, and scalene muscles (anterior, middle, and posterior).

TABLE 4.1: Intercostal muscles

Muscle	Origin (O) and Insertion (I)	Action	Innervation	Blood Supply	Additional Notes
External intercostal	O: inferior border of the rib above I: superior border of the rib below	Elevate and protract the ribs on forceful inhalation	Intercostal nerves	Intercostal and internal thoracic vessels	Most superficial muscle of the three The muscle fibres run **inferoanteriorly** (downwards and forwards) Anteriorly, they continue as the **anterior intercostal membrane**
Internal intercostal	O: inferior border of rib above I: superior border of ribs below	Depress and retract the ribs on forceful exhalation	Intercostal nerves	Intercostal and internal thoracic vessels	In between external and innermost Muscle fibres are in the **inferoposterior** orientation (downwards and backwards) Posterior to the angles of the ribs, they are continuous with the **posterior intercostal membrane**
Innermost intercostal	O: inferior border of rib above I: superior border of ribs below (Same as internal)	Depress the ribs on forceful exhalation	Intercostal nerves	Intercostal and internal thoracic vessels	Deepest muscle of the three Muscle fibres are in the **inferolateral** orientation (downwards and towards the sides) **The neurovascular bundle runs in between the internal and innermost muscle layers**

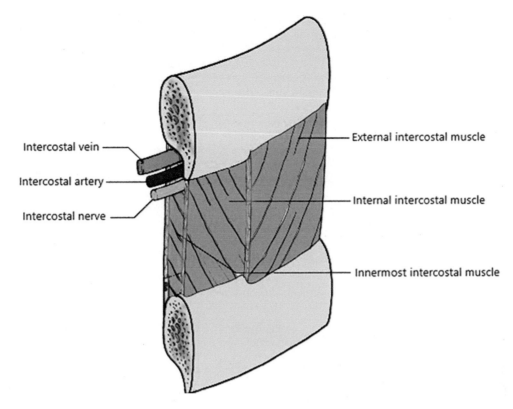

FIGURE 4.7 Intercostal muscles and intercostal neurovascular bundle. (Courtesy of Vamsi Thammandra.)

The **endothoracic fascia** separates the ribs and intercostal muscles from the parietal pleura. Superiorly, the fascia is continuous as the thicker **suprapleural membrane**, which covers the lung apex covered by the cervical pleura.

Vasculature and Innervation of the Thoracic Wall

The thoracic wall has a rich vasculature and receives blood from several sources. There is a lot of variation from person to person, but understanding the common anatomy is imperative to appreciate any differences.

The arteries and veins of the thoracic wall (i.e., the intercostal spaces) are segmental, as different regions are supplied by different sources. Arterial supply to the intercostal spaces is divided into the **posterior** and **anterior intercostal arteries.**

There are **11 posterior intercostal arteries** in which:

- The **upper two** arise from the superior intercostal branch of the **costocervical trunk of the subclavian artery.**
- The **lower nine** arise from the **descending thoracic aorta.**

There are **nine anterior intercostal arteries** of which:

- The **upper six** arise from the **internal thoracic artery** (branch of first part of the subclavian artery,) which descends vertically about one fingerbreadth from the lateral margin of the sternum. The internal thoracic artery divides into the superior epigastric (see **Section 5**, Abdomen) and musculophrenic artery, which also supplies the diaphragm.
- The **lower three** arise from the **musculophrenic artery.**

The venous drainage is also split into anterior and posterior intercostal veins:

- There are 9 anterior intercostal veins, which follow the same path as the anterior intercostal arteries and **drain into the internal thoracic veins**, which ultimately join the **brachiocephalic veins.**
- The 11 posterior intercostal veins utilise the azygos and hemiazygos venous system (**Figure 4.8**).

Due to this, there is some variation between the venous drainage of the right and left side of the thorax (**Table 4.2**).

TABLE 4.2: Venous drainage of the posterior intercostal veins

Posterior Intercostal Veins	Right Side	Left Side
First	Right brachiocephalic vein	Left brachiocephalic vein
Second and third	Join to form right superior intercostal vein, which drains into the azygos vein	Join to form left superior intercostal vein and drains into left brachiocephalic vein
Fourth to eighth	Azygos vein	Accessory hemiazygos vein
Ninth to eleventh	Azygos vein	Hemiazygos vein

The **azygos vein** is formed by the union of the right ascending lumbar vein and the right subcostal vein and enters the thorax through the aortic hiatus. It receives the lower eight right posterior intercostal veins and the right bronchial vein.

The **accessory hemiazygos vein** is formed from the union of the left fourth to eighth posterior intercostal veins. The left bronchial vein drains into it.

The **hemiazygos vein** is the continuation of the left ascending lumbar vein and passes upwards under the left crus of the diaphragm. It receives the 9th to 11th posterior intercostal veins in addition to the left subcostal vein.

Note that the accessory hemiazygos and hemiazygos drain into the azygos vein at the levels of T8 and T9, respectively. The azygos then arches forward over the right main bronchus to drain into the superior vena cava (creating an impression on the right lung). An interesting variation is the azygos lobe, which is when the azygos vein loops around the right lung, creating a small lobe, rather than a groove. The azygos system may also act as a continuation of the inferior vena cava, as it directly drains into the superior vena cava, bypassing the inferior aspect. This does lead to a dilated azygos, but in most cases, it is asymptomatic.

Note: Azygos is from *zyg*, "paired" in Latin, and *a* meaning "not".

branch continues as the first intercostal nerve, within the first intercostal space, and continues anteriorly as the first cutaneous branch.

A branch of the second intercostal nerve joins the medial cutaneous nerve of the arm to form the intercostobrachial nerve that supplies the skin of the axilla and medial side of the upper arm. This nerve may be sacrificed during axillary node clearance for treatment of metastatic cancer in the axillary lymph nodes, commonly from breast cancer. Therefore, patients should be well informed of the possibility of loss of skin sensation after surgery.

The anterior rami from **nerves T7–T11** also supply the anterior abdominal wall and supply the skin, muscles, and parietal peritoneum (remember T10 supplies the skin at the level of the umbilicus). T12 is the subcostal nerve (runs below the 12th rib).

The intercostal nerves give rise to the lateral and anterior cutaneous branches.

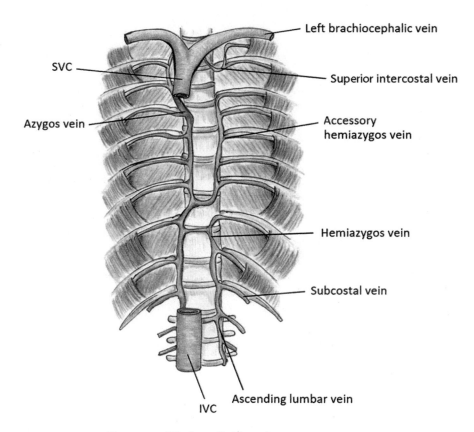

FIGURE 4.8 Azygos venous system. (Courtesy of Kathryn DeMarre.)

Innervation of the Chest Wall

Each spinal nerve emerges from an intervertebral foramen and divides into anterior (ventral) and posterior (dorsal) rami. The intercostal nerves, which run in the most inferior position in the neurovascular bundle, are the anterior rami of the spinal nerves in the thoracic region from T1 to T11. The **upper six intercostal nerves** run in the intercostal spaces to supply the chest wall (skin, intercostal muscles, periosteum of the ribs, and parietal pleura).

The first thoracic nerve contributes a large branch to the brachial plexus (see **Section 3**, Upper Limb). Another small

The **posterior rami** supply the skin, muscles, and bony structures of the midback.

Lymphatic Drainage of the Chest Wall

Lymphatic drainage of the skin of the anterior and posterior chest wall is to the anterior and posterior axillary nodes, respectively. The lymphatic drainage of the intercostal spaces is anteriorly to the internal thoracic nodes and posteriorly to the posterior intercostal nodes and then to the para-aortic lymph nodes in the posterior mediastinum.

CLINICAL NOTES

THORACIC WALL

Auscultation is an important skill that will need to be learnt for any clinical examination. Using a stethoscope, there are points on the chest wall that can be used to listen to every valve of the heart opening and closing (first and second heart sounds in addition to murmurs) and breath sounds (inspiratory and expiratory and abnormal sounds like rhonchi and crepitations).

Another commonly practised test is an **electrocardiogram** (ECG), which requires six chest leads placed at specific areas that can be identified using bony landmarks on the chest wall.

The costal cartilages allow the thoracic wall to be durable and resilient to trauma that could damage the chest wall. For example, during cardiopulmonary resuscitation (CPR), the ability to press down on the chest without breaking the ribs is due to the presence of the sturdy but flexible costal cartilages. However, in the elderly, the cartilages lose their elasticity and become brittle, making them more prone to fractures. The costal cartilages may calcify and become radio-opaque.

Another clinical condition associated with the cartilage is **costochondritis** (also known as **Tietze's syndrome**) which is inflammation of the costal cartilage and presents as localised pain at the site of inflammation. This can lead to confusion, as women presenting with localised chest pain may be erroneously referred to a breast clinic (although breast cancer is usually painless, *vide infra*) or to the cardiology clinic for suspicion of anginal chest pain.

Pectus excavatum is a congenital deformity in which the sternum and the ribs abnormally grow inward, forming a depression of the sternum. In severe cases it can cause cardiopulmonary symptoms.

Pectus carinatum (pigeon chest) is a less common deformity than excavatum, and it is the opposite, where the anterior chest wall protrudes forward, and is more of a cosmetic rather than a clinical problem. However, it could be part of another genetic problem such as Marfan's syndrome.

CERVICAL RIB

This is an extra rib which arises from the transverse process of the seventh cervical vertebra. Cervical ribs occur in approximately 0.5% of the population and are more common in females. The rib is normally asymptomatic, but can cause **thoracic outlet syndrome**, as the rib can compress the subclavian vessels and lower trunk of the brachial plexus. This can present clinically as pain and numbness on the medial (ulnar) aspect of the forearm and hand and sometimes even wasting of the small muscles of the hand (T1 spinal segment distribution). The compression of the subclavian artery can result in arm ischaemia.

RIB FRACTURES

One of the most common forms of injuries that ribs encounter are fractures. These are mostly following blunt chest trauma. Although rib fractures alone are rarely serious, it may be an external marker for severe internal injury inside the chest and upper abdomen. As the 7th to 10th ribs are the

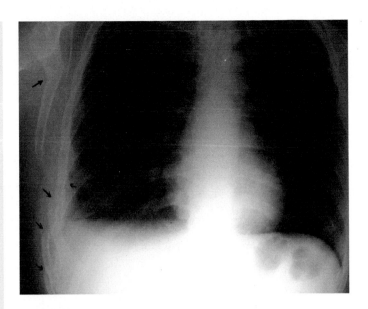

FIGURE 4.9 Chest X-ray showing fractures of right-sided ribs and scapula. (Courtesy of Abdel-Aziz Abdel-Ghany.)

most commonly fractured, the lungs are prone to problems such as a bruised lung (pulmonary contusion) or collapsed lung (due to pneumothorax with or without the accumulation of blood in the pleural cavity, a haemothorax) that may need the insertion of a chest drain (**Figure 4.9**).

If the lower ribs are fractured, abdominal organs, such as the liver or the spleen, may also sustain damage. A ruptured spleen or liver is a medical emergency and can be lethal if not detected early, due to their rich blood supply and hence rapid blood loss. Along with the other organs, the diaphragm may also be ruptured. Since the pressure is higher in the abdominal cavity than in the chest cavity, rupture of the diaphragm is almost always associated with herniation of abdominal organs into the chest cavity, which is called a **traumatic diaphragmatic hernia**. This herniation can interfere with breathing, and the blood supply to the organs that herniate through the diaphragm can be cut off, damaging them. This rupture may be undiagnosed for many months and present with problems, such as bowel obstruction, in the future (**Figures 4.10** and **4.11**).

(Continued)

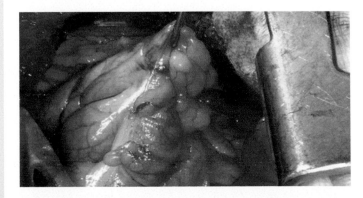

FIGURE 4.10 Herniation of the colon into the left chest due to ruptured left dome of the diaphragm. (Courtesy of Waleed M. Hussen.)

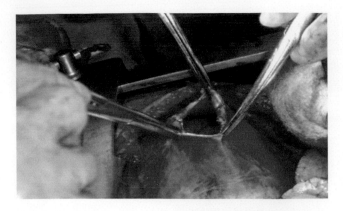

FIGURE 4.11 Thoracic view of tear of the left dome of the diaphragm. (Courtesy of Waleed M. Hussen.)

A **flail chest** can occur if several adjacent ribs (at least three) fracture in more than one place and the chest wall separates. This makes ventilating very painful, and the patient is breathless due to paradoxical respiration (area of injury "sinks in" with inspiration and expands with expiration (opposite of normal chest wall mechanics).

A **thoracotomy** is a surgical procedure that can be used to gain access to the thoracic cavity to deal with problems like excision of lung cancer or to stop severe bleeding inside the thoracic cavity. This procedure involves making an incision in between the ribs, usually at the fourth or fifth intercostal space on the lateral aspect close to the upper border of the rib (to avoid the neurovascular bundle), and incising the pleura to get access to the thoracic cavity. This procedure is sometimes combined with exploration of the abdomen (laparotomy) to deal with severe liver trauma or for the management of cancers, e.g., excision of oesophageal cancer (the Ivor-Lewis procedure).

Intercostal nerve block provides local anaesthetic infiltration to numb the intercostal nerves in the subcostal groove before the origin of the lateral cutaneous nerve at the midaxillary line. This procedure is usually performed by the anaesthetist to alleviate pain from, for example, fractured ribs. The main complication is puncture of the pleura leading to a pneumothorax.

The **sternum** is used for many examinations and procedures. Examples include:

- **Bone marrow biopsy** is sometimes taken from the sternum to diagnose haematological disorders (due to abundance of red bone marrow); the other alternative is the iliac crest (see **Section 6**, Pelvis and Pericardium).
- **Fracture of the sternum** is rare and needs a high-impact force such as high-speed vehicle accidents. The underlying heart enclosed by the pericardium is at risk of injury, which can be fatal (see below, cardiac tamponade).
- In heart surgery, a **sternotomy** is commonly used to gain access. This involves cutting the sternum in half vertically with a bone saw. Procedures such as coronary artery bypass graft (CABG) and heart valve surgery are common examples for using this approach. At the end of surgery, the sternum is joined back together using metal wires.

Thoracic Spine

The vertebral bodies increase in size from T1 to 12 due to increased weight from above. Wedge vertebral fracture is most common at T12, due to the abrupt transition of thoracic to lumbar characteristics. In general, the vertebral column is the third most common site for metastasis (following the lung and liver) due to its abundant blood supply. Cancers which most frequently metastasise here are breast, lung, and prostate. Osteoporosis, cancer, and infections (e.g., tuberculosis) cause weakening in the vertebrae, which can result in vertebral compression fractures.

T4 is an important level in the thorax. It is the level of the sternal angle, which divides the mediastinum into superior and inferior parts (vide infra).

Scoliosis is a condition resulting in a lateral S-shaped curvature of the spine.

Kyphosis (from the Greek, "hump") is excessive convex curvature of the spine.

Kyphoscoliosis is a combination of both conditions.

Lordosis is excessive inward curvature of the spine, usually in the cervical and the lumbar parts of the spine.

Adolescent idiopathic scoliosis (AIS) is the most common type of scoliosis. It affects children (more commonly girls) in early adolescence. The aetiology is not fully understood. Severe cases may require surgery (**Figure 4.12a**).

Muscles of the Back

There are superficial, intermediate, and deep muscles of the back (**Figure 4.12b**). **Table 4.3** summarises some of the important muscles of the back.

CLINICAL NOTE

Latissimus dorsi (LD) can be used as a flap during breast reconstructive surgery. Injury to the rhomboid major can result in winging of the scapula; another cause is damage to the long thoracic nerve, paralysing the serratus anterior.

The Diaphragm

The **diaphragm is the major muscle of respiration** and consists of peripheral muscular parts and a central tendinous part at the level of the xiphisternal joint (T9). The diaphragm contracts upon inspiration to move down and create a larger surface area and lower pressure in the thorax. The diaphragm has two domes, or cupolae (right and left), which can reach the fifth rib (**Figure 4.13**).

Embryology

The diaphragm develops from the septum transversum at the level of C2 (mesodermal origin) and takes its origin from the

TABLE 4.3: Muscles of the back

Name	Attachments	Innervation	Actions
Trapezius	*Origin:* nuchal ligament and cervical spinous processes *Insertion:* external occipital protuberance, clavicle, acromion, spine of scapula	Accessory nerve –motor C3–C4 fibres for proprioception	Rotation, retraction, elevation, and depression of the scapula
Latissimus dorsi	*Origin:* T6–12 spinous processes, thoracolumbar fascia, iliac crest, inferior four ribs, inferior angle of scapula *Insertion:* bicipital groove of humerus	Thoracodorsal nerve	Adduction, extension, and internal rotation of the arm
Rhomboid major	*Origin:* T2–T5 spinous processes *Insertion:* medial border of scapula	Dorsal scapular nerve	Retracts and rotates the scapula to depress it
Rhomboid minor	*Origin:* C7–T1 spinous processes *Insertion:* medial border of scapula	Dorsal scapular nerve	Retracts and rotates the scapula
Spinalis*	*Origin:* spinous processes of lumbar vertebrae *Insertion:* spinous processes of thoracic and cervical vertebrae	Dorsal ramus of spinal nerve	Laterally flexes head and neck Bilaterally extends vertebral column
Longissimus*	*Origin:* transverse processes of lumbar vertebrae *Insertion:* transverse processes of cervical and thoracic vertebrae	Dorsal ramus of spinal nerve	Laterally flexes head and neck Bilaterally extends vertebral column
Iliocostalis*	*Origin:* sacrum, spinous processes of lumbar vertebrae, iliac crest *Insertion:* ribs	Dorsal ramus of spinal nerve	Laterally flexes vertebral column Bilaterally extends vertebral column
Psoas major	*Origin:* T12–L5 transverse processes *Insertion:* lesser trochanter of femur	L1–L3 nerves from lumbar plexus	Flexion of hip
Quadratus lumborum	*Origin:* iliac crest and iliolumbar ligament *Insertion:* last rib and transverse processes of lumbar vertebrae	Anterior rami of T12–L4	Unilateral: lateral flexion of vertebral column Bilateral: depression of the rib cage, fixes 12th rib

* Indicates the muscles supplied by the posterior rami of the spinal nerves, collectively known as erector spinae.

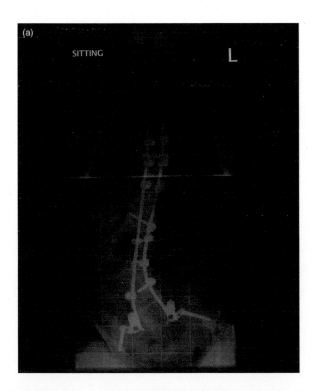

FIGURE 4.12A Anteroposterior (AP) postoperative X-ray showing fixation of rods from T1 to L5 to correct severe kyphoscoliosis in a 15-year-old girl. (Courtesy of Philip J. Adds.)

third, fourth, and fifth cervical myotomes, hence the phrenic nerve origin from C3, C4, and C5 spinal segments, which follows the descent of the diaphragm to divide the thorax from the abdomen. The other part is the growth of the pleuroperitoneal membranes medially from the body wall.

The diaphragm's motor innervation is by the phrenic nerve ("C3, 4, 5 keeps the diaphragm alive").

The phrenic nerve also supplies sensory fibres to the diaphragmatic pleura over the domes and the diaphragmatic peritoneum lying beneath the dome. The sensory supply of the peripheral parts of the diaphragmatic pleura is via the lower six intercostal nerves.

An accessory phrenic nerve may also be observed as an anatomical variant, seen in around one-third of patients.

Occasionally, the C5 part of the phrenic nerve originates from the nerve to the subclavius.

The diaphragm has several attachments. The main attachments are:

- Lower costal cartilages and ribs 7 to 12
- Xiphoid process (posterior surface)
- Lumbar vertebrae (L1–L3 and their intervertebral discs) and arcuate ligaments

Two main tendinous structures arise from the vertebrae:

- *Left crus:* starts from L1 to L2 (overlapping their intervertebral discs).

(b)

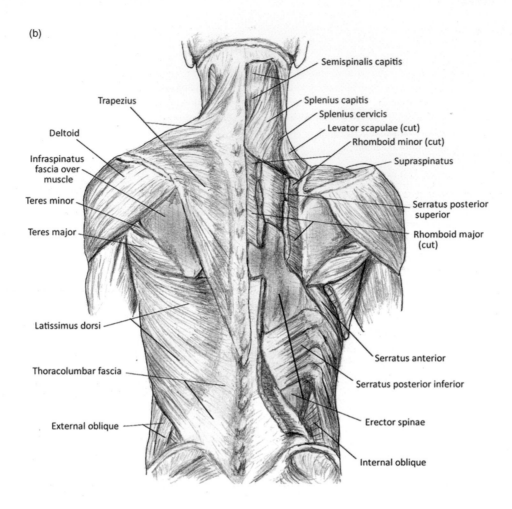

FIGURE 4.12B   Diagram showing the muscles of the back. (Courtesy of Gabriela Barzyk.)

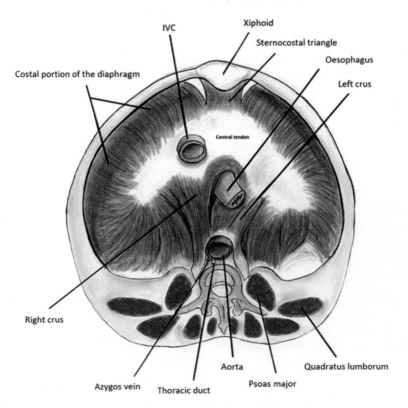

FIGURE 4.13   Abdominal surface of the diaphragm. (Courtesy of Kathryn DeMarre.)

- *Right crus:* starts from L1 to L3 (overlapping the inter-vertebral discs). **A few muscular fibres surround the oesophageal sphincter and help to prevent reflux**.

Three ligaments are formed by the attachments of the diaphragm:

- The **median arcuate ligament** is formed in between the right and left crura. This encloses the aorta and thoracic duct.
- The **medial arcuate ligament** is situated between the median and lateral arcuate ligaments. The psoas major passes posterior to it.
- The **lateral arcuate ligament** is the most lateral ligament; the quadratus lumborum passes posterior to it.

Openings

a. *Aortic:* the **descending aorta** passes through the aortic hiatus at **T12**, with the thoracic duct and azygos vein.
b. *Oesophageal:* the **oesophagus passes** through the right crus at **T10**, in addition to the right and left vagus nerves and the oesophageal branches of the left gastric vessels.
c. *Caval:* the inferior vena cava (IVC) passes through at **T8**. It passes through the **central tendon** of the diaphragm – this allows the hiatus to remain open even in inspiration to ensure constant blood flow back to the heart.

How to remember: *aortic hiatus* **has 12 letters,** *oesophagus* **has 10, and** *vena cava* **has 8.**

Learning Point

During normal respiration, the diaphragm is the only muscle that contracts to inflate the lungs and relaxes to deflate the lungs. The accessory muscles are used to further expand and collapse the lungs during *forceful* inspiration and expiration, e.g., during exercise.

During forced inspiration, the external intercostal muscles and diaphragm increase the volume of the thorax when they contract. This creates a negative pressure in the thoracic cavity, which causes air to move into the lungs, allowing them to fill. The lungs themselves cannot expand!

The opposite happens during forced expiration (i.e., the diaphragm relaxes and the internal intercostals contract to decrease thoracic volume and hence increase pressure). These forces air out of the cavity, causing exhalation.

CLINICAL NOTES

Pain from the irritation of diaphragmatic peritoneum due to acute cholecystitis (inflammation of the gallbladder) can be felt in the right shoulder, which is innervated by the supraclavicular nerves, sharing the same spinal segments as the diaphragm (referred pain).

Congenital diaphragmatic hernia (rare) can occur due to the persistence of the pleuroperitoneal membrane.

Paralysis of the phrenic nerve can follow involvement of the nerve in malignant tumours in the neck or thorax and, rarely, due to injury to the nerve in the neck. The hemidiaphragm on the involved side moves upwards on inspiration.

THE THORACIC CAVITY

The thoracic cavity is divided into three main compartments: **right** and **left pleural cavities** and the **mediastinum**.

The mediastinum (**Figure 4.14**) is divided into **superior** and **inferior** compartments through an imaginary **transverse plane** at the vertebral level of **T4–T5** at the manubriosternal joint.

The **superior mediastinum** is bounded superiorly by the superior border of the manubrium, the first thoracic vertebra (T1), and the first ribs and their costal cartilages; inferiorly by the transverse thoracic plane (T4–T5); and laterally by the upper lungs and pleura. The manubrium forms its anterior border, whilst the first four thoracic vertebrae form its posterior border.

The **inferior mediastinum** can be further subdivided into anterior, middle, and posterior compartments. The anterior, middle, and posterior mediastina are bounded by the same superior, inferior, and lateral boundaries.

The **anterior mediastinum** is bounded superiorly by the transthoracic plane (T4–T5), inferiorly by the thoracic surface of the diaphragm, and laterally by the lungs and the mediastinal pleura. The body of the sternum forms its anterior surface, whilst the anterior surface of the pericardium forms its posterior surface. The anterior and posterior surfaces of the pericardium form the respective anterior and posterior borders of the middle mediastinum. The **posterior mediastinum** is also bounded anteriorly by the posterior surface of the pericardium and posteriorly by the bodies of T5–T12 vertebrae.

Contents of the Mediastinum

Superior Mediastinum
Many structures can be found within the superior mediastinum, including blood vessels, nerves, the trachea, the oesophagus, the thoracic duct, and the thymus gland sitting on top of the aortic arch.

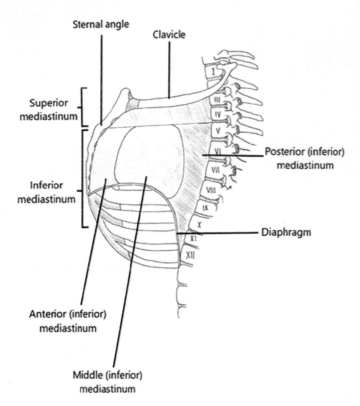

Sternal angle
Clavicle
Superior mediastinum
Inferior mediastinum
Posterior (inferior) mediastinum
Diaphragm
Anterior (inferior) mediastinum
Middle (inferior) mediastinum

FIGURE 4.14 Sagittal view of the thorax. (Courtesy of Ming Zhu.)

Blood vessels within the superior mediastinum include:

- *The arch of the aorta (which divides into its respective branches*: brachiocephalic trunk, left common carotid, and left subclavian arteries)
- The superior vena cava, which drains the right and left brachiocephalic veins and the azygos system

Nerves include **right and left phrenic nerves**, which descend anterior to the anterior scalene muscles before entering the superior mediastinum via the superior thoracic aperture. The phrenic nerves run in the superior and then the middle mediastinum.

The **right phrenic nerve** runs lateral to the right brachiocephalic vein and superior vena cava (SVC). It then passes anterior to the root of the right lung and descends to the right side of the fibrous pericardium, which it supplies, in addition to the mediastinal pleura. It finally supplies the muscle of the right dome of the diaphragm, in addition to supplying sensory fibres to the diaphragmatic pleura, and diaphragmatic peritoneum, via branches which pass through the caval opening of the diaphragm.

The **left phrenic nerve** runs lateral to the left subclavian artery to cross the left side of the aortic arch. Like the right phrenic nerve, it passes **in front** of the root of the left lung to continue over the left side of the pericardium (where it supplies both the mediastinal pleura and pericardium with sensory

fibres) to terminate by supplying the left dome of the diaphragm and sending sensory fibres to the peritoneum of the undersurface of the diaphragm and the pleura covering the central diaphragm.

The course of the **right and left vagi** in the neck is related to their respective carotid sheaths, along with the common carotid artery and the internal jugular vein.

The **right vagus nerve** enters the superior mediastinum lateral to the trachea to pass **behind** the root of the right lung (where it supplies parasympathetic fibres to the pulmonary plexus). It continues in the posterior mediastinum posterior to the oesophagus to take part in the oesophageal plexus (it supplies the oesophageal branches). Note that the **right recurrent laryngeal nerve** loops around the right subclavian artery in the root of the neck to ascend in the tracheo-oesophageal groove to supply structures in the neck, mainly the larynx. The right vagus contributes parasympathetic innervation to the cardiac plexus.

The **left vagus nerve** enters the thorax between the left common carotid and left subclavian arteries to cross the left side of the aortic arch (note the left vagus is crossed by the left phrenic nerve). It passes posterior to the root of the left lung (sending parasympathetic branches to the pulmonary plexus). The left vagus nerve then passes in the posterior mediastinum, anterior to the oesophagus, to contribute to the oesophageal plexus and passes through the oesophageal opening of the diaphragm to supply parasympathetic fibres to the anterior surface of the stomach (see **Section 5**, Abdomen). The **left recurrent laryngeal nerve** arises in the thorax as the vagus crosses the aortic arch. It then loops around the arch of the aorta at the site of the ligamentum arteriosum and ascends to the neck in the tracheo-oesophageal groove (see **Section 2**, Head and Neck).

Thoracic Sympathetic Trunks

Each trunk is composed of a chain of 11 to 12 ganglia and lies posteriorly on the heads of the ribs to leave the thorax at the T12 level by passing beneath the medial arcuate ligament (see the discussion on the anatomy of the diaphragm). It continues upwards and downwards as the cervical sympathetic and lumbar sympathetic trunks, respectively. The sympathetic trunk is connected to the spinal nerves via white and grey rami communicates. The sympathetic paravertebral ganglia receive the pre-ganglionic white fibres (T1–L2) along the ventral rami of the spinal nerves to either synapse at the same level, ascend, descend, **or pass without synapsing to the prevertebral ganglia (coeliac, superior mesenteric, inferior mesenteric**, and the **adrenal medulla**). The post-ganglionic fibres (grey) are longer than the pre-ganglionic fibres and run along all the spinal nerves to different parts of the body.

The upper thoracic ganglia give rise to post-ganglionic fibres to the:

- **Cardiac plexus** (sympathetic stimulation causes tachycardia and increased cardiac muscle contractility and dilatation of the coronary arteries); afferent pain fibres pass with the sympathetic nerves to the central nervous system (CNS) (see below, The Heart). There are superficial and deep cardiac plexuses. The superficial plexus lies anterior to the arch of the aorta and medial to the ligamentum arteriosum, whereas the deep plexus lies anterior to the trachea and posterior to the arch of the aorta.

- **Pulmonary plexus** (for bronchodilation).
- **Aorta and oesophagus**.

The splanchnic nerves on each side (greater, lesser, and least) arise from the lower eight thoracic ganglia and enter the abdominal cavity through the right and left crura of the diaphragm. The **greater splanchnic nerves** arise from T5 to T9, contributing to the nerve supply of the foregut; the **lesser splanchnic nerves** arise from T10 to T11 to join the aorticorenal ganglion and supply the midgut; and the **least splanchnic nerves** arise from T12, supplying the kidneys (see **Section 5, Abdomen**).

The **stellate ganglion** ("star-shaped") is formed by the fusion of upper thoracic and lower cervical ganglia opposite the head of the first rib (see discussion on Horner's syndrome).

Endoscopic thoracic sympathectomy is a form of minimal-access surgery targeting the upper thoracic sympathetic chain to treat excessive sweating (hyperhidrosis) when other non-invasive measures fail to relieve it.

Other structures within the superior mediastinum include the trachea (which divides into two bronchi at the carina) oesophagus, thymus gland, and thoracic duct.

Anterior Mediastinum

The thymus gland and the phrenic nerves (see earlier) continue into the anterior mediastinum.

The **thymus gland** is a triangular-shaped, bilobar organ located on the superior surface of the heart. It is positioned posterior to the body of the sternum. Each lobe consists of three distinctive regions (superficial to deep): fibrous capsule, cortex, and medulla. It is a primary lymphoid organ which is involved in T-lymphocyte maturation. It is most prominent in size during childhood and atrophies during puberty.

Middle Mediastinum

The middle mediastinum contains the heart, surrounded by the pericardium. The roots of the great vessels, i.e., the ascending aorta, the pulmonary trunk, and the SVC, pass through the pericardium to, or from, the heart.

Posterior Mediastinum

The oesophagus and the vagi continue from the superior mediastinum and into the posterior mediastinum (see earlier).

The **oesophagus** runs posterior to the trachea and anterior to the thoracic aorta. It pierces the diaphragm through the oesophageal hiatus at the vertebral level of T10.

Thoracic Oesophagus

The oesophagus is a fibromuscular tube approximately 25 cm long extending from the cricoid cartilage (C6) down to the stomach.

The oesophagus enters the superior mediastinum posterior to the trachea. It then passes to the left behind the left bronchus and the left atrium down to the posterior mediastinum, where it passes anterior to the bodies of the thoracic vertebrae. The thoracic descending aorta is posterior to the lower oesophagus (see the discussion on the relations of the right and left vagi).

The oesophagus consists of three parts: cervical, thoracic (the longest), and the short intra-abdominal.

The wall of the oesophagus contains two types of muscles: longitudinal (outermost) and circular (innermost). It is also composed of a combination of skeletal and smooth muscle with different innervations.

The oesophagus has three anatomical constrictions, one in the neck and two in the thorax (some sources give four constrictions – including both aortic and left bronchi separately):

- *Upper/pharyngeal constriction*: in the neck. It is constricted by the upper oesophageal sphincter (the cricopharyngeus muscle).
- *Middle/aortobronchial constriction*: in the thorax. It is constricted first by the aorta then by the left main bronchus at the level of T4, where the bronchus passes anterior to the oesophagus.
- *Inferior/diaphragmatic constriction*: as it passes through the diaphragm at T10.

The three anatomical narrowings of the oesophagus are the most likely places for foreign bodies to lodge. They are 15 cm, 25 cm, and 40 cm from the upper incisor teeth, respectively.

Blood supply of the thoracic oesophagus is from the descending thoracic aorta for the middle third. The lower third is supplied by the oesophageal branches of the left gastric artery (a branch of the coeliac trunk). For the cervical part of the oesophagus, see (**Section 2**, Head and Neck).

The venous drainage is via the azygos system and left gastric veins (portal system) (see **Section 5**, Abdomen).

Lymphatic drainage of the middle and lower thirds is to the mediastinal lymph nodes and coeliac lymph nodes (along the left gastric vessels). This is of surgical importance in the treatment of oesophageal cancer.

The **aortic arch** continues as the descending thoracic aorta at the level of the transthoracic plane (T4–T5). The thoracic aorta gives rise to its respective branches, which include the bronchial arteries, posterior intercostal arteries, oesophageal arteries, pericardial arteries, and superior phrenic arteries. It enters the abdomen at T12 via the aortic hiatus to become the abdominal aorta (**Figure 4.15**).

The **thoracic duct** is the largest lymphatic vessel in the human body, and it can also be found within the posterior mediastinum. The thoracic duct arises from the cisterna chyli in the abdomen at the vertebral level of L1. It enters the thorax through the aortic opening of the diaphragm, initially on the right of the midline, but crosses to the left around the vertebral levels of T4–T6. It continues to ascend on the left side of the thoracic cavity and drains at the junction between the left internal jugular vein and left subclavian vein. It drains three-fourths of the body's lymph; the upper right quadrant of the body is drained by the right lymphatic duct.

The azygos system of veins is also found within the posterior mediastinum (see earlier).

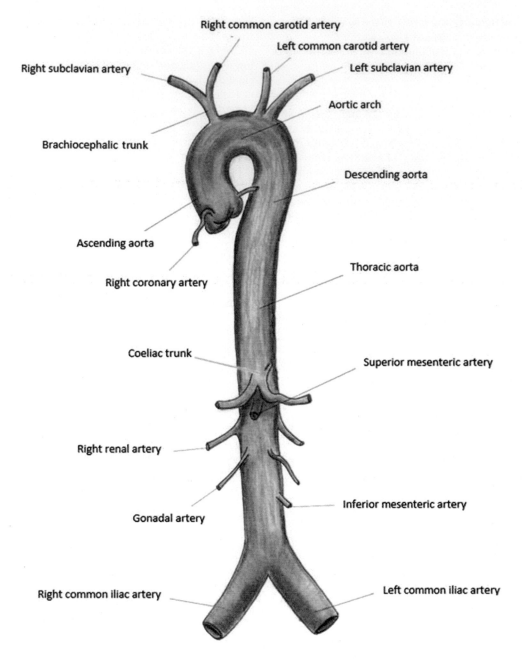

FIGURE 4.15 The aorta. (Courtesy of Kathryn DeMarre.)

CLINICAL NOTES

LANDMARKS IN RELATION TO THE MEDIASTINAL VISCERA RELATIVE TO POSITION

Supine (lying down) position

- The tracheal bifurcation occurs at the carina at the transthoracic plane.
- The arch of the aorta lies superior to the plane.

- The central tendon of the diaphragm is located at the level of the xiphisternal junction and T9 vertebra.

Standing up

- The tracheal bifurcation lies inferior to the plane.
- The arch of the aorta lies at the plane.
- The central tendon falls to the level of the middle xiphoid process opposite the T9–T10 intervertebral disc.

Mediastinal Tumours

Mediastinal tumours are rare and are typically found in middle-aged patients. However, they can develop in patients of all ages.

Mediastinal tumours occurring in children are often benign in nature and are usually found in the posterior mediastinum. Neurogenic neoplasms (peripheral nerve sheath tumours, paragangliomas, and tumours related to the sympathetic ganglia) are the most common type of tumours found within the posterior mediastinum.

In contrast, tumours found in middle-aged patients usually occur in the anterior mediastinum and tend to be malignant, such as thymic carcinoma, which is the most common pathology; germ cell tumours; and lymphoma.

Some patients are asymptomatic, and therefore may not be diagnosed until later stages. If a patient does present with symptoms, it is often due to the compression of surrounding structures, e.g., the trachea. These patients will therefore present with symptoms such as dyspnoea, wheezing, stridor, or hoarseness of the voice, which occur due to the compression of the recurrent laryngeal nerve.

Retrosternal goitre is an enlarged thyroid gland extending down into the superior mediastinum and tends to displace the trachea (**Figure 4.16**) (see **Section 2**, Head and Neck).

Mediastinal masses can be indicated on a chest X-ray via a widened mediastinum. Computed tomography (CT) scans are used more commonly to define the extent of these masses. A widened mediastinum can also be indicative of other pathologies as well, including aortic aneurysms.

Technical factors such as patient positioning (when carrying out an X-ray of the chest) may exaggerate the width of the mediastinum, so ensure that this is ruled out before making a diagnosis.

Mediastinitis is inflammation of tissues, mostly due to bacterial infection, within the mediastinum and can be dangerous because of its close proximity to essential organs.

Common causes include infection following cardiovascular surgery, such as median sternotomy, and perforation of the oesophagus following endoscopic procedures or dehiscence of oesophageal anastomosis following oesophageal resection (e.g., Ivor-Lewis operation). Perforated oesophagus is a rare but serious condition with a high mortality rate if the diagnosis is delayed. Therefore, early diagnosis is vital. Subcutaneous emphysema at the root of the neck, due to leakage of air, is an important clinical feature.

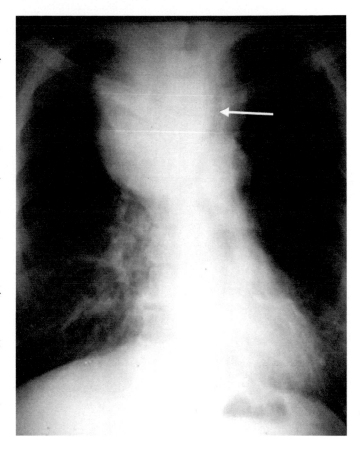

FIGURE 4.16 Chest X-ray showing large retrosternal goitre compressing the trachea to the left side *(arrow)*. (Courtesy of Qassim F. Baker.)

Mediastinoscopy is the passing of an endoscope to the superior mediastinum by making a small incision above the suprasternal notch and taking a biopsy from the lymph node at the carina to exclude metastatic spread, for example, from lung cancer.

Endobronchial ultrasound bronchoscopy (EBUS bronchoscopy) is a procedure where transbronchial biopsies are taken from mediastinal and hilar lymph nodes. Confirming involvement of these lymph nodes secondary to lung cancer is crucial for the proper staging and planning of treatment, as early-stage lung cancer can still be treated with surgery.

THE LUNGS

These air-filled organs lie on either side of the mediastinum. Their main function is for gas exchange, allowing oxygen from the air to enter the blood and carbon dioxide, a product of metabolism, to be removed from the blood (**Figure 4.17**, **Table 4.4**).

Gross Appearance of the Lungs

The typical appearance of the lung of a healthy, non-smoking individual is pink. However, it may appear dark on the cadaver if the lungs have been exposed to pollution (as seen in urban environments) or due to irritants such as tobacco smoke.

Each lung is made up of:

Apex: the most superior point, covered by the cervical pleura and the suprapleural membrane.
Surfaces: three main surfaces including diaphragmatic (base), mediastinal (surface on which the hilum is present), and costal (outer surface exposed to the ribs and costal cartilages).

TABLE 4.4: Comparison of right and left lungs

Right Lung	Left Lung
Has three lobes known as the upper, middle, and lower lobes	Has two lobes known as the upper and lower lobes
Horizontal fissure runs from the fourth costal cartilage to meet with the oblique fissure at the midaxillary line, usually visible on PA chest x-ray. The middle lobe is bounded by the horizontal and oblique fissures	Left lung lacks a horizontal fissure and also lacks a middle lobe
Oblique fissure runs lateral to the spine of the fourth thoracic vertebra down to the sixth costochondral junction. Can be seen on lateral chest X-ray	Oblique fissure runs lateral to spine of fourth thoracic vertebra down to sixth costal cartilage
Groove for superior vena cava and azygos vein are visible on the right lung only	Cardiac notch and groove for arch of aorta are visible on the left lung only
Occasionally on the right lung, an extra fissure is formed from the indentation of the **azygos vein** as it arches over the apex of the lung. This occurs in around 1% of people	Lingula (Latin, "little tongue"), refers to the projection of the upper lobe of the left lung only

Lobes: the right lung has three lobes, upper, middle, and lower (**Figure 4.17**). The left lung has two lobes, upper and lower – this is to allow room for the heart which lies on its cardiac impression.

Borders: the three main borders are anterior, posterior, and inferior. The anterior border of the right lung extends from behind the sternoclavicular joint vertically to the xiphisternal joint, at the junction of the costal and the mediastinal surfaces. The anterior border of the left lung differs by deviating laterally at the fourth costal cartilage, forming the cardiac notch, to accommodate the heart.

The inferior border separates the base of the lung from the costal surface and corresponds to the same course as the pleura. The rounded posterior border of each lung lies beside the vertebral column, about 4 cm from the midline and vertical from the spinous process of C7–T10.

Note that the **pleura crosses the 12th rib posteriorly**, and this of surgical importance in operations such as nephrectomy when 12th rib resection is needed to improve access.

It is possible to identify which lobe is involved in pneumonic process by looking at a chest X-ray (CXR) and using the silhouette sign, which refers to the loss of the radiological borders between thoracic structures on chest radiograph.

Root and Hilum of the Lungs

The root of the lung contains several structures that enter or leave the lung from the mediastinum of the thorax surrounded by a sleeve of pleura, where the mediastinal and visceral pleurae meet. The hilum is a depression on the mediastinal surface of the lung which extends from T5 to T7 (**Figure 4.18**) (compare with the porta hepatis of the liver **Section 5**, Abdomen).

The **pulmonary ligament**, a sleeve of pleura made up of both parietal and visceral layers, is located inferior to the hilum of the lungs and attaches the lungs medially to the mediastinum by attaching to the parietal pleura. Its function is to allow the expansion of lung tissue during inspiration.

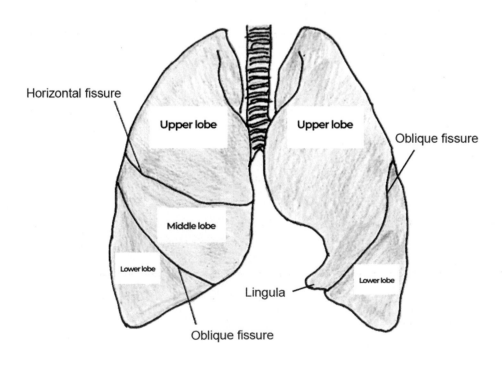

FIGURE 4.17   Lobes of the lungs. (Courtesy of Hannah Katmeh.)

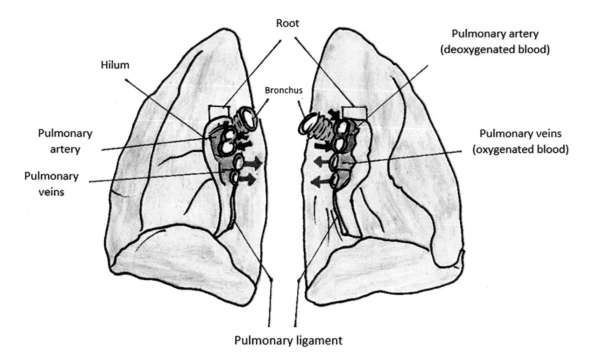

FIGURE 4.18   Root and hilum of right and left lung. (Courtesy of Hannah Katmeh.)

Each root is made up of **one** pulmonary artery, **two** pulmonary veins, a bronchus (with C-shaped cartilaginous rings to prevent collapsing), bronchial vessels, various plexuses of nerves, and numerous groups of lymph nodes.

Learning Point

(LUNG ROOT)

Arteries Above the veins and Bronchus at the Back!
Note that there is only *ONE* pulmonary artery but *TWO* pulmonary veins.
Arteries = Carry blood *AWAY* from the heart.
Veins = Carry blood *TO* the heart.

The Respiratory Tree (Tracheobronchial Tree)

The **trachea** is a continuation of the larynx and begins at **C6**. It is about 12 cm in length and is made up of incomplete C-shaped cartilaginous rings. This is because posterior to the trachea lies the oesophagus, and hence the C-shape allows the bolus of food to move freely down. The C-shape also protects and maintains the airways. The trachealis muscle fills the gap between the ends of the cartilaginous rings and is supplied by sympathetic nerves. Sensory supply is via the vagal and the recurrent laryngeal nerves.

The trachea is centrally located in the suprasternal notch, so it can be easily felt. In the superior mediastinum, the trachea lies posterior to the aortic arch.

The trachea bifurcates at the **carina**, which lies at the level of **T4**, into the left and right principal bronchi. The right bronchus is **more vertical, shorter, and wider** than the left (**Figures 4.19** and **4.20**). Any object aspirated is more likely to get lodged in the right side than in the left. The right bronchus is about 1 inch long, while the left bronchus is about 2 inches long.

Each of these bronchi continues distally until it enters the lungs at the hilum. The airways then divide in a dichotomous branching to 23 generations; down to 16 generations represent the conducting zone, and the remaining form transitional and respiratory zones (**Figure 4.21**).

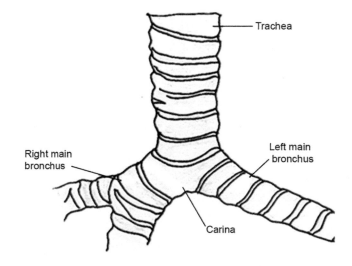

FIGURE 4.19   The bifurcation of the trachea. (Courtesy of Hannah Katmeh.)

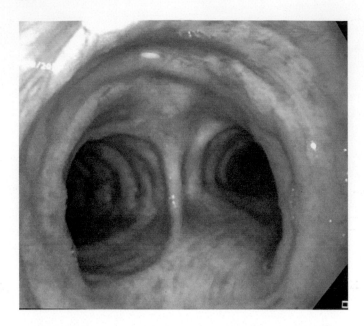

FIGURE 4.20 Bronchoscopy showing the bifurcation of the trachea and the carina. (Courtesy of Mohammed Al Janabi.)

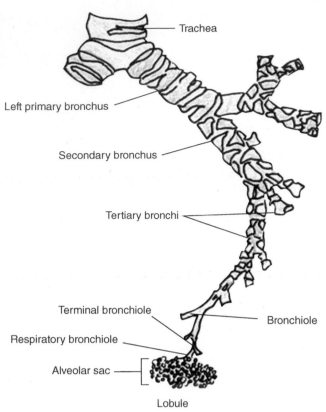

FIGURE 4.21 Tracheobronchial tree. (Courtesy of Hannah Katmeh.)

The right bronchus gives rise to the superior lobar bronchus before entering the hilum to supply the upper lobe. Then it divides into the middle and inferior lobar bronchi. The left bronchus enters the hilum and divides into a superior and an inferior lobar bronchus.

Each lobar bronchus subdivides into smaller branches (segmental or tertiary bronchi), which pass to part of the lung forming a functionally independent unit with its own blood supply, autonomic nerves, and lymphatic drainage (i.e., segmental division). The tributaries of the pulmonary veins lie in the connective tissues between the segments.

The smallest bronchi give rise to bronchioles, which lack cartilaginous rings and are lined by ciliated columnar epithelium and have smooth muscle fibres in their walls.

The terminal or respiratory bronchioles end by branching into the alveolar ducts, where alveolar sacs contain the alveoli (with a combined surface area of 40 to 80 m^2). Gaseous exchange takes place between the air in the alveoli and blood in the capillaries surrounding the alveoli. Oxygen diffuses into the blood in exchange for carbon dioxide. The terminal bronchioles, alveolar ducts, and alveoli constitute the respiratory zone of the tracheobronchial tree.

The clinical importance of **bronchopulmonary segments** (10 in the right lung and 8 to 10 in the left lung) is relevant to diseased segments (cancer, tuberculosis [TB]), which can be removed individually without removing the whole lobe or lung. Compare with the liver segments (see **Section 5**, Abdomen).

Deoxygenated blood enters the right atrium and then the right ventricle. Contraction of the ventricle pumps blood to the pulmonary trunk, which bifurcates into two pulmonary arteries, one entering each lung at the hilum. Oxygenated blood leaves via two pulmonary veins from each lung. Thus, the left atrium receives blood from four pulmonary veins in total.

The **control of breathing** is modulated by higher centres and feedback from sensors such as peripheral chemoreceptors, located near the bifurcation of the common carotid artery at the carotid body, and central chemoreceptors located near the ventral surface of the medulla. The rostral ventrolateral medulla (RVLM) of the brainstem is split into the dorsal and ventral respiratory groups and governs the pattern and rate of breathing.

The **bronchial arteries** are branches of the **descending thoracic aorta** and carry **oxygenated blood** to the bronchi and connective tissues of the lungs, including the visceral pleura.

The **bronchial veins** provide venous drainage of the pulmonary tissues. Veins from the right lung drain into the azygos vein, whilst the left lung drains into the accessory hemiazygos vein, which will subsequently drain into the azygos vein.

Innervation of the Lungs

The pulmonary plexuses run both anterior and posterior to the hilum of the lungs. These plexuses are made up of fibres from the vagus nerve joined by sympathetic nerves. The sympathetic nerves have bronchodilator and vasoconstrictor actions. Parasympathetic stimulation leads to bronchoconstriction, vasodilatation, and an increase in glandular secretion.

Lymphatic Drainage of the Lungs

There are no lymphatic vessels in the alveolar walls. The lymphatic drainage of the lungs collects at the bronchopulmonary lymph nodes at the hilum of each lung. From there, lymph passes to the tracheobronchial nodes at the carina and then to the bronchomediastinal lymph trunks. **This is of special importance when resecting lung cancer.** Suspicious lymph nodes can be biopsied with the bronchoscope to stage cancer or to diagnose other pathologies, e.g., infections.

The Pleura

Surrounding the lungs is a serous membrane, the pleura, which is composed of two layers:

- *Parietal:* the parietal pleura adheres to the rib cage, mediastinum, and diaphragm.
- *Visceral:* the visceral pleura covers the lung itself and extends into the depth of the interlobar fissures.

The parietal and visceral pleurae are continuous at the hilum of the lung (see the earlier discussion on the pulmonary ligament).

The **pleural cavity** or pleural space lies between the parietal and visceral layers, at a **sub-atmospheric pressure** of around minus 4 mm Hg, due to the opposing elastic forces of the chest wall and the recoil of the lungs. This negative pressure in the pleural cavity allows the lungs to be pulled, and hence inflated, when the chest wall expands up and out.

The parietal pleura can be further split into four parts:

- Cervical, which is attached to the under-surface of the suprapleural membrane at the root of the neck
- Costal, related to the ribs
- Diaphragmatic, related to the domes of the diaphragm
- Mediastinal, related to the mediastinal surfaces of the lungs

Nerve Supply of the Pleura

The parietal pleura is sensitive to pain, touch, and temperature. Its sensory innervation comes from:

- *Costal pleura:* intercostal nerves
- *Mediastinal pleura:* phrenic nerve
- Diaphragmatic pleura over the domes is supplied by the phrenic nerve, while the peripheral part is supplied by the intercostal nerves

Visceral pleura is sensitive only to touch and is supplied by the pulmonary plexus (from the autonomic nervous system).

Note: Compare the arrangement of the nerve supply with that of the peritoneum (see **Section 5**, Abdomen).

Pleural Recesses

During forced inspiration, the lungs fill the pleural cavities; however, during quiet respiration there are some parts that do not get filled. These are the pleural recesses, of which we have two:

- Costodiaphragmatic (a potential space between the costal and diaphragmatic pleura)
- Costomediastinal (a potential space between the mediastinal and costal pleura)

Pleural effusion tends to collect in these recesses.

CLINICAL NOTES

LUNGS

Chronic obstructive pulmonary disease (COPD): a collective term which includes both chronic bronchitis and emphysema. It is a chronic, progressive, and irreversible disease, mostly linked to cigarette smoking and air pollution. It is characterised by chronic inflammation of the airways and damage to the lung parenchyma and alveoli. The main symptoms are shortness of breath and productive cough. Chronic hypoxaemia and hypercapnia, with the need for supplemental oxygen, and pulmonary hypertension are some of the complications of COPD.

Asthma: a common intermittent chronic condition that affects the airway. In contrast to COPD, it represents a reversible bronchoconstriction. It causes intermittent wheezing (caused by bronchospasm due to spasmodic contraction of the smooth muscle of the airways); cough (increased mucus production), although unlike COPD, the cough is usually dry; and difficulty in breathing. It is the most common chronic condition in childhood.

Pneumonia: an inflammatory condition of the lung caused by infections, mainly affecting the alveoli. This condition may prove serious, especially in the extremes of life and in the immunosuppressed patient and may need admission to an intensive care unit (ICU) for mechanical ventilation. It is usually treated by administrating antibiotics and oxygen therapy.

Pulmonary oedema: fluid pushed into the alveoli, resulting in restricted oxygen exchange between the lungs and blood. This is often caused by congestive heart failure, mainly left-sided heart failure.

Acute respiratory distress syndrome (ARDS): a life-threatening condition caused by inflammation of the lungs due to sepsis or severe injury. This inflammation causes fluid from small blood vessels to leak into the alveoli, leading to non-cardiogenic pulmonary oedema restricting the rate of oxygen transfer from the lungs to the blood. Ultimately, this will affect other major organs such as the kidneys and brain, as they will be receiving less oxygen, so symptoms can escalate quickly and become life-threatening (**Figure 4.22**).

Coronavirus disease 2019 (COVID-19): a highly infectious disease caused by the novel severe acute respiratory syndrome coronavirus 2 (SARS-CoV-2). The virus primarily affects the respiratory system with a heterogeneous presentation of lower respiratory tract symptoms ranging

(Continued)

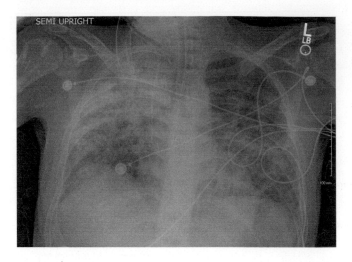

FIGURE 4.22 Chest X-ray showing acute respiratory distress syndrome (ARDS). Note the bilateral heterogeneous appearance. (Courtesy of Mohammed Al Janabi.)

from mild, dry cough and fever to significant hypoxia with ARDS (**Figure 4.23**). Although the pathophysiology is not fully understood, the virus binds to the angiotensin-converting enzyme 2 (ACE2) receptor, which is abundant in the lung as well as other organs (e.g., heart, kidney, bladder), making it susceptible to invasion and subsequent inflammation. Overall, inflammation in this region results in a variety of respiratory symptoms which ultimately contribute to complications such as hypoxia, subsequent multiorgan failure, and septic shock.

Pulmonary embolism (PE): an obstruction in the pulmonary artery, commonly due to a clot that has travelled from elsewhere in the body. Deep vein thrombosis (DVT) is often the main cause of PE, as clots in the deep veins of the legs get dislodged and can travel up towards the heart. If the DVT arises above the level of the knee, it is more likely

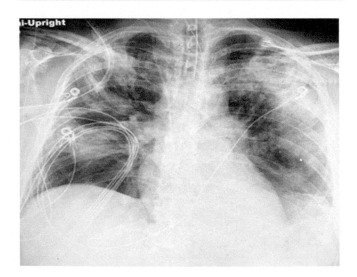

FIGURE 4.23 Chest X-ray of a patient with typical features of COVID-19 infection: bilateral multifocal areas of consolidation, predominantly peripheral rather than perihilar. (Courtesy of Mohammed Al Janabi.)

to cause PE. The thrombus travels up into the right atrium via the inferior vena cava and into the pulmonary artery. If it obstructs a smaller branched vessel of the pulmonary artery, the outcome is not immediately serious. However, if the obstruction is in one of the main branches, it can cause immediate death due to a lack of lung perfusion leading to a decrease in blood oxygenation, and blood will build up in the right ventricle. Other substances blocking the pulmonary artery can include fat and air. The symptoms are non-specific; therefore, the diagnosis needs a high index of suspicion and should be based on pre-test probability. Prophylactic measures to combat DVT, and hence PE, are taken seriously in the management of all surgical patients, especially those who are immobile after surgery or injury.

Lung cancer: primary lung cancer is one of the most common cancers in both males and females and is mainly related to smoking. Secondary lung cancer (metastatic) may spread to the lungs from the breast, the kidney (renal cell carcinoma), the placenta (choriocarcinoma), the prostate, or the gastrointestinal (GI) tract (**Figure 4.24**).

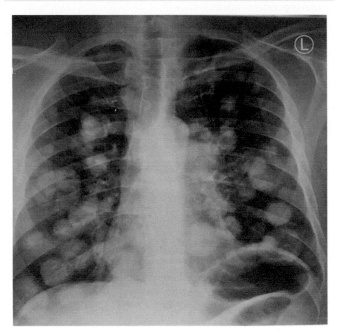

FIGURE 4.24 Cannonball metastatic lung cancer in 50-year-old male diagnosed with colon cancer 2 years previously. (Courtesy of Hamza Al Sabah.)

Pancoast syndrome: also known as cancer of the apex of the lung. Due to its location, the tumour can cause compression and invasion of the structures at the thoracic inlet and lower brachial plexus (thoracic outlet syndrome). It can also cause Horner's syndrome if the cervical sympathetic trunk becomes compressed. Horner's syndrome presents with a triad of symptoms: ptosis (drooping eyelid due to loss of innervation of the superior tarsal muscle), miosis (constricted pupil), and ipsilateral anhidrosis (absence of sweating of the face); enophthalmos (sinking of the eyeball) may be noticed as well.

PLEURA

The cervical pleura protrudes through the superior thoracic aperture and is the covering of the apex (or cupola) of the lung. It can extend to about 2.5 cm into the root of the neck, especially on the left side, above the clavicle, in a curved line, which extends from the sternoclavicular joint to the junction of the medial and middle thirds of the clavicle. This is clinically significant if there is a wound in the root of the neck, and upon inserting a central line into the subclavian vein or internal jugular vein, sometimes it can pierce the cervical pleura as it protrudes above the clavicle. For this reason, CXRs are recommended after a central line has been inserted to exclude iatrogenic pneumothorax.

Pneumothorax (air in the pleural cavity): this can occur as a result of puncturing the pleura surrounding the lungs, e.g., due to rupture of emphysematous bullae (spontaneous pneumothorax), or due to penetrating thoracic injuries (traumatic pneumothorax) and iatrogenic (perioperative pneumothorax), or due to insertion of central venous lines in the subclavian or internal jugular vein. Air enters the pleural space and the lung collapses (**Figure 4.25**).

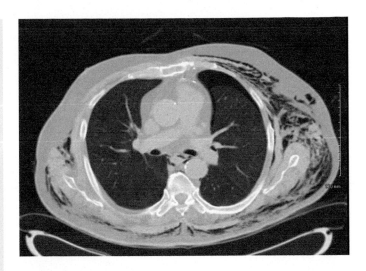

FIGURE 4.26 CT scan of the chest showing left-sided pneumothorax, pneumomediastinum, and diffuse subcutaneous emphysema. (Courtesy of Mohammed Al Janabi.)

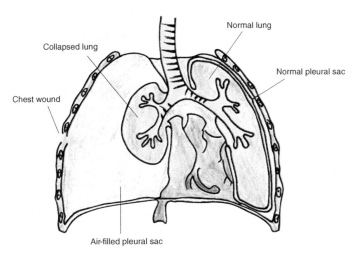

FIGURE 4.25 Diagram illustrating right-sided traumatic pneumothorax. (Courtesy of Hannah Katmeh.)

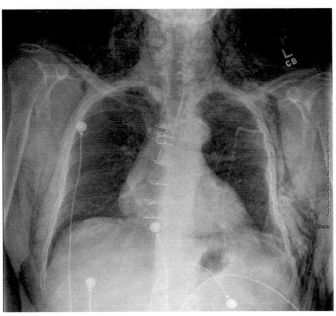

FIGURE 4.27 Chest X-ray after insertion of small pig-tail catheter in the left second intercostal space, which resolved the patient's pneumothorax and emphysema. (Courtesy of Mohammed Al Janabi.)

A 76-year-old male patient sustained blunt trauma to the left chest wall after falling on the stairs. He developed chest pain, shortness of breath, and diffuse subcutaneous emphysema extending superiorly to the neck and inferiorly to the abdominal wall. Computed tomography (CT) of the chest showed non-displaced fractures of the fifth to eighth ribs and left pneumothorax (**Figures 4.26** and **4.27**).

Tension pneumothorax: a life-threatening condition in which the air is trapped in the pleural cavity under pressure. The one-way valve mechanism allows air to get in but not to return. This causes an increase in pressure within the pleural space that can rapidly lead to a collapsed lung and deviation of the mediastinum towards the unaffected side, occluding the venous return to the heart. Patients in

(Continued)

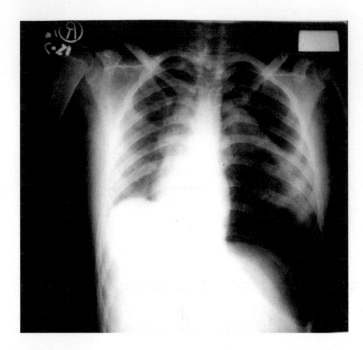

FIGURE 4.28 Chest X-ray showing left tension pneumothorax, with collapsed left lung and downward displacement of the left dome of the diaphragm. (Courtesy of Qassim F. Baker.)

ICUs can develop tension pneumothorax (**Figure 4.28**) due to positive-pressure mechanical ventilation, and therefore should be monitored carefully.

In clear-cut cases (i.e., shock, respiratory distress, cyanosis, distended neck veins, reduced breath sounds, deviated trachea), **needle thoracostomy** can be lifesaving. A large IV cannula size, 14 to 16 G, is usually inserted through the second intercostal space in the midclavicular line. An immediate rush of air is typical of tension pneumothorax if the tip of the IV cannula is sited correctly in the pleural cavity.

Pleural effusion: fluid accumulating in the pleural space is known as a pleural effusion. There are various types of pleural effusion, dependent on the nature of the fluid entering the pleural space, such as **haemothorax** (blood), **chylothorax** (chyle), **hydrothorax** (water), and **pyothorax** (pus). It can be divided into inflammatory exudate, e.g., parapneumonic, due to lung infections, or non-inflammatory transudate. The most common cause of transudate is right-sided heart failure. Other important causes include metastatic cancers such as lung and breast cancer and pulmonary TB.

A sample of fluid can be aspirated from the pleural cavity and sent for analysis mainly for protein content and lactate dehydrogenase (both high in exudate) to differentiate exudate from transudate. Other tests include Gram stain, culture and sensitivity, glucose, pH (both low in empyema), cell count and differential, and cytology (looking for malignant cells, especially for haemorrhagic non-traumatic effusion).

Pleural effusion can be aspirated below the inferior angle of the scapula at the level of the spinous process of T7.

The insertion of the needle into the pleural cavity **should be on the superior border of the rib** to avoid injury to the intercostal vessels and subsequent bleeding (the intercostal neurovascular bundle runs along the inferior border of the rib). The procedure is preferably done with ultrasound guidance to avoid injury to the intrathoracic organs.

Chest drains can be inserted into the pleural space to remove the fluid. For this procedure, the patient needs to be leaning forward, or lying down with head of the bed elevated and their arm outstretched at 90 degrees and the hand resting behind their head, or in the supine position, for example, in the resus room or theatre. The insertion site, known as the **safe triangle**, must be identified (**Figure 4.29**).

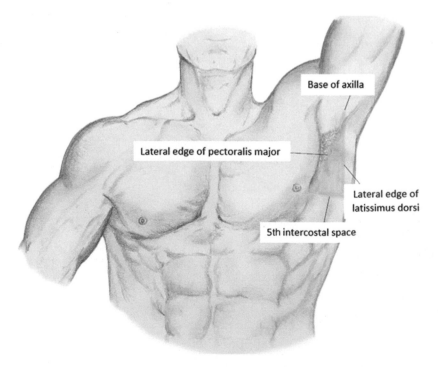

FIGURE 4.29 Boundaries of the safe triangle. (Courtesy of Kathryn DeMarre.)

There are several techniques used to insert the tube (e.g., the Seldinger technique, for more details see **Section 7, Lower Limb**), and a chest X-ray is normally taken to confirm placement and position. The tube is attached to an underwater seal.

CLINICAL CASE

Read the following clinical case and relate it to the imaging to aid in your understanding.

Presenting complaint: a 75-year-old male with a history of malignant melanoma treated with surgical excision presented with shortness of breath and a dry cough of 2 weeks' duration.

CXR: large right-sided pleural effusion. Note that air appears dark on a CXR and CT (**Figures 4.30**, **4.31**, and **4.32**).

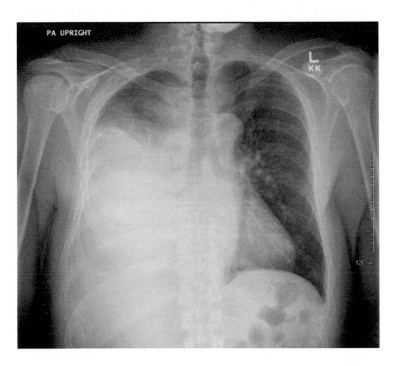

FIGURE 4.30 Chest X-ray showing massive right pleural effusion. (Courtesy of Mohammed Al Janabi.)

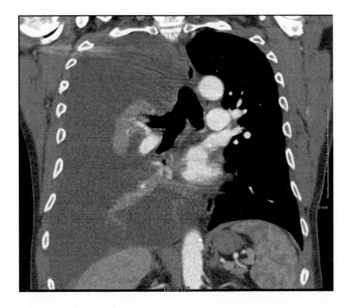

FIGURE 4.31 CT chest with contrast, coronal view: Large right-sided pleural effusion with massive right pulmonary atelectasis (partial collapse of the lung). (Courtesy of Mohammed Al Janabi.)

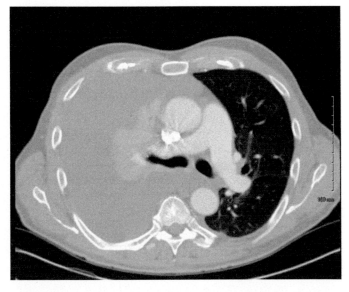

FIGURE 4.32 CT chest with contrast, axial view: Large right-sided pleural effusion with massive right pulmonary atelectasis (partial collapse of the lung). (Courtesy of Mohammed Al Janabi.)

THE HEART

Introduction

This muscular organ is complex and has many functions, which are all responsible for sustaining life. Many pathologies are associated with this organ, and while it is vital for normal function, its failure can be fatal.

Surface Anatomy

The heart is situated in the middle mediastinum and is orientated so that the right atrium forms the right border and the left ventricle forms most of the left border (**Figure 4.33**).

The right and left ventricles are separated by the anterior and posterior interventricular sulci.

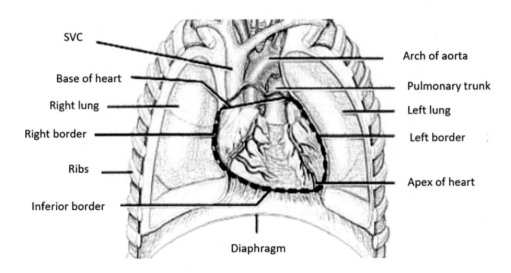

FIGURE 4.33   Borders of the heart. (Courtesy of Kathryn DeMarre.)

The surfaces and borders of the heart are:

- *Right border:* right atrium.
- *Left border:* left ventricle and a small part of the left atrium superiorly to the apex inferiorly.
- *Superior border:* atria and the great vessels (ascending aorta and pulmonary trunk).
- *Inferior surface:* most of the left ventricle and some of the right ventricle in close association with the central tendon of the diaphragm; the inferior border consists mainly of the right ventricle and a small contribution from the left ventricle.
- *Base:* consists of the posterior surface of the left atrium.
- *Anterior surface:* consists of the right atrium, right ventricle, and some of the left ventricle.

The atria and the ventricles are separated by a grooved sulcus, the atrioventricular sulcus.

The Pericardium

The pericardium is the sac that surrounds the heart and the roots of the great vessels entering or leaving the heart and helps to stabilise the heart within the thoracic cavity.

The pericardium consists of two layers:

- An outer fibrous layer, which prevents excessive dilation of the heart, especially during sudden rises in blood volume
- An internal, serous double layer

The internal serous layer of the pericardium consists of the:

- Parietal pericardium (found on the inside of the fibrous layer).
- Visceral pericardium, or epicardium (this is directly attached to the myocardium – the heart muscle).
- **Pericardial cavity, which is a potential space between the visceral and the parietal layers of the serous pericardium.** It contains pericardial fluid (normally about 25 mL), which

is secreted by the inner visceral layer. The pericardial fluid acts as a lubricant to reduce friction on the cardiac surface during systole and diastole, thereby allowing smooth cardiac contraction (**Figure 4.34**).

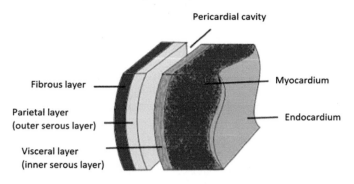

FIGURE 4.34 Layers of the heart and pericardium. (Courtesy of Aditya Mavinkurve.)

Pericardial Sinuses

There are two pericardial sinuses:

- Oblique pericardial sinus
- Transverse pericardial sinus

These are located on the posterior surface of the heart and are formed by the reflection of the serous pericardium.

The transverse pericardial sinus can be found posterior to the origin of the ascending aorta and the pulmonary trunk and anterior to the superior vena cava (SVC). It can be used to apply a clamp or pass a ligature to the aorta and pulmonary trunk during coronary artery bypass graft (CABG) surgery or other cardiac surgical procedures in order to temporarily divert the circulation (extracorporeal circulation).

The oblique sinus lies behind the left atrium.

A surgeon may insert their index finger through the transverse pericardial sinus and use their thumb to massage the great vessels to control the cardiac output of the heart (**Figure 4.35**).

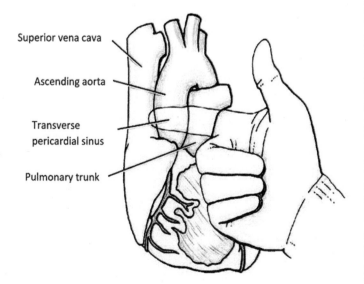

FIGURE 4.35 Transverse pericardial sinus. (Courtesy of Vamsi Thammandra.)

Blood Supply of the Pericardium

The pericardium is supplied by the pericardiophrenic artery (a branch of the internal thoracic) in addition to branches from the musculophrenic, bronchial, oesophageal, and superior phrenic arteries.

Venous drainage is via the azygos venous system.

Innervation of the Pericardium

The phrenic nerves supply the fibrous layer and the parietal layer of the serous pericardium.

The visceral layer of the serous pericardium has autonomic innervation (vagus and sympathetic fibres).

CLINICAL NOTES

Pericarditis refers to inflammation of the pericardium. Common causes include post-viral infections, bacterial infections like tuberculosis (TB) (which is more common in developing countries), and kidney failure. Some cases are also idiopathic in nature. The condition is more common in men than in women and is more prevalent in adults than in children.

Acute pericarditis usually the presents with acute chest pain along with fever, chills, dyspnoea, dysphagia, and excessive sweating. An important physical sign for this condition is **pericardial rub**, which is the sound produced by rubbing of the inflamed visceral and parietal layers on auscultation.

Chronic pericarditis, e.g., due to TB, can take a slower course and end up with fibrosis and even calcification of the pericardium (constrictive pericarditis).

Pericardial effusion is the abnormal accumulation of fluid within the pericardial cavity. Common causes include pericarditis, congestive heart failure, chest trauma, aneurysm of the thoracic aorta, kidney failure, and lung cancer. Pericardial effusion is potentially life-threatening but may be treated by performing **pericardiocentesis**. This involves inserting a needle at Larry's point* into the pericardial cavity and aspirating the fluid from that region.

* *Note:* **Larry's point** is at 45 degrees to the skin, at the junction between the xiphoid process and costal margin. The needle must be aimed towards the left shoulder, and the procedure must be carried out under ultrasound guidance.

Cardiac tamponade occurs due to build-up of fluid, such as blood (haemopericardium) in the pericardial cavity. Fluid build-up exerts pressure on the heart, which reduces normal expansion of the ventricles. This prevents appropriate contraction of the heart. As a result, cardiac output declines, causing reduced perfusion to target organs, which can subsequently lead to organ failure and death. Common symptoms include acute chest pain which radiates to neck, shoulders, back, or abdomen (see "Innervation of the Pericardium"). Other symptoms and signs include dyspnoea, tachycardia, tachypnoea, pallor

(Continued)

(due to low cardiac output)/blue (cyanosis) skin discolouration, excessive sweating, and fainting.

Three clinical signs which are collectively referred to as **Beck's triad** are used to help identify cardiac tamponade (the "three Ds"). These signs are:

- *Muffled heart sounds:* the extra fluid in the pericardial cavity acts to insulate, and therefore reduce, the amplitude of the heart sounds detected by auscultation.
- *Hypotension:* a result of reduced cardiac output (remember, blood pressure is the product of cardiac output and total peripheral resistance).
- *Raised jugular venous pressure:* blood accumulates in the veins leading to a pressure rise within, since the heart is unable to pump the blood that returns to the heart via these veins.

Beck's Triad of Acute Cardiac Tamponade

3 Ds
- Distant or muffled heart sounds
- Decreased arterial blood pressure
- Distended jugular veins

Heart Tissue

The heart is primarily composed of the epicardium, myocardium, and endocardium.

Epicardium forms the outermost layer and is synonymous with the serous visceral pericardium. It is made up of loose fatty connective tissue, nerves, and blood vessels, including coronary arteries.

Myocardium consists of cardiac myocytes (involuntary striated muscle), which is involved in carrying out cardiac contractions.

Endocardium is the thinnest and innermost layer which lines the heart valves. It consists of endothelial cells and collagen. It is rich in Purkinje fibres, which are essential for conduction of electrical impulses. (Purkinje fibres are modified cardiac myocytes, not nerves.)

Coronary Circulation

The heart receives oxygen and nutrients via the **coronary arteries**. The coronary arteries are functionally end arteries; however, during coronary occlusion, coronary collaterals are a potential alternative blood supply in areas of ischaemia.

The coronary arteries arise from the ascending aorta (coronary arteries are the first branches of the aorta). The two main branches are the **right** and **left** coronary arteries.

Right coronary artery:

- Arises from the anterior aortic sinus of the ascending aorta and runs initially between the right atrial appendage and the pulmonary trunk.

- Descends in the right atrioventricular groove and wraps around the diaphragmatic surface of the heart to the cardiac crux (the junction between the interatrial and interventricular grooves) to become the **posterior (inferior) interventricular artery**, supplying the posterior one-third of the interventricular septum and atrioventricular (AV) node. This is called **right dominance** and occurs in about 60% of people. Left dominance is where the posterior interventricular artery originates from the circumflex artery (**Figure 4.36**). This occurs in about 30% of people. In about 10% of the population the right coronary artery and the circumflex artery contribute to the posterior interventricular artery.
- The right coronary artery supplies branches to the right atrium and ventricle, and its marginal branch runs on the lower border of the heart toward the apex.
- Also supplies the artery of the sinuatrial (SA) node (the pacemaker of the heart). Therefore, inferior myocardial infarction (MI) results in bradycardia or AV block.

Left coronary artery

- Arises from the left posterior sinus of the ascending aorta and runs in the left AV groove. After a short course it branches into the circumflex and left anterior descending (LAD) arteries. It provides most of the blood supply to the left atrium and ventricle.
- Its calibre is larger than the right coronary artery.
- **The LAD artery (left anterior interventricular)** runs in the anterior interventricular groove and is directed towards the apex of the heart. The LAD provides the main blood supply to the left ventricle and the anterior two-thirds of the interventricular septum. It may continue in the interventricular groove to meet the terminal branches of the posterior interventricular artery.
- **The circumflex artery** runs in the AV groove posteriorly, after winding around the left border of the heart. It supplies branches to the left atrium and ventricle. **Left dominance** is where the posterior interventricular artery originates from the circumflex artery (**Figure 4.36**).

Cardiac perfusion is limited to diastole, because the aortic valve opens during systole, its cusps cover the ostia that lead to the coronary arteries, which prevents blood flow into the coronary arteries. Furthermore, the rapid ejection of blood limits the amount of time blood can pool around the ostia and enter the coronaries.

The blood supplied is drained by the coronary veins. These veins drain into the **coronary sinus**, which lies in the **posterior cardiac sulcus** located posteriorly in the atrioventricular groove (**Figure 4.37**).

The coronary sinus is formed by the junction of the **great cardiac vein** (which runs from the apex of the heart through the anterior interventricular groove and drains both the ventricles and the left atrium) and the oblique vein of the left atrium.

Two main veins drain into the **coronary sinus**:

- *Middle cardiac vein:* runs in the posterior interventricular groove. It drains the posterior aspect of the heart.
- *Small cardiac vein:* runs in the posterior AV groove and drains the right atrium and right ventricle.

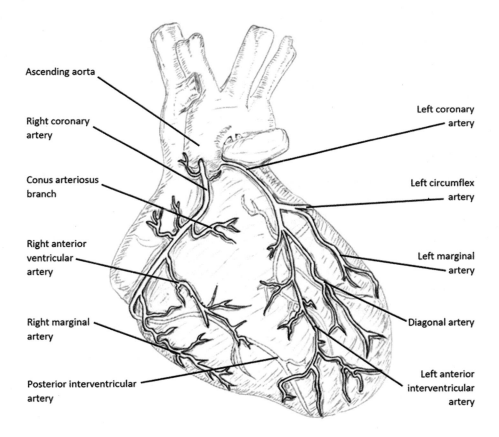

FIGURE 4.36   Coronary arteries of the heart. (Courtesy of Alina Humdani.)

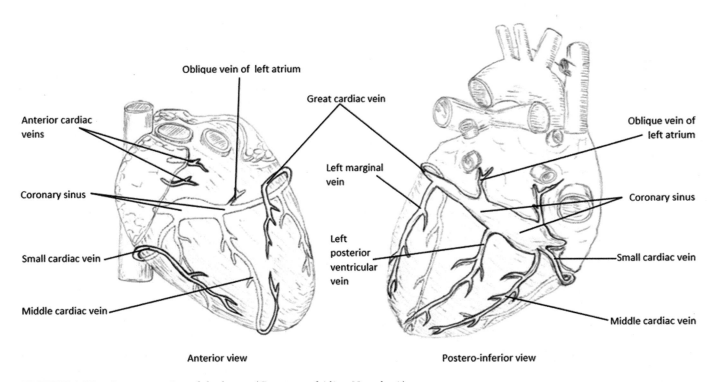

FIGURE 4.37   Coronary veins of the heart. (Courtesy of Alina Humdani.)

Blood in the coronary sinus drains into the right atrium via an opening between the tricuspid valve and the inferior vena cava (IVC).

CLINICAL NOTES

MYOCARDIAL INFARCTION

Commonly known as a heart attack. This condition is caused by lack of perfusion to heart tissue, which is usually due to thrombosis secondary to atherosclerosis of the coronary arteries. With massive MI, sudden death can occur before reaching the hospital.

The most serious MIs are caused by occlusion of the LAD artery, which therefore had the infamous nickname of "the widow maker".

MI is clinically manifested in most patients as severe central chest pain, which may radiate to the arms, neck, or even the jaw. The **afferent pain fibres**, activated by a reduced arterial blood supply, reach the central nervous system **via the sympathetic nerves of the cardiac plexus** within the upper four thoracic spinal nerves. The pain is felt in the skin areas supplied by those nerves (T1–T4).

MI of the diaphragmatic surface of the heart may be misdiagnosed as due to gastric causes. MI should be part of the differential diagnosis of patients with epigastric pain and, if suspected, electrocardiogram (ECG) and plasma troponin estimation should be requested.

ANGINA PECTORIS

Angina is chest pain caused by temporary cardiac ischaemia (lack of oxygen supplied to the cardiac tissue). It is characterised by pain on exertion and relieved by rest (compare with intermittent claudication of the lower limb muscles). It is indicated by an ST depression in an ECG. By contrast, an MI is indicated by an ST elevation.

   NSTEMI: non-ST elevation MI is caused by partial obstruction of coronary arteries.
   STEMI: sT elevation MI is caused by complete obstruction of coronary arteries.

Coronary angiogram: a special X-ray procedure under fluoroscopic control which delineates the coronary arteries for blockage by injecting a radio-opaque dye through a long catheter inserted into the femoral artery at the groin or the radial artery at the wrist. The tip of the catheter is carefully threaded into the coronary arteries through their ostia. This procedure is performed as a matter of urgency, before irreversible death of the cardiac muscle (MI) occurs.

Occlusions are treated by using **balloon angioplasty**, a technique where an inflatable balloon is used to widen the artery. A **stent** may then be placed to hold the artery open. Coronary angiography and catheterization plus interventions (balloon angioplasty and stenting) are major advances in treating myocardial ischaemia and aid in early revascularisation of the cardiac muscle before irreversible damage occurs.

Coronary artery bypass graft (CABG): if the blockage in the coronary arteries or their main branches is not amenable to balloon angioplasty, open surgery is indicated to bypass the blockage using a segment of vein (commonly the long saphenous vein), which is harvested from the leg, or occasionally, the internal thoracic artery can be used instead.

Nerve Supply of the Heart

The heart is myogenic in nature; however, the autonomic nervous system is also involved in controlling both the rate and the force of contraction. The nerve supply to the heart is by both preganglionic sympathetic nerve fibres (upper four thoracic nerves – remember T1 is part of the brachial plexus) that synapse in the upper thoracic ganglia or ascend to synapse in the cervical ganglia and by the parasympathetic nerve fibres originating from the vagus nerve on each side. The sympathetic and parasympathetic innervation form the cardiac plexus.

Both are regulated by the cardioregulatory centre in the medulla and have opposite actions on the **SA node**. Sympathetic innervation increases the heart rate and contractility. However, the SA node can function autonomously by depolarising the cardiac muscles.

Ischaemic pain afferent fibres pass with the sympathetic fibres through the upper four thoracic nerves, so the pain is typically felt as band-like pain anteriorly and can radiate to the upper arm through T1.

Conductive System of the Heart

For the heart to contract, both nodal and non-nodal action potentials are required. These pacemaker potentials are generated at the SA node, which is located at the top of the right atrium, at the **crista terminalis** (the embryonic junction between the venous part and the right atrium proper). The impulses spread across the right and left atria simultaneously, down to the **AV node** found in the floor of the right atrium. The nodes (SA and AV) are specialised cardiac muscle fibres that are continuous with the rest of the organ.

Bachmann's bundle is a broad band of myocytes which passes from the right atrium between the SVC and the ascending aorta to the wall of the left atrium. Its function is to provide a preferential path for electrical activation of the left atrium, allowing it to contract simultaneously with the right atrium.

Pacemaker potentials produced by the SA node are delayed at the AV node to allow proper ventricular filling during late diastole. Nodal action potentials are then transmitted via the **bundle of His** towards the apex of the heart. Impulses are then released via **Purkinje fibres** leading to the contraction of the ventricles **from the apex upwards** (towards the base).

The bundle of His is a collection of heart muscle cells which transmit the electrical signal of the heart. It is located along the interventricular septum before branching further into right and left bundles which give rise to the thin Purkinje fibres, which distribute the electrical impulses to the ventricular muscles (**Figure 4.38**).

Electrical Conduction Diagnosis and Disorders

ECG: a diagnostic tool that shows electrical activity of the heart and any possible disorders (**Figure 4.39**).

   * *P wave:* atrial contraction
   * *QRS complex:* ventricular contraction + atrial relaxation
   * *T wave:* ventricular relaxation
   * *PR segment:* atrial nodal delay
   * *ST interval:* time during which ventricles are contracting and emptying (systole)
   * *TP interval:* time during which ventricles are relaxing and refilling (diastole)

ECG is part of the investigations to diagnose cardiac ischaemia and conductive heart problems such as heart block.

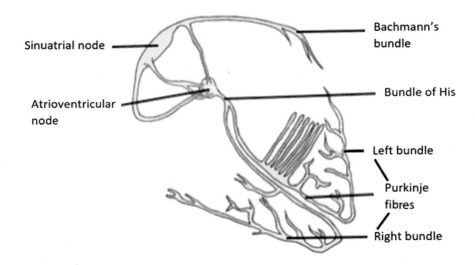

FIGURE 4.38 Electrical conduction system of the heart. There are several pathways that the impulses may take; however, the standard path is shown here. (Courtesy of Calum Harrington-Vogt.)

FIGURE 4.39 Normal sinus wave, which represents electrical cardiac conductance.

Heart Block

This is a common condition which is caused by the destruction or desensitisation of conductive pathways. It leads to an abnormal heart rhythm as the electrical signals are not transmitted, leading to unsynchronised contractions of different regions of the heart.

There are three types of heart block, each with increasing levels of severity.

Atrial Fibrillation

Atrial fibrillation (AF) is a rhythm characterised by uncoordinated, irregular, and rapid contractions of the atrial walls. Rapid contractions lead to pooling of blood within the atria. This can lead to the formation of a thrombus and the possible spread of emboli in the arterial system leading to ischaemia (e.g., cerebral, lower limb, or mesenteric ischaemia). Clinically, the pulse is irregularly irregular. The ECG shows typical features.

Virchow's triad refers to the three main factors that contribute to clot formation and mainly applies to venous thrombosis. Stasis of blood flow is of particular concern in AF (**Figure 4.40**).

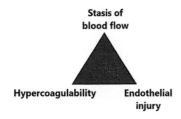

FIGURE 4.40 Virchow's triad.

Ventricular Fibrillation

Ventricular fibrillation (VF) is characterised by uncoordinated, irregular, and fast contraction of the ventricles. This condition normally results in cardiac output dropping to zero and can be fatal if not attended to immediately. There are several causes of VF, most commonly coronary artery disease (CAD). VF can be diagnosed by an ECG, which should show an increase in irregular QRS complexes without distinct P waves. This is commonly seen before the onset of MI and hence is a valuable diagnosis.

Internal Cardiac Anatomy

The heart has **four chambers: two atria and two ventricles**. The right atrium receives blood that is returned to the heart from the rest of the body via the superior and inferior vena cavae. It also receives blood from the coronary circulation (see earlier).

Atria

The right atrium is covered by an **appendage** called the **right auricle** (or right atrial appendage) which serves to increase the storage volume for blood and plays a minor role in the contraction of that chamber. The right atrium is anterior and to the right of the left atrium. The left atrium also has an **auricle** (left atrial appendage), although this appendage is much longer, narrower, and smaller in size.

The SVC enters the dome of the right atrium, while the IVC enters posteroinferiorly.

The wall of the right atrium is lined with **musculi pectinati** (Latin, "like a comb"), which gives it a rough appearance. The pectinate muscle ends at the **crista terminalis**, which is a C-shaped fibromuscular ridge, at which point the wall becomes smoother in nature and is formed by the junction of the embryonic sinus venosus and primitive right atrium. The crista terminalis marks the boundary between the right atrium proper and its appendage and the venous sinus. The musculi pectinati are parallel muscular fibres that extend anterolaterally from the crista terminalis to the auricle. On the external aspect of the right atrium, and corresponding to the crista terminalis, is a groove, the **sulcus terminalis**, which is the groove between the right atrium and right auricle. **The SVC, IVC, and coronary sinus open into the venous sinus** (represents the embryological sinus venosum). The entrance of the SVC has no valve, in contrast to the opening of the IVC which is guarded by the flap-like eustachian valve (or valve of the IVC), which is well developed in embryonic life to direct blood from the right atrium to the left atrium through the foramen ovale.

The **fossa ovalis** is an oval depression seen on the septal wall of the right atrium. During fetal development, the fossa ovalis is open and is called the foramen ovale. This foramen allows blood to be shunted into the left atrium in order to bypass the lungs, as they are still developing, and the pulmonary circulation is not functional at birth. Once born, this foramen is sealed shut, preventing blood flow into the left atrium, as the lungs are now functional and can oxygenate the blood.

The venous component of the left atrium has four openings for the pulmonary veins (left and right superior and inferior), returning oxygenated blood to the heart. The mitral valve allows the oxygenated blood to flow into the left ventricle (**Table 4.5**). The musculi pectinati are fewer and smaller in the left atrium.

TABLE 4.5: Differences between the right and the left atrium

Right Atrium	Left Atrium
Auricle is larger	Auricle is smaller
Venous return via SVC, IVC, and coronary sinus	Venous return via four pulmonary veins
Blood leaves through TRICUSPID VALVE into right ventricle	Blood leaves through BICUSPID/ MITRAL VALVE into left ventricle
Venous blood is deoxygenated	Venous blood is oxygenated

Atrial septal defect (ASD), also known as **patent foramen ovale**, is a condition which is characterised by the failure of the foramen ovale to close after birth. This results in diversion of blood from left to right due to the difference in pressure gradient, leading to the enlargement of the right atrium, right ventricle, and pulmonary trunk. Usually, this condition is asymptomatic, as in most cases, the patent foramen ovale is too small to cause haemodynamic disturbances.

Ventricles

The **ventricles** are the largest chambers with the most cardiac muscle. It is important to note that the left ventricle has a thicker myocardium than the right, as the left side pumps blood to the entire body, while the right-side pumps blood only to the lungs. The internal structure of the ventricles is similar.

The ventricle wall has a rough lining of muscle called **trabeculae carneae** (meaty ridges), which is equivalent to **musculi pectinati** found in the atria. The **papillary muscles** are part of the trabeculae carneae attached to both mitral and tricuspid valves via **chordae tendineae** (tendinous chords or "heart strings"). Papillary muscles contract **before ventricular systole** which allows the chordae tendineae to become **taut** and maintain tension when the ventricles contract. This tension prevents the valves from prolapsing, thus preventing backflow of blood into the atria.

Each ventricular wall becomes smooth leading up to the aortic and pulmonary valves (in the right ventricle, this area is called the **infundibulum** or **conus arteriosus**). The ventricles pump blood through the semilunar valves into the aorta and pulmonary trunk. The right ventricle contains the **moderator band** (or septomarginal trabecula), which spans between the interventricular septum and the anterior papillary muscle. This transmits the right branch of the AV bundle. The **tricuspid valve**

(right atrioventricular valve) is located in between the right atrium and the right ventricle.

> ### Learning Point
>
> Both ventricles have the same cardiac output, but the pressure of ejection is far greater on the left than on the right.

CLINICAL NOTES

VENTRICULAR SEPTAL DEFECT

This represents about 25% of all congenital heart defects. Ventricular septal defect (VSD) is an opening which is present in the interventricular septum that leads to shunting of blood from left to right, causing pulmonary hypertension and right heart failure.

TETRALOGY OF FALLOT

This is a congenital defect and one of the most common causes of cyanotic heart disease consisting of four separate defects (tetralogy) (**Figure 4.41**):

- VSD
- Pulmonary stenosis (right ventricular outflow tract obstruction [RVOTO])
- Overriding aorta (aorta is located over the VSD in between the right and left ventricles)
- Right ventricular hypertrophy

The cause of this condition is not known; however, it is common in people with Down's syndrome.

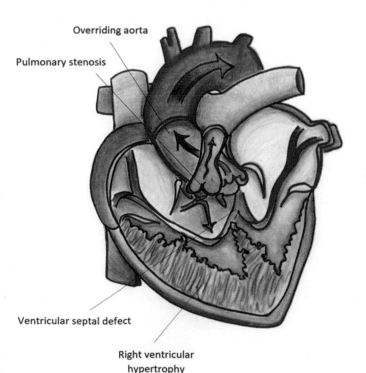

FIGURE 4.41   Tetralogy of Fallot. (Courtesy of Kathryn DeMarre.)

Heart Valves

The valves consist of **tendinous rings** (or annulus) of collagen and elastic fibres, which ensure that the valves do not collapse, with cusps (leaflets) that allow blood to flow in one direction only.

The aortic and pulmonary valves (semilunar valves) both have three cusps and allow blood flow into the great vessels (aorta and pulmonary trunk, respectively). The tricuspid valve is composed of three cusps: anterior, posterior, and septal.

The **mitral valve** (from the Latin *mitra*, "headdress" – a mitre is a bishop's hat, which is two-sided) is the **only bicuspid valve in the heart**. This valve has a single cusp and a conjoined cusp. The space between each cusp is called the **commissure (Figure 4.42)**.

The first and second heart sounds are caused by opening and closing of the valves.

Heart Valvular Disease

Dysfunction of valves can be separated into two categories:

- *Regurgitation:* leakage of the valves due to incomplete closure. Retrograde flow reduces cardiac output.
- *Stenosis:* narrowing of valve cusps, which is usually caused by inflammation; this increases the workload for the heart and can lead to reduced blood flow to the body or the lungs.

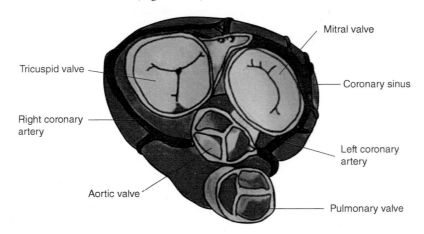

FIGURE 4.42 Cross-section of the heart at the level of T6. (Courtesy of Aditya Mavinkurve.)

The four valves can be auscultated superficially as shown (**Figure 4.43**):

- *Aortic valve:* second intercostal space, right sternal edge
- *Pulmonary valve:* second intercostal space, left sternal edge
- *Tricuspid valve:* fourth intercostal space, left sternal edge
- *Mitral valve:* left fifth intercostal space, midclavicular line

Heart murmurs are abnormal sounds heard on auscultation due to turbulent blood flow through stenosed or leaking valves. Echocardiography can be used to visualise the irregular flow as a non-invasive form of imaging and assessment. Other investigations include transthoracic echocardiography and transoesophageal echocardiography (TEE), which allows a description of the anatomical relation of the left atrium to the oesophagus,

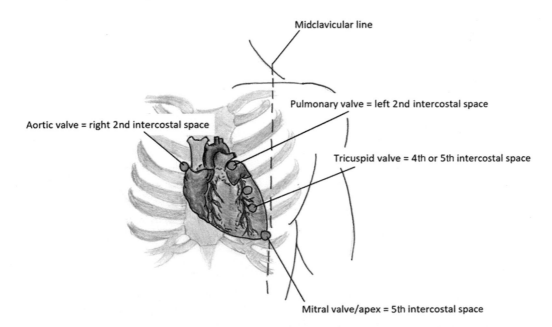

FIGURE 4.43 Locations of auscultation of the different heart valves. (Courtesy of Kathryn DeMarre.)

which is very important. Also, TEE is the best way to visualise the mitral valve.

Causes of valvular disease

- **Age-related calcification of a normal valve** occurs as a result of cumulative "wear and tear" due to valve movement over many years, which leads to endothelial and fibrous damage, causing gradual calcification and stenosis of an otherwise normal valve.
- **Bicuspid aortic valve** is a congenital abnormality whereby the valve is made up of only two leaflets. It occurs in approximately 1% to 2% of the population and has a strong association with aortic coarctation. Years of turbulent flow across this abnormal valve causes continual disruption of the endothelial and collagen matrix, resulting in gradual calcification. This develops by approximately 30 years of age with progressive stenosis.
- **Rheumatic heart disease** can arise from rheumatic fever, which is an inflammatory disease that develops after a streptococcal infection. It is the most common paediatric cardiovascular condition in developing countries. This inflammatory disease affects various connective tissues, especially the heart valves (with predilection to the mitral valve), joints, and skin. As the heart valves become inflamed and scarred over time, they lead to stenosis or regurgitation.
- **Vegetations** (mass of platelets, fibrin, and microcolonies of microorganisms). Infections by bacteria such as streptococci or fungi can cause vegetations to grow on the valve cusps, leading to conditions like **subacute infective endocarditis**, where vegetations get detached and spread via the bloodstream to different body organs and cause further complications (infective emboli). Infection may be introduced during brief periods of having bacteria in the bloodstream, such as after dental work, colonoscopy, and other similar procedures.

Great Vessels

The **superior vena cava** (SVC) is responsible for venous return from the thorax, the head and neck, and both upper limbs. It is formed by the union of the right and left brachiocephalic (innominate) veins.

Each brachiocephalic vein is formed by the union of the subclavian and the internal jugular veins at the root of the neck. The SVC drains blood into the right atrium, and **this junction is NOT guarded by any valves – it is almost continuous**. The azygos vein also drains into the SVC before the latter enters the pericardium. The azygos system connects the IVC and SVC outside the right atrium, giving a path for blood to return to the right atrium if either vena cava is blocked. Its main function is to drain the intercostal spaces and the posterior thoracic wall.

The **aorta** is the largest artery in the body (see **Figure 4.15**) and is split into four sections:

- *Ascending aorta*: this part arises from the left ventricle and immediately gives rise to the right and left coronary arteries. A dissecting aneurysm is formed when the inner layer (the intima) separates from the middle layer and allows the blood to pass between them. The dissection can extend proximally (in this case compromising the origin of the coronary arteries), or distally. Both are life-threatening conditions requiring immediate attention. Aortic dissection is mostly related to hypertension and Marfan's syndrome.

  In the past (pre-antibiotic era) aneurysms of the ascending aorta correlated to syphilis (syphilitic aortitis), but nowadays this is very rare.
- *Arch of the aorta*: starts and ends at the level of T4, in front of the trachea, and arches to the left to continue as the descending aorta. The aortic arch gives rise to three branches: the brachiocephalic trunk, the left common carotid artery, and the left subclavian artery.
- *Thoracic descending aorta*: runs posterior to the oesophagus, through the posterior mediastinum. It gives rise to small arteries that supply the thoracic wall (posterior intercostal arteries) on both sides and several paired branches as it descends. In descending order, these include the bronchial, mediastinal, oesophageal, pericardial, and superior phrenic arteries.
- *Abdominal aorta*: the thoracic aorta becomes the abdominal aorta at the level of **T12** when it passes through the diaphragm via the aortic hiatus. The abdominal aorta terminates at the level of L4, at which point it bifurcates to form the two common iliac arteries (see **Section 5** for further details).

The **pulmonary trunk** arises from the right ventricle and divides into the right and left pulmonary arteries, which carry deoxygenated blood to the lungs for oxygenation. The right pulmonary artery runs posterior to the ascending aorta and SVC, while the left pulmonary artery runs below the aortic arch and anterior to the descending aorta on its way to the root of the left lung.

CLINICAL NOTES

COARCTATION OF THE AORTA

Coarctation of the aorta is a congenital narrowing of the aorta, limiting the blood flow to the inferior part of the body. The narrowing most commonly occurs near the point of attachment of the ligamentum arteriosum. If the coarctation is inferior to this site, it is possible for the development of a collateral circulation to bypass the stenotic aorta through the intercostal and internal thoracic arteries.

PATENT DUCTUS ARTERIOSUS

Patent ductus arteriosus (PDA) is the persistence of the ductus arteriosus, which connects the left pulmonary artery to the aortic arch in embryonic life to bypass the lungs. PDA leads to highly pressured blood flow from the aorta to the pulmonary artery, leading to pulmonary hypertension. Normally, after birth, the ductus arteriosus is closed and replaced by the ligamentum arteriosum (remember the relation of the left recurrent laryngeal nerve to this structure).

THE BREAST

Introduction

The breast refers to the collection of tissue that lies anterior to the pectoralis major muscle and is a distinguishing feature of the class Mammalia. It develops as an epidermal appendage (ectodermal tissue) derived from the apocrine glands. Understanding the anatomy of the breast is incomplete without studying the anatomy of the axilla (see **Section 3**, Upper Limb).

Boundaries

About two-thirds of the breast are located superficial to the pectoralis major and pectoral fascia, which covers the pectoralis major. The rest of the breast lies laterally over part of the serratus anterior (this is important when placing subpectoral breast implants into the retromammary space during breast augmentation).

The breast extends horizontally from the lateral border of the sternum to between the anterior and midaxillary lines. This is of surgical importance when performing a mastectomy. Vertically it extends from the second to sixth ribs.

The axillary tail of the breast extends superiorly and laterally, pierces the deep fascia at the lateral border of the pectoralis major, and enters the axilla (**Figures 4.44** and **4.45**).

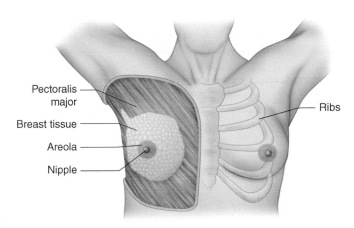

FIGURE 4.44   Anterior view of the breast and thorax. (Courtesy of Calum Harrington-Vogt.)

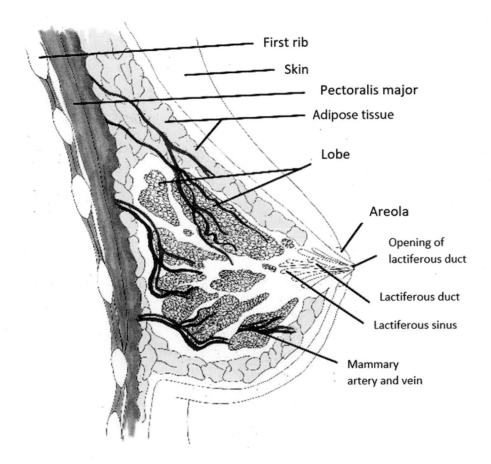

FIGURE 4.45   Sagittal section of the breast showing the lobes and lactiferous ducts. (Courtesy of Calum Harrington-Vogt.)

The **nipple-areola complex** (**NAC**) is usually located at the level of the fourth intercostal space and is therefore supplied by the T4 dermatome. This location alters with age, as the breast begins to sag (breast ptosis). The NAC comprises the **nipple** (a larger central projection that becomes more prominent during arousal and cold weather), surrounded by the **areola**, a pigmented circular area of skin, which includes smaller projections, called Montgomery's tubercles. The total diameter of the NAC usually spans 4 cm; however, this is variable. Appreciating the normal anatomy is important for recognising symptoms of breast cancer, e.g., recent inversion of the nipple, which may suggest the development of breast cancer in the lactiferous ducts underneath the NAC.

The smallest functional units of the breast are the acini. These contain secretory cells, which empty into ducts. About 10 to 100 acini form a lobule, and 20 to 40 lobules form a lobe. The breast is made up of 15 to 20 lobes embedded in fat. These drain via lactiferous ducts (15 to 20 from each lobe) into the nipple.

Cooper's ligaments are bands of connective tissue which support the breast in its upright position on the chest wall and run through the breast tissue to the dermis overlying the breast. Involvement of the ligaments by malignant cells causes skin dimpling. This becomes more evident by asking the patient to raise their arms.

Blood Supply

Arterial supply (Figure 4.46)

- Medially by perforating branches from the internal thoracic (mammary) artery (a branch of the subclavian artery which runs along the internal aspect of the internal thoracic wall, lateral to the sternum) and small branches from the anterior intercostal arteries.
- The greatest contribution is from the perforating branches.
- Laterally by the pectoral branch of the thoracoacromial artery, the external mammary branch of the lateral thoracic artery, and branches from the subscapular artery.
- Perforating branches from the second, third, and fourth intercostal arteries.

Venous drainage

- Veins accompany the arteries and drain mainly to the axillary and subclavian veins.

Lymphatic drainage

- Ninety to ninety-five per cent drains to axillary lymph nodes (this is of surgical importance when assessing lymph node status (*vide infra*, sentinel node biopsy); 5% to 10% drains to the internal mammary lymph nodes (thoracic chain) and to the contralateral breast.
- Axillary lymph node levels: see **Table 3.14**, **Section 3**, Upper Limb.

Nerve supply of the breast: anterior and lateral cutaneous branches of the second to the sixth intercostal nerves.

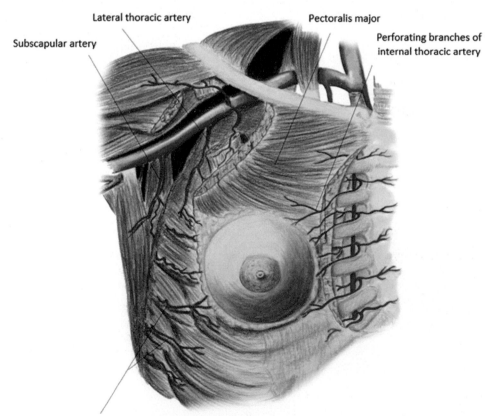

FIGURE 4.46 Arterial supply of the breast. (Courtesy of Kathryn DeMarre.)

Breast Cancer

Breast cancer is the most common cancer in females in the United Kingdom. There are around 56,000 new diagnoses of breast cancer in the UK each year according to Breast Cancer UK, which is over 150 cases diagnosed every day. Worldwide, it is estimated that more than 2.3 million women were diagnosed with breast cancer in 2020, and there were 685,000 deaths.

CLINICAL NOTES

- Interference with lymphatic drainage due to malignancy can cause skin oedema (*peau d'orange*).
- A rare but more aggressive type of breast cancer mimics mastitis (inflammation of breast tissue) and is called inflammatory cancer (**Figure 4.47**).
- One of the clinical pitfalls is diagnosing Paget's disease of the nipple as nipple eczema (**Figure 4.48**).
- Breast cancer often metastasises to axillary lymph nodes, bone, lungs, pleura, liver, and skin.
- Breast cancer in males (**Figure 4.49**) tends to infiltrate deep to the pectoral fascia, pectoralis major, and axillary lymph nodes, and therefore has a poor prognosis. Breast cancer in males is about 1% the rate in females; this is probably due to the fact that the volume of breast tissue in males is roughly 100 times less than in females. Another factor contributing to its poor prognosis is that men are generally not aware that it is possible and ignore symptoms, whereas women are more suspicious of lumps in their breast.

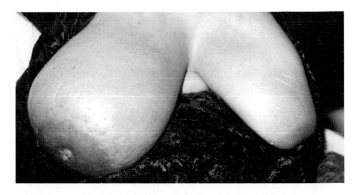

FIGURE 4.48 Advanced cancer of the right breast (Paget's disease of the nipple) showing erosion of the nipple, skin changes (*peau d'orange*), and increased size. (Courtesy of Qassim F. Baker.)

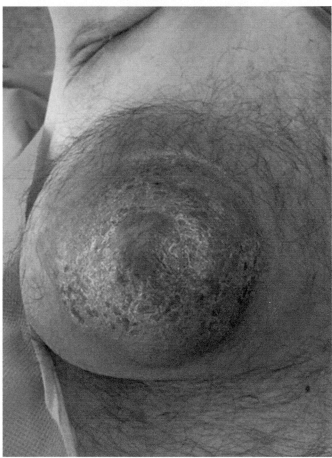

FIGURE 4.49 Advanced right breast cancer in a 63-year-old male. (Courtesy of Ali M. Hasan.)

Triple assessment is the term used in the assessment of breast problems and involves:

- *Clinical assessment:* history taking and examination of both breasts and axillae in addition to other body areas, if needed.
- *Pathological:* core biopsy of suspicious areas sent for histopathological examination; this procedure can be ultrasound-guided for small or impalpable lesions.

(Continued)

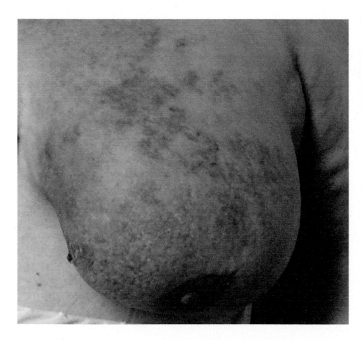

FIGURE 4.47 Inflammatory cancer of the left breast. (Courtesy of Qassim F. Baker.)

- *Radiological:* mammogram and/or ultrasound of the breast. Usually two views are taken: craniocaudal (CC) and mediolateral oblique (MLO). Ultrasound of the axilla may be added as well to check for suspicious lymph nodes (**Figures 4.50** and **4.51**).

The American College of Radiology introduced its original report on the Breast Imaging Reporting and data System (BI-RADS) in 1993 as a universal quality assurance tool to standardise breast imaging reporting and facilitate outcome monitoring. It utilizes a score of 0 to 6 to assess breast imaging (Magny et al., 2021).

Mastectomy: removal of whole breast tissue for treatment of breast cancer or as a risk-reducing procedure (rather than the old terminology of prophylactic mastectomy) in patients with a genetic predisposition to breast cancer. In 2013, Hollywood actress Angelina Jolie underwent a double mastectomy to reduce her chances of getting breast cancer (*BBC News*, 2013).

Lumpectomy: also known as wide local excision (WLE), this is removal of the cancerous area in addition to a free margin around it as a part of breast-conserving surgery (BCS).

Sentinel lymph node biopsy: surgical removal of axillary nodes closest to the tumour and most likely affected if the tumour spreads. This can be achieved by either injection of blue dye or radioactive isotope, or both, in the breast (**Figure 4.52**). This procedure is intended to avoid unnecessary removal of lymph nodes, which can result in lymphoedema of the upper limb.

Axillary node dissection or clearance: removal of lymph nodes affected by the cancer spread, usually for level 1 and 2 lymph nodes.

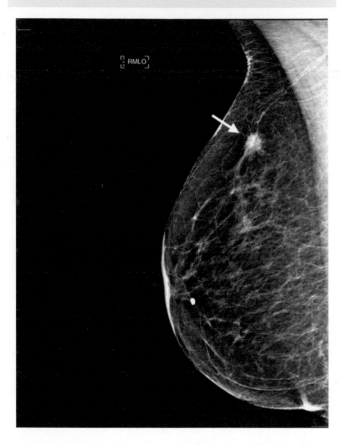

FIGURE 4.50 Right breast MLO view mammogram showing suspicious opacity *(arrow)* in the upper part of the breast. (Courtesy of Thomas Marsh.)

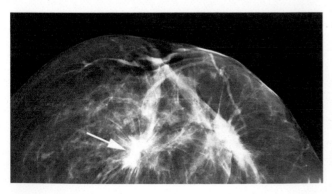

FIGURE 4.51 Mammogram showing spiculated mass *(arrow)* and nipple retraction due to cancer invasion of the lactiferous ducts. (Courtesy of Ali M. Hasan.)

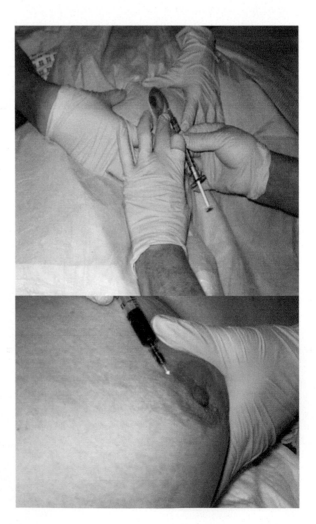

FIGURE 4.52 Injection of the radioisotope in the X-ray department *(top)* and blue dye in the theatre (patient is anaesthetised). (Courtesy of Qassim F. Baker.)

Revision Questions

The Thoracic Wall

Q1. The second costal cartilage can be located by palpating the:
a. Costal margin
b. Sternal angle
c. Sternal notch
d. Sternoclavicular joint
e. Xiphoid process

Q2. The tubercle of the seventh rib articulates with which structure?
a. Body of vertebra T6
b. Body of vertebra T7
c. Body of vertebra T8
d. Transverse process of vertebra T6
e. Transverse process of vertebra T7

Q3. The serratus anterior is innervated by which nerve?
a. Intercostal nerves
b. Lateral pectoral nerve
c. Long thoracic nerve
d. Medial pectoral nerve
e. Nerve to subclavius

Q4. What is the order of the intercostal muscles from anterior to posterior?

Q5. What type of rib is the fourth rib, and list three differences between this rib and the first rib?

Divisions of the Thoracic Cavity

Q1.

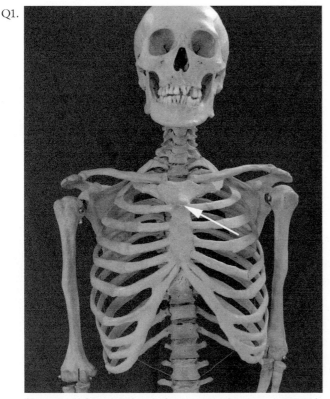

(Courtesy of Department of Anatomical Sciences, SGUL.)

Q1A. What is this joint called?
a. Costochondral
b. Manubriosternal
c. Sternoclavicular
d. Sternocostal
e. Xiphisternal

Q1B. Between which two vertebral levels is this structure located?
a. C7 and T1
b. T2 and T3
c. T4 and T5
d. T5 and T6
e. T6 and T7

Q2.

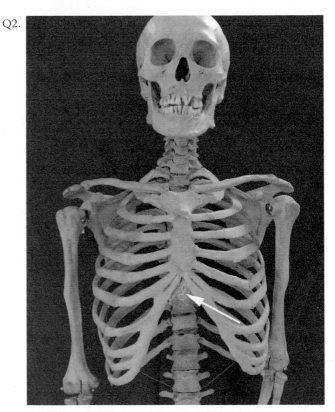

Q2A. What structure is shown by the arrow?
a. Angle of Louis
b. Body of sternum
c. Costal angle
d. Floating rib
e. Xiphoid process

Q2B. The junction between the structure shown and the body of the sternum corresponds to which two vertebrae?
a. T7 and T8
b. T8 and T9
c. T9 and T10
d. T10 and T11
e. T11 and T12

Q3.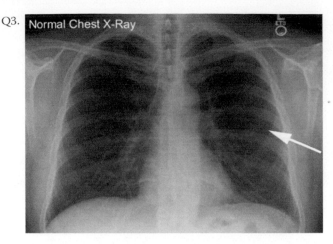

Normal Chest X-Ray

The Heart

Q1.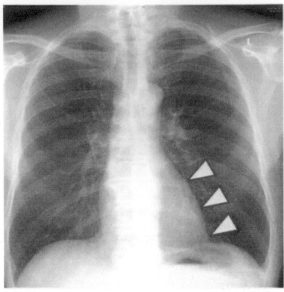

(Courtesy of Department of Anatomical Sciences, SGUL.)

Q3A. What nerve innervates the region marked by the arrow?
a. Intercostal nerve
b. Long thoracic nerve
c. Phrenic nerve
d. Sympathetic trunk
e. Vagus nerve

Q3B. What does damage of this nerve lead to?
a. Bradycardia
b. Hemidiaphragm
c. Hoarse voice
d. Paralysis of intercostal muscles
e. Winged scapula

Q1A. Which of the following best describes the structure outlined by the arrowheads?
a. Aorta
b. Left atrium
c. Left ventricle
d. Right atrium
e. Right ventricle

Q1B. Which of the following best describes the sensory nerve supply to the region indicated by the arrowheads?
a. Left cardiac sympathetic plexus
b. Left phrenic
c. Left vagus
d. Right phrenic
e. Right vagus

Q4.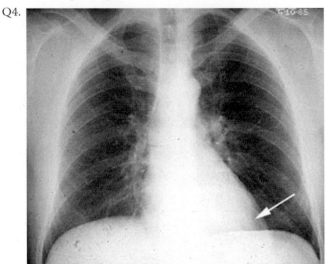

Q4A. What structure is indicated by the arrow?
a. Left atrium
b. Left ventricle
c. Right atrium
d. Right auricle
e. Right ventricle

Q4B. In which anatomical compartment can this structure be found?
a. Anterior mediastinum
b. Middle mediastinum
c. Pleural cavity
d. Posterior mediastinum
e. Superior mediastinum

Q2.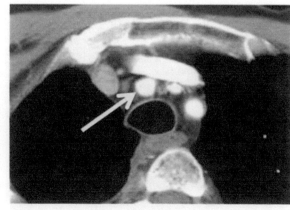

Q2A. Identify the vessel indicated by the arrow.
a. Brachiocephalic trunk
b. Left common carotid artery
c. Left subclavian artery
d. Right common carotid artery
e. Right subclavian artery

Q2B. Which of the following best describes the regions supplied by the vessel indicated by the arrow?
    a.   Left head and neck
    b.   Left upper limb
    c.   Right head and neck
    d.   Right upper limb
    e.   Right upper limb and head and neck

Q3.

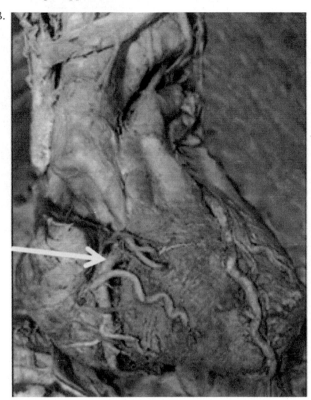

Q3. Which of the following best describes the artery indicated by the arrow?
    a.   Anterior descending
    b.   Circumflex
    c.   Marginal
    d.   Nodal
    e.   Right coronary

The Lungs

Q1. What nerve runs posterior to the hilum of the lung?
    a.   Accessory nerve
    b.   Phrenic nerve
    c.   Posterior intercostal nerve
    d.   Sympathetic trunk
    e.   Vagus nerve

Q2. List three clinical signs of Horner's syndrome.
Q3. What is the term used to describe the embryological origin of the ligamentum arteriosus?
Q4. What is the normal pressure of the pleural cavity at the end of inspiration?
Q5. How many pleural recesses are present in the thorax, and what are their names?
Q6. What is the surface marking of the oblique fissure?
Q7. What is the function of the pulmonary ligament?
Q8. What is the average length of the adult trachea?
Q9. What are the accessory muscles of respiration?

The Breast

1. What is the main contributor to arterial blood supply of the breast?
2. What is the significance of the levels of the axillary lymph nodes?
3. What is the concept of sentinel node biopsy in the treatment of early breast cancer?
4. What is meant by Cooper's ligaments of the breast, and what is their clinical significance?

Answers

The Thoracic Wall
A1. b
A2. e
A3. c
A4. External intercostals, internal intercostals, and innermost intercostals.
A5. True rib, first rib has scalene tubercle, first rib has no costal groove, and the first rib is joined to the sternum by a fibrous joint. The fourth rib has no scalene tubercle, has a costal groove, and the rib is joined to the sternum by a synovial joint.

Divisions of the Thoracic Cavity
A1A. b
A1B. c
A2A. e
A2B. c
A3A. a
A3B. d
A4A. b
A4B. b

The Heart
A1A. c
A1B. b
A2A. a
A2B. e
A3. e

The Lungs
A1. e
A2. Ptosis, miosis, enophthalmos
A3. Ductus arteriosus
A4. −0.5 kpa
A5. Two, the costodiaphragmatic and costomediastinal recesses.
A6. From the tip of the T3 or T4 spinous process posteriorly to the fifth intercostal space at the midaxillary line down to the sixth costal cartilage anteriorly.
A7. Its function is to allow the expansion of lung tissue during inspiration.
A8. Approximately 12 cm; the range is 10 to 13 cm in adult males and shorter in females
A9. The sternocleidomastoid, pectoralis major, and scalene muscles: anterior, middle, and posterior.

The Breast
A1. The main contributors to arterial blood supply are the perforating branches of the internal thoracic artery.
A2. The significance of the levels of the axillary lymph nodes is to assess the extent of lymph node involvement.

A3.   Sentinel node biopsy entails removal of the closest axillary lymph nodes to the cancer without removing the whole nodes, in the old days risking the development of arm lymphoedema.

A4.   These are strands of fibrous tissue which connect the skin overlying the breast to the pectoral fascia and are responsible for keeping the shape of the breast and preventing sagging (breast ptosis).

Further Reading

The Thoracic Wall

Intercostal Drain (Chest Drain/Pleural Drain) Insertion – Oxford Medical Education [Internet]. Oxford Medical Education. Available from: http://www.oxfordmedicaleducation.com/clinical-skills/procedures/intercostal-drain/

Rib Fracture: Practice Essentials, Pathophysiology, Epidemiology [Internet]. Emedicine.medscape.com. Available from: http://emedicine.medscape.com/article/825981-overview

Scoliosis

Farhaan Altaf F, et al. Clinical review: Adolescent idiopathic scoliosis *BMJ* (2013) 346:f2508 doi: https://doi.org/10.1136/bmj.f2508

The Mediastinum

Abu-Omar Y, et al. European Association for Cardio-Thoracic Surgery expert consensus statement on the prevention and management of mediastinitis. *Eur J Cardio-Thorac Surg* (2017)51(1): 10–29. doi: 10.1093/ejcts/ezw326.

Jabłoński S, et al. Acute mediastinitis: Evaluation of clinical risk factors for death in surgically treated patients. *ANZ J Surg* (2013) 83(9).

Jilani TN, Siddiqui AH. Mediastinal Cancer. StatPearls Publishing (2020) Available from: https://www.ncbi.nlm.nih.gov/books/NBK513231/

McNally PA, Arthur ME. Mediastinoscopy. [Updated 2020 Sep 19]. In: StatPearls [Internet]. Treasure Island (FL): StatPearls Publishing (2020) Available from: https://www.ncbi.nlm.nih.gov/books/NBK534863/

Wackerman L, Gnugnoli DM. Widened Mediastinum. In: StatPearls [Internet], StatPearls Publishing; (2020) Available from: https://www.ncbi.nlm.nih.gov/books/NBK539890/

Warren WA, et al. Endobronchial ultrasound bronchoscopy: current uses, innovations and future directions. *AME Medi J* (2018) 3:70. doi: 10.21037/amj.2018.06.

The Lungs

D'Silva K. Pancoast Syndrome: Practice Essentials, Pathophysiology, Etiology [Internet]. Emedicine.medscape.com (2017) Available from: http://emedicine.medscape.com/article/284011-overview

Furlow, PW, Mathisen DJ. Surgical anatomy of the trachea. *Ann Cardiothorac Surg* (2018) 7(2), 255–260. https://doi.org/10.21037/acs.2018.03.01

Horner's Syndrome – NORD (National Organization for Rare Disorders) [Internet]. Available from: https://rarediseases.org/rare-diseases/horners-syndrome/

Lowe R. Muscles of Respiration – Physiopedia [Internet]. Available from: http://www.physio-pedia.com/Muscles_of_Respiration

Tewfik T. Trachea Anatomy: Overview, Development of the Human Trachea, Gross Anatomy [Internet]. Emedicine.medscape.com (2015) Available from: http://emedicine.medscape.com/article/1949391-overview#a5

The Breast

BBC News, 2013. Available from: https://www.bbc.co.uk/news/world-us-canada-22520720 (accessed 26/12/21)

Breast Cancer UK. Available from: https://www.breastcanceruk.org.uk/about-breast-cancer/facts-figures-and-q-as/facts-and-figures/

Magny SJ, et al. Breast Imaging Reporting and Data System. In: StatPearls [Internet]. Treasure Island (FL): StatPearls Publishing (2021) Available from: https://www.ncbi.nlm.nih.gov/books/NBK459169/

5

ANATOMY OF THE ABDOMEN

Reviewed by Qassim F. Baker and David Sunnucks

Learning Objectives

- *Anterior abdominal wall*: rectus sheath, umbilical and para-umbilical hernia
- The peritoneal cavity (greater and lesser sac) and peritonitis
- Major blood vessels (abdominal aorta and its branches, inferior vena cava, portal vein)
- *Foregut*: coeliac axis, lower oesophagus, stomach, liver, biliary system, spleen and pancreas
- *Midgut*: superior mesenteric artery, small bowel
- *Hindgut*: inferior mesenteric artery and colon
- Posterior abdominal wall and the retroperitoneal space
- Kidneys and the adrenal glands
- Revision questions

What Is Meant by the Anterior Abdominal Wall?

The anterior abdominal wall refers to the area bounded above by the costal margins and the xyphoid process between them, laterally by the midaxillary lines, inferiorly by the anterior part of the iliac crests, the junction of the groin (including the inguinal canals) with the upper thighs, and the upper part of the symphysis pubis.

Divisions of the Anterior Abdominal Wall

The anterior abdominal wall can be divided into four quadrants (right upper, right lower, left upper, and left lower) by a midline vertical line and a horizontal line which bisects the umbilicus. Clinically, we speak about pain in the upper right quadrant due to, for example, gallstones, or right lower quadrant pain due to, for example, acute appendicitis.

The anterior abdominal wall can also be divided into nine regions by two imaginary horizontal (transpyloric and intertubercular) and two imaginary vertical (midclavicular) lines (**Figure 5.1**).

- **Transpyloric (Addison's) plane** is an imaginary plane midway between the jugular (suprasternal) notch and the upper border of the symphysis pubis. It passes through the pylorus of the stomach at the vertebral level of L1.
- **Intertubercular plane** passes between the tubercles of the iliac crests, which corresponds to the vertebral level of L5.

Layers of the Anterior Abdominal Wall

The anterior abdominal wall is composed of several layers. From superficial to deep, it includes:

- Skin
- Superficial fascia
- Muscles and their fascia

- Transversalis fascia
- Extraperitoneal tissue
- Peritoneum

Skin

Sensory supply is from the ventral rami of spinal nerves T7–L1. The umbilicus is present between the vertebral levels of L3 and L4 and at the dermatomal level of T10.

Superficial Fascia

The superficial fascia can be divided into two main layers:

- The outer fatty layer, referred to as **Camper's fascia**, continues downwards to the scrotum, where there is very little adipose tissue, and which contains the dartos muscle (continues to the labia majora in females).
- The inner membranous layer, called **Scarpa's fascia**, continues inferiorly into the perineal region, including the external genitalia, as the **superficial perineal fascia** (Colles' fascia), which attaches to the deep fascia of the thigh (fascia lata), about 1 inch below the groin and posteriorly to the perineal body and the posterior margin of the perineal membrane (see **Section 6**). This layer becomes thinner in the upper abdomen.

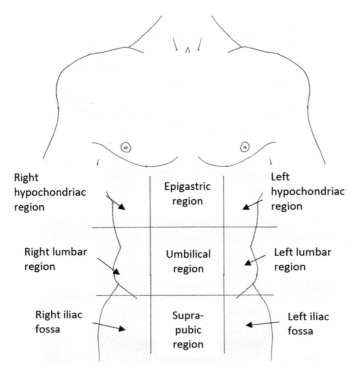

FIGURE 5.1 Divisions of the anterior abdominal wall. (Courtesy of Calum Harrington-Vogt.)

DOI: 10.1201/9781003312895-6

Muscles

Muscles in the anterior abdominal wall can be divided into two categories: vertical muscles and flat muscles (**Figure 5.2**).

- *Vertical muscles:* rectus abdominis on each side (*vide infra*) and pyramidalis (which is sometimes absent)
- *Flat muscles:* external oblique, internal oblique, and transversus abdominis

Rectus Abdominis

Anteriorly, the two recti are present within the rectus sheath. They are vertically aligned muscles which run parallel to each other. On each side, the rectus abdominis originates from the symphysis pubis and pubic crest. It inserts into the fifth, sixth, and seventh costal cartilages and xiphoid process. There are **three tendinous intersections** across the rectus muscle, which give rise to the six- pack appearance in thin individuals, which are adherent to the anterior aspect of the rectus sheath. The tendinous intersections are situated at the level of the umbilicus, xyphoid process, and midway between them. The **semilunar line** (linea semilunaris) is the lateral margin of the rectus abdominis.

The rectus abdominis muscle is supplied by the lower six thoracic nerves (T7–T12).

Action: flexor of the trunk.

Pyramidalis

A triangular-shaped muscle located anterior to the inferior aspect of the rectus abdominis. It arises from the pubic crest and symphysis and inserts into the linea alba. It is missing in some people.

The **linea alba** (Latin: "white line") is a midline fibrous structure that binds the two rectus sheaths together and extends from the xyphoid process to the symphysis pubis and the pubic crest. It is formed by decussation of the aponeuroses of the two oblique muscles and the transversus abdominis (*vide infra*, the **midline incision**).

The **umbilicus** (navel or belly button) is a cicatrix (scar from a healed injury) sited almost in the middle of the linea alba and represents the fusion of embryonic structures. In embryonic life it transmits the umbilical cord and the urachus. After birth, the urachus is closed and forms the median umbilical ligament (if it stays open, it forms a fistula between the bladder and the umbilicus). Other causes of umbilical fistulas include patent omphalomesenteric duct (see the embryology of the gut and Meckel's diverticulum).

- The left umbilical vein becomes the round ligament (ligamentum teres) of the liver after birth. The right umbilical vein starts to disappear at the fourth week of intrauterine life.
- The right and left medial umbilical ligaments are formed from the obliterated umbilical arteries.

The site just inferior to the umbilicus is the most common site for the insertion of ports in laparoscopic surgery (*vide infra*, umbilical hernia).

Rectus Sheath

The rectus sheath wraps around the vertical muscles. It is made up of the aponeuroses of external oblique, internal oblique, and transversus abdominis.

The aponeurosis of the external oblique unites with part of the aponeurosis of the internal oblique to form the anterior wall of the rectus sheath.

The other part of the internal oblique aponeurosis unites with that of the transversus abdominis to form the posterior wall of the sheath.

This arrangement of the aponeuroses changes midway between the umbilicus and the pubic symphysis, as all the aponeuroses unite anterior to the rectus muscles. At this point, the rectus muscle is now in direct contact with the transversalis fascia behind it. The point at which this change occurs is referred to as the **semi-circular fold of Douglas, or the arcuate line** (arcuate means bent like an arc or bow). The arcuate line is at the level of the anterior superior iliac spine (ASIS) (**Figure 5.2**).

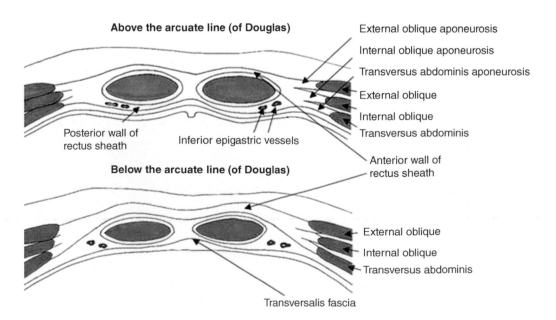

FIGURE 5.2 Arrangement of the rectus sheath above and below the arcuate line. (Courtesy of Calum Harrington- Vogt.)

The **inferior epigastric vessels** enter the rectus sheath at the arcuate line.

The **transversalis fascia** is the fascia which is deep to the transversalis muscle and outside the extraperitoneal tissue.

The **deep inguinal ring** is an opening in the transversalis fascia to transmit the spermatic cord in the male and the round ligament of the uterus in the female (see **Section 6** for more details).

The **extraperitoneal fat** is the layer between the transversalis fascia and the parietal peritoneum.

Flat Muscles

Laterally, there are three muscular layers (external oblique, internal oblique, and transversus abdominis); each muscle ends in a strong aponeurosis to form the rectus sheath on each side (**Table 5.1**).

External oblique:

- Fibres run medially and inferiorly towards the anterior aspect of the body ("hands in pockets" direction) (**Figure 5.3**).
- Fans out into a large aponeurosis, the **lower margin of which is the inguinal ligament** which runs between the ASIS and the pubic tubercle; see **Section 6**, Pelvis and Perineum.

The **conjoint tendon** is the union of the lower fibres of the internal oblique and the tendinous part of the transversus abdominis, which is attached to the pubic crest and the pectineal line.

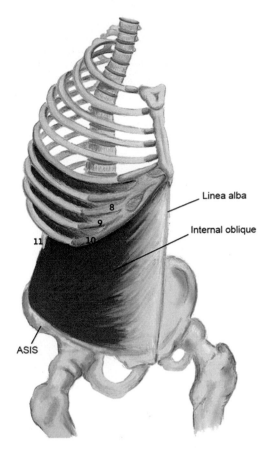

FIGURE 5.4 The right internal oblique muscle. (Courtesy of Kathryn DeMarre.)

The fibres of the **transversus abdominis** run horizontally from the back to the rectus sheath (**Figure 5.5**).

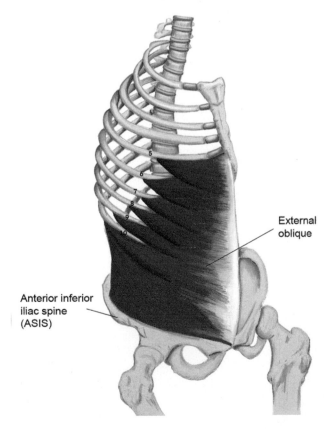

FIGURE 5.3 Origin of the right external oblique muscle. (Courtesy of Kathryn DeMarre.)

Internal oblique (**Figure 5.4**): fibres run medially and superiorly towards the anterior aspect of the body, i.e., at right angles to those of the external oblique.

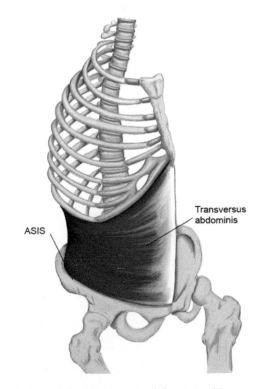

FIGURE 5.5 The right transversus abdominis. (Courtesy of Kathryn DeMarre.)

TABLE 5.1: Flat muscles of the lateral abdominal wall

Muscle	Origin	Insertion	Nerve Supply	Function
External oblique	Arises from the lower 8 ribs (ribs 5–12), interdigitating with the lower fibres of serratus anterior and latissimus dorsi muscles	Rectus sheath, pubic tubercle, anterior half of the outer lip of the Iliac crest	• Intercostal nerves T7–T11 • Subcostal nerve T12	• Contralateral rotation of torso • Compression of abdominal contents and increasing the intra-abdominal pressure (during forced expiration, defaecation, and vomiting) • Flexor of the trunk when contracting bilaterally
Internal oblique	Thoracolumbar fascia, anterior two-thirds of iliac crest, and to the iliopectineal arch (thickened fascia between the ASIS and the iliopectineal eminence)	• Ribs 10–12 and their costal cartilages, xiphoid process, anterior and posterior layers of rectus sheath, and conjoint tendon • The superior margin of the aponeurosis is attached to costal cartilages of seventh, eighth, and ninth ribs	Intercostal nerves (T7–T11) Subcostal nerve (T12) Iliohypogastric nerve and ilioinguinal nerve (L1)	• Ipsilateral rotation of torso • Compression of abdominal contents
Transversus abdominis	Anterior two-thirds of the inner lip of the iliac crest,7th–12th costal cartilages (interdigitating with the diaphragm) and from iliopectineal arch (deep to the lateral one-third of the inguinal ligament)	Anterior and posterior layers of the rectus sheath and conjoint tendon	• Intercostal nerves (T7–T11) • Subcostal nerve (T12) • Iliohypogastric and ilioinguinal nerves (L1)	Compression of abdominal contents

Blood Supply

Blood supply of the rectus sheath is via the **superior epigastric artery** (one of the terminal branches of the internal thoracic artery, from the first part of the subclavian artery) and the **inferior epigastric artery** (branch of the external iliac artery and has the largest contribution). The inferior epigastric vessels form an important landmark in laparoscopic inguinal hernia repair surgery (see **Section 6**).

These arteries form a **free anastomosis** between the subclavian and external iliac arteries.

Lymphatic drainage of the skin above the umbilicus is via axillary lymph nodes, whilst lymphatic drainage below the umbilicus is via inguinal lymph nodes.

CLINICAL NOTES

Infections around the umbilicus can spread towards both the axillary and the inguinal lymph nodes. However, oedema of the abdominal wall can be caused by obstruction of the lymphatic vessels by malignant cells. Rarely, the cause is intrapelvic malignancy, such as ovarian cancer (**Figure 5.6**). (For teaching purposes, a female patient who opted to have a vaccination around the umbilicus for cosmetic reasons, ended up with swollen axillary and inguinal lymph nodes.)

The abdominal wall used to be the site for rabies vaccine prophylaxis and is one of the favourite sites for insulin injection in patients with diabetes mellitus type 1 (insulin dependent).

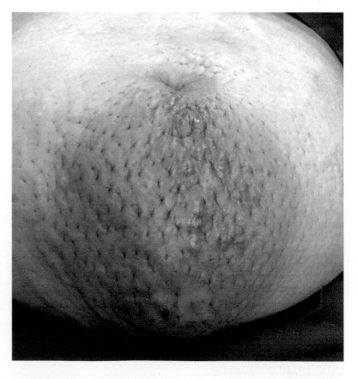

FIGURE 5.6 Oedema of the lower anterior abdominal wall due to lymphatic spread from advanced ovarian cancer in a 35-year-old patient. (Courtesy of Mohammed M. Habash.)

ANOMALIES OF THE ANTERIOR ABDOMINAL WALL

Omphalocele is a birth defect of the anterior abdominal wall, with evisceration of bowel loops and other intra-abdominal organs that are covered with peritoneum and the amnion.

Gastroschisis is similar to omphalocele with evisceration of the intra-abdominal organs through a defect near to the umbilicus where the organs are not covered by membranes.

ABDOMINAL WALL HERNIAS

A hernia is an abnormal protrusion of peritoneum (sac) and viscera (e.g., small bowel and omentum) through an opening in the abdominal wall (external hernia) or through an opening inside the abdominal cavity, e.g., a hole in the mesentery (internal hernia).

Hernias of the groin (inguinal and femoral hernias) are the most common type of abdominal wall hernias (see **Sections 6** and **7**).

VENTRAL HERNIAS

Hernias that occur at the anterior or lateral abdominal wall are referred to as ventral hernias. Examples of ventral hernias include umbilical, paraumbilical, epigastric, incisional, and Spigelian hernias.

Umbilical hernias are the most common types of ventral hernias. They can be both congenital and acquired. Umbilical hernias can arise after birth if the rectus sheath fails to close properly during embryological development.

Epigastric hernia is the protrusion of extraperitoneal fat through a defect in the linea alba above the umbilicus, which can present as a tender lump.

Paraumbilical hernia is an acquired condition which is more prevalent in females and occurs as a result of a defect in the rectus sheath, usually around the umbilicus. It is liable to strangulation of its contents (omentum, bowel); this constitutes a medical emergency (**Figures 5.7** and **5.8**).

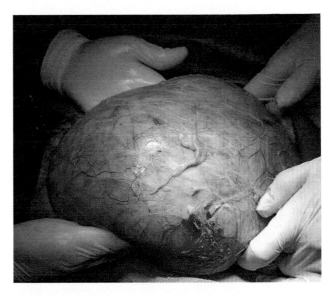

FIGURE 5.8 The sac of the paraumbilical hernia contains small and large bowels; this is the same patient as in **Figure 5.**7. (Courtesy of Omar M. Khalaf.)

Incisional hernia is a complication of abdominal surgery. It occurs through the scar at the site where an incision was previously made, including insertion of ports in laparoscopic surgery (port-site hernia).

Spigelian hernia is a rare type of hernia that occurs in an area of weakness at the semilunar line, commonly at the level of the arcuate line. This type of hernia is easily missed during a clinical examination (especially in obese patients) because the hernia is typically small (**Figure 5.9**).

(Continued)

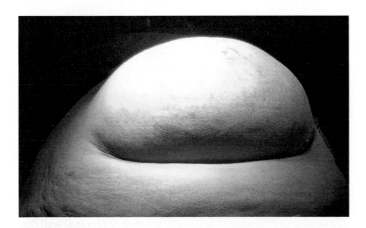

FIGURE 5.7 Huge obstructed paraumbilical hernia in an 80-year-old female. (Courtesy Omar M. Khalaf.)

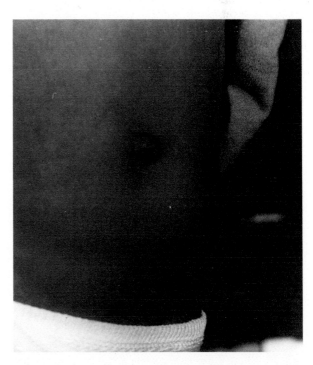

FIGURE 5.9 Left Spigelian hernia. (Courtesy of Qassim F. Baker.)

NECROTISING FASCIITIS

Necrotising fasciitis is a serious, **rapidly spreading infection** of the fascia and is characterised by thrombosis of the cutaneous blood vessels resulting in the development of gangrene of the skin and subcutaneous tissue (Baker & Aldoori, 2009). It can be caused by several types of aerobic and anaerobic bacteria, including group A haemolytic streptococcus and Bacteroides. It is more common in immunocompromised patients, e.g., diabetic, alcoholic, cancer patients on chemotherapy, and HIV patients.

Patients with this condition will present with symptoms such as red/purplish skin pigmentation and ulceration, skin gangrene, and systemic manifestations of sepsis.

If it occurs on the scrotum and the perineum, it is called **Fournier's gangrene**.

Early diagnosis and treatment are of prime importance, as these infections are associated with high complications and mortality. The treatment includes radical wound debridement, which may need repeating after 24 hours (second-look surgery), in addition to vigorous systemic antibiotic therapy and resuscitation.

A **TRAM flap** (transverse rectus abdominis myocutaneous flap) is a **pedicled flap** of the skin, subcutaneous fat, and rectus abdominis muscle, used to reconstruct the breast following mastectomy.

A **DIEP flap** (deep inferior epigastric perforator) is a **free flap** of the skin and subcutaneous fat (but without harvesting the rectus abdominis muscle). It is transferred from the lower abdomen to the anterior chest wall, following mastectomy. This is a lengthy operation, using a microsurgical technique to anastomose the deep inferior epigastric vessels to blood vessels in the anterior chest, e.g., the internal thoracic vessels.

RECTUS SHEATH HAEMATOMA

- Bleeding within the rectus sheath, usually unilateral.
- Follows strenuous contraction and rupture of the epigastric vessels.
- May cause clinical confusion because this condition is an uncommon cause of abdominal pain, and therefore may be misdiagnosed. Imaging with ultrasound scan (USS) or computed tomography (CT) scan helps in reaching a diagnosis and avoiding unnecessary explorative laparotomy.
- Patients undergoing anticoagulant therapy are at higher risk, due to larger haematoma formation and comorbidities.

COMMON SURGICAL INCISIONS

With the advances in keyhole surgery (minimally invasive surgery), fewer open procedures are being performed. Open abdominal surgery remains an important part of emergency surgery for different indications, however, such as trauma and acute abdomen.

Midline incision

Midline incision, **through the linea alba**, gives excellent access to the abdominal cavity. It is relatively easy to perform (and to extend, if needed) and causes minimal blood loss; this is ideal for emergency surgery.

The skin incision skirts the umbilicus to avoid wound contamination and difficult wound closure.

Gridiron incision

Gridiron (McBurney's) incision is located one-third of the distance between the ASIS and the umbilicus.

It entails incising the aponeurosis of the external oblique along the wound and splitting the internal oblique and transversus muscle fibres to access the peritoneal cavity.

McBurney's incision is classically used for open appendectomy (Figure 5.10).

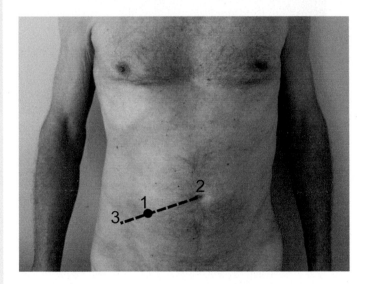

FIGURE 5.10 McBurney's point (1), umbilicus (2), ASIS (3). (Courtesy of Philip J. Adds.)

Lanz's incision is a modification of the gridiron incision, being in the crease line of the skin; it provides better cosmetic results.

Other incisions, such as subcostal (Kocher's incision), paramedian, and transverse, are less commonly performed.

Nowadays there is more emphasis on laparoscopic (keyhole) surgery to avoid unnecessary damage to the abdominal wall, less postoperative pain, quicker postoperative recovery, and shorter hospital stays.

Closure of abdominal incisions can be followed by complications of wound failure, e.g., wound infection, burst abdomen, and incisional hernia.

BURST ABDOMEN

Burst abdomen is one of the complications that can follow laparotomy, as the abdominal wound opens up. It can be complete dehiscence or partial (**Figures 5.11** and **5.12**).

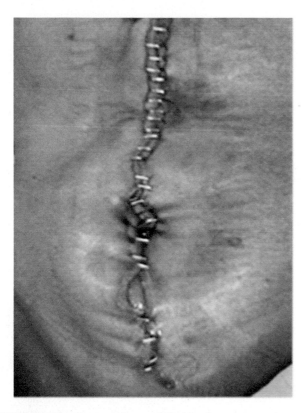

FIGURE 5.11 Burst abdomen following laparotomy via a midline incision, with knuckle of small bowel protruding. (Courtesy of Wan Khamizar.)

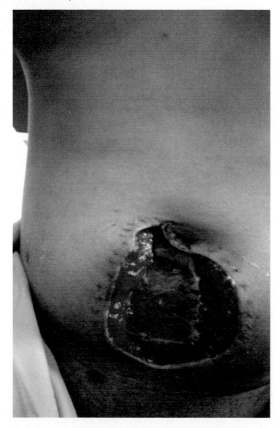

FIGURE 5.12 Partial abdominal wall dehiscence following lower midline incision laparotomy for perforated appendix. Note the exposed rectus abdominis muscle. (Courtesy of Qassim F. Baker.)

Peritoneum

Visceral and Parietal Layers

The peritoneum is a serous membrane (single layer of mesothelial cells on a connective tissue base) which covers the abdominal cavity and its contents. It is composed of two continuous layers: the visceral and parietal layers.

The **visceral layer** surrounds the viscera in the abdominopelvic cavity, whilst the **parietal layer** covers the internal surface of the abdominal wall.

Embryologically, the parietal layer arises from the somatic mesoderm, whilst the visceral layer arises from the splanchnic mesoderm.

Due to its embryological origin, the parietal layer receives the same blood and lymphatic and somatic nerve supply as the region of the abdominal wall it covers, whilst the visceral layer receives the same neurovascular supply as the organs that it covers.

The parietal peritoneum is sensitive to changes in pressure, temperature, and stretching, whilst the visceral peritoneum is only sensitive to distension and chemical irritation. The parietal peritoneum of the abdominal cavity is supplied by the same somatic nerves that supply the overlying skin (T7–L1), except for the central part of the diaphragmatic peritoneum, which is supplied by the phrenic nerve, while the peripheral part is still supplied by T7. The pelvic peritoneum is supplied by branches from the obturator nerve (L2–L4).

Somatic pain felt from irritation of the parietal peritoneum is well localised, whilst visceral pain felt from damaging the visceral peritoneum is poorly localised and is referred to areas of the skin that are supplied by the same nerve root.

Peritoneal Cavity

The peritoneal cavity is a potential space which exists between the visceral and parietal layers of the peritoneum. It contains a small amount of fluid, which is important for lubrication of the two layers, *vide infra*, ascites.

The abdominal cavity is the largest serous cavity of the human body. The total surface area of the peritoneum in adults approximates the surface area of skin (1.5 to 2 m²).

The parietal peritoneum comprises about 30% of the whole peritoneum and receives its blood supply from the blood vessels of the abdominal wall.

The visceral peritoneum represents the rest of the whole peritoneal surface, and its arterial supply comes from the three arteries of the gut (coeliac trunk, superior mesenteric, and inferior mesenteric arteries).

Do not confuse the abdominal cavity with the peritoneal cavity, as the abdominal cavity is composed of both the peritoneal cavity and the space behind it (the retroperitoneal space).

Intraperitoneal Organs versus Retroperitoneal Organs

Intraperitoneal organs are present within the peritoneal cavity and are attached to the abdominal wall via a mesentery (e.g., the jejunum, ileum, and transverse and sigmoid colon) or greater and lesser omenta (the stomach and first inch of the duodenum). The liver is an intraperitoneal organ, except for the bare area posteriorly (see later). The spleen is an intraperitoneal organ.

Retroperitoneal organs are present behind the peritoneal cavity, such that the anterior surface of the respective organ is covered by parietal peritoneum. Examples include the kidneys, suprarenal glands, ureters, bladder, and upper rectum. The abdominal aorta, including its terminal divisions (the common iliac and external and internal iliac arteries), inferior vena cava (IVC), and common and internal and external iliac veins are all retroperitoneal.

Secondary retroperitoneal organs are organs which were originally intraperitoneal. However, during embryological development, the mesentery of these organs became fused with the posterior abdominal wall, causing these organs to become retroperitoneal in nature. Examples include most of the duodenum, the pancreas, and ascending and descending colon (mnemonic: PCD for pancreas, colon, and duodenum).

Peritoneal Attachments

A peritoneal attachment is a double fold of peritoneum. Three types of peritoneal attachments can be found (mesentery, omentum, and peritoneal ligaments) (**Figure 5.13**).

A **mesentery** is a peritoneal attachment that usually connects an organ to the posterior abdominal wall. Examples include small bowel (jejunum and ileum), transverse mesocolon, and sigmoid mesocolon. It is important to note that mesenteries are important in transmitting neurovascular structures and lymphatics to their respective organs.

An **omentum** is a peritoneal attachment which connects the greater and lesser curvatures of the stomach to the transverse colon and liver, respectively.

Other examples of peritoneal folds are **peritoneal ligaments**, including the falciform ligament, coronary, and triangular ligaments (*vide infra*).

Greater Omentum

The greater omentum is an apron-like fold of peritoneum which arises from the greater curvature of the stomach and rolls up to the transverse colon. It hangs from the transverse colon and forms part of inflammatory masses, such as the appendicular mass in the right iliac fossa (RIF). This is why it is referred to as the "abdominal policeman", because it helps to localise infection, preventing its spread across the peritoneal cavity.

- It can be divided into three main components (gastrocolic, gastrosplenic, and gastrophrenic ligaments) depending on its attachment point.

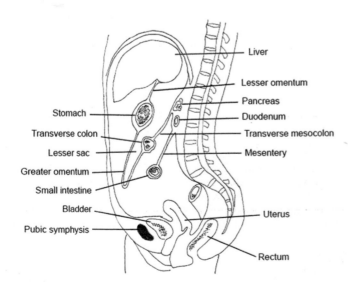

FIGURE 5.13 Sagittal section of the abdomen showing the arrangements of the peritoneum in a female. (Courtesy of Ho Chun.)

- It serves as a site for the storage of fatty deposits and is also involved in producing an immune response against foreign material (contains a macrophage collection).

Lesser Omentum

The lesser omentum is a double fold of peritoneum which arises from the lesser curvature of the stomach and the first inch of the first part of the duodenum and extends to the liver.

The lesser omentum is composed of two ligaments: the hepatogastric and hepatoduodenal ligaments.

Three important structures pass in the free margin of the lesser omentum:

- Common bile duct (CBD)
- Common hepatic artery (anteriorly)
- Portal vein (posteriorly)

Bleeding from the gallbladder during cholecystectomy can be controlled by gentle bidigital pressure or after applying a soft clamp to the free border of the lesser omentum through the epiploic foramen (of Winslow) and is traditionally known as **Pringle's manoeuvre**.

Divisions of the Peritoneal Cavity

The peritoneal cavity can be divided into greater and lesser sacs.

The greater sac forms the largest portion of the peritoneal cavity. It is divided into two compartments (supracolic and infracolic) by the mesentery of the transverse colon (the transverse mesocolon).

The two compartments communicate with each other via the right and left paracolic gutters.

The infracolic compartment is further subdivided into right and left infracolic compartments by the mesentery of the small intestines.

The lesser sac (omental bursa) is the space behind the lesser omentum and the stomach. It is the smaller of the two sacs.

Epiploic Foramen

The lesser sac communicates with the greater sac via the epiploic foramen or aditus to the lesser sac, which is **located posterior to the free edge of the hepatoduodenal ligament**.

Boundaries of the epiploic foramen are:

- *Anterior:* hepatoduodenal ligament (medial part of the lesser omentum)
- *Posterior:* parietal peritoneum, which covers the IVC
- *Superior:* visceral peritoneum, which covers the caudate lobe of the liver
- *Inferior:* visceral peritoneum, which covers the first part (superior aspect) of the duodenum

CLINICAL NOTES

Pseudocyst *vide infra*, anatomy of the pancreas.

Paracolic gutters are recesses between the lateral aspects of the ascending and descending colon and the lateral abdominal wall.

These gutters form pathways for the flow of ascitic fluid and intraperitoneal infections (e.g., following perforation of the appendix or a hollow viscus such as perforated duodenal ulcer).

PERITONITIS

Peritonitis is inflammation of the peritoneum which, in the majority of cases, follows the spread of infection from:

- Abdominal organs such as the vermiform appendix (acute appendicitis is still the most common cause of acute abdomen that needs surgical intervention).
- Perforated hollow viscera such as the stomach and duodenum (peptic ulcers), colon (colonic cancer, diverticulitis), ruptured gallbladder, and intraperitoneal urinary bladder rupture.
- Infection may spread from female genital organs (see **Section 6**).

Peritonitis and pus collection may stay localised to one part of the peritoneal cavity, such as the pelvis (pelvic peritonitis), or it may spread to a larger area (generalised peritonitis), which carries a poor prognosis due to septicaemia (absorption of bacterial toxins into the circulation) and the development of liver abscesses through the spread of infection via the portal vein (portal pyaemia).

Chemical peritonitis follows spillage of irritant substances such as gastric juices, including hydrochloric acid, with early perforated gastric or duodenal ulcer; bile (ruptured gallbladder or liver trauma); or urine (intraperitoneal bladder rupture) into the peritoneal cavity.

Blood collection in the peritoneal cavity (haemoperitoneum) causes peritoneal irritation.

Common causes of haemoperitoneum include:

- Bleeding from ruptured viscus (injury to solid organs, e.g., the liver or spleen)
- Ruptured ectopic gestation
- Vascular accidents such as ruptured aortic abdominal aneurysm

Symptoms of peritonitis include abdominal pain, nausea, vomiting, abdominal distension, and constipation or the passage of loose stools in pelvic peritonitis.

On examination, localised or generalised tenderness and rigidity of the abdomen can be noted. Bowel sounds (borborygmi) may be absent on auscultation of the abdomen.

Since abdominal pain becomes more intense with movement, patients often lie still (in contrast to patients with biliary or ureteric colic) and may flex their knees and hips in an attempt to alleviate their pain.

Ascites is excessive fluid collection in the peritoneal cavity. General causes include liver cirrhosis (the most common cause), heart failure, and constrictive pericarditis. Local causes commonly include metastatic spread from gastrointestinal (GI) and ovarian cancers, inflammatory causes like tuberculosis (TB), and pancreatitis. Aspiration of ascitic fluid (paracentesis) can be done for diagnostic and therapeutic reasons. In classical medical teaching remembering the 5Fs helps in reaching a clinical diagnosis of distended abdomen (Fat, Fluid, Flatus, Faeces, and Fetus).

PERITONEAL DIALYSIS (PD)

Due to the large surface area of the peritoneum, it can work as one of the options in treating chronic kidney disease (CKD). Commonly, haemodialysis is performed through a vascular fistula between the radial artery and a suitable vein, such as the cephalic vein, at the wrist. PD starts with the instillation of pre-packaged fluid (dialysate), through a Tenckhoff catheter into the peritoneal cavity. The dialysis occurs between the capillaries of the peritoneum on one side and the dialysate on the other side across the semipermeable membrane (the peritoneum).

Mesenteries

Mesentery of the small intestine (mesentery proper) begins at the duodenojejunal junction, and ends at the ileocaecal junction, attaching the jejunum and ileum to the posterior abdominal wall.

The colon is primarily intraperitoneal. Only the ascending and descending colon are (secondarily) retroperitoneal, and therefore without a mesentery. The caecum is intraperitoneal, but usually lacks a mesentery.

Mesoappendix is the mesentery of the appendix. The appendicular artery (a branch of the ileocolic artery) passes through the mesoappendix. Functionally, it is an end artery, and therefore thrombosis of the appendicular artery due to acute appendicitis will lead to ischaemia and gangrene of the appendix, leading to localised or generalised peritonitis.

Transverse mesocolon and **sigmoid mesocolon** are the respective mesenteries of the transverse and sigmoid colon.

The transverse mesocolon transmits the middle colic artery, whilst the sigmoid mesocolon transmits both the sigmoidal arteries (from the inferior mesenteric artery) and the superior rectal artery (a continuation of the inferior mesenteric artery).

The **transverse mesocolon** is attached to the posterior abdominal wall and runs obliquely from the lower pole of the right kidney, across the second part of the duodenum and the pancreas, to be attached to the upper pole of the left kidney, in close proximity to the lower pole of the spleen, as often there is a ligament which connects the two structures.

The root of the **sigmoid mesocolon** forms an inverted V shape. Its apex is anterior to the left ureter and is near the division of the common iliac artery. The mobility of both the transverse and sigmoid colon helps to bring them outside the abdominal cavity when creating a stoma (colostomy).

Peritoneal Ligaments

The **falciform** (Latin: "sickle-shaped") **ligament**, a double peritoneal fold, attaches the ventral surface of the liver to the anterior abdominal wall. It is derived from the ventral mesentery of the fetus (ventral mesogastrium).

Along with the coronary ligament, it helps to divide the liver into **right and left anatomical lobes**. The falciform ligament splits into two layers. The right layer forms the upper layer of the coronary ligament and the right triangular ligament at its right corner. The left layer forms the upper layer of the left triangular ligament, which attaches the lateral part of the liver to the diaphragm.

The **round ligament** (ligamentum teres) runs along the inferior free edge of the falciform ligament. It is a remnant of the left umbilical vein which delivers oxygenated blood from the placenta to the growing fetus.

The **ligamentum venosum** is a fibrous remnant of the ductus venosus, a vein which shunts blood from the left umbilical vein to the IVC to bypass the liver sinusoids in fetal life. Note that the ligamentum venosum is not a peritoneal ligament.

The **coronary (crown-like) ligament** has anterior and posterior layers which converge on the right and left sides of the superior surface of the liver to form the **right and left triangular ligaments**, respectively. The area between the peritoneal layers of the coronary ligament is called the **bare area** of the liver (lymphatics from this area drain to the posterior mediastinal lymph nodes) (see **Figure 5.33**).

The liver can be mobilised during relevant surgical procedures by dividing these ligaments.

Umbilical Folds

Elevations of the peritoneum, referred to as folds, can found on the deep surface of the anterior abdominal wall.

A median fold, made up of the falciform ligament, can be found superior to the umbilicus.

One median, two medial, and two lateral folds can be found inferior to the umbilicus.

The median fold contains a remnant of the urachus (**median ligament**). The urachus is a canal that connects the bladder to the umbilicus in fetal life. This canal usually becomes obliterated after the 12th week of gestation to be replaced by the median ligament. Failure to do so leads to a patent urachus. Patients with this condition may leak out urine via their umbilicus.

The two medial folds contain medial umbilical ligaments which are remnants of umbilical arteries.

The two lateral folds are formed by the course of the inferior epigastric vessels toward the rectus sheath.

Blood Supply of the Abdominal Cavity

- *Arterial:* abdominal aorta and its branches
- *Venous:* IVC and hepatic portal vein

Abdominal Aorta

The descending thoracic aorta enters the abdomen through the aortic hiatus of the diaphragm at the level of T12 (tip: "aortic hiatus" has 12 letters). The aorta gives origin to:

- *Paired arteries:* middle suprarenal, renal, lumbar, inferior phrenic, and gonadal.
- *Unpaired arteries:* coeliac trunk (T12 level), superior mesenteric artery (SMA) (L2 level) and inferior mesenteric artery (IMA) (L3 level), and the small median sacral artery.

The IVC is to the right of the abdominal aorta, and both lie on the posterior abdominal wall.

The **abdominal aorta divides at the level of L4** into right and left common iliac arteries.

True aneurysm involves dilatation of all three layers of the arterial wall (intima, media, and adventitia). Subdivisions of true aneurysms include fusiform and saccular aneurysms, according to the shape. The main cause of abdominal aortic aneurysm (AAA) is atherosclerosis.

The common clinical problem which affects the abdominal aorta is leaking or ruptured AAA, most commonly infrarenal, i.e., below the origin of the renal arteries.

False or pseudoaneurysm is caused by leakage of the blood following a breach in the arterial wall but contained within the adventitia, commonly following a puncture of the wall – for example, false aneurysms of the femoral artery following intra-arterial catheterisation and injections in the groin in IV drug abusers.

Learning Point

AAA should be always looked for in patients above 60 years old who clinically present with abdominal, loin, or back pain. On examination it manifests as pulsatile supraumbilical swelling. Clinicians who overlook this condition risk the main danger of aneurysmal rupture with high morbidity and mortality. With advances in interventional radiology, most uncomplicated aneurysms are repaired with endovascular stenting (endovascular aneurysm repair [EVAR]). However, the open approach may still be necessary.

Inferior Vena Cava

The IVC is the biggest vein in the body and is formed from the union of the right and left common iliac veins **at the level of L5**.

It does not receive the corresponding veins of the coeliac trunk, SMA, and IMA, which drain to the portal vein, while the IVC receives veins corresponding to the paired arteries (see above).

The three hepatic veins drain into the IVC.

The IVC leaves the abdomen through the central tendon of the diaphragm **at the level of T8** (tip: "vena cava" has eight letters) to immediately join the right atrium.

Embryology of the Gut

The gut originates from the yolk sac. The endoderm contributes to the development of the epithelial layer, including the glands. The mesoderm forms the muscular layers and the serous layers.

The **stomach** is a dilated part of the foregut and originally has right and left surfaces related to the right and left vagus, respectively, and ventral and dorsal mesenteries. With progressive growth of the liver, the stomach rotates to the right, and the left surface becomes anterior and the right surface posterior. With the new position of the stomach, the stomach mesenteries become the greater and lesser omenta.

The **duodenum shares an origin from the foregut and midgut**. Originally, it has a dorsal mesentery, which later disappears, except for a small part at the duodenojejunal junction that forms the **suspensory ligament of Treitz**. The first part and a portion of the second part have a ventral mesentery, but only a small bit will remain as part of the lesser omentum that attaches to the first inch of the first part of the duodenum.

The midgut forms a loop to which the vitelline duct is attached. This loop is forced to herniate through the umbilical cord and leave the coelomic cavity because of the rapidly enlarging liver.

This loop has a cephalic part (jejunum and most of the ileum) and caudal part (rest of the ileum, caecum, vermiform appendix, ascending colon, and transverse colon as far as the splenic flexure). The midgut rotates around the supplying artery (SMA) a total of **270 degrees anticlockwise** (90 degrees initially and 180 degrees after returning to the abdominal cavity). The caecum and appendix are initially under the liver but later descend to the right iliac fossa, and the ascending colon is formed. The transverse colon is formed anterior to the SMA and the second part of the duodenum, but the SMA passes over the third part of the duodenum (see later discussion on superior mesenteric syndrome).

The omphalomesenteric duct connects the midgut to the yolk sac. Failure of the duct to obliterate results in Meckel's diverticulum (see later), or umbilical fistula (see later discussion on the umbilicus), or rarely, the presence of a band that connects the ileum to the umbilicus, which may allow small bowel loops to twist around it and cause small bowel obstruction.

The mesenteries are related to most of the duodenum, and the ascending and descending colon fuse with the parietal peritoneum of the posterior abdominal wall. This explains why surgeons mobilise these parts during operative procedures, such as reflecting the duodenum medially (Kocherisation).

The gut is divided into three parts according to its arterial supply:

- *Foregut*: **coeliac trunk (also known as the coeliac axis)**
- *Midgut*: **SMA**
- *Hindgut*: **IMA**

Foregut
The foregut, anatomically speaking, includes the lower oesophagus, stomach, liver, spleen, pancreas, and duodenum down to the major duodenal papilla. The foregut originally extends from the buccopharyngeal membrane to the second part of the duodenum. It is the caudal portion that gives rise to the distal end of the oesophagus, liver, pancreas, spleen, stomach, and biliary system, which all appear during weeks 4 to 5 of fetal life. **All these structures are supplied by the branches of the coeliac trunk (Figure 5.14)**.

The coeliac trunk can get compressed by the median arcuate ligament, which binds the left and right diaphragmatic crura. This can cause chronic abdominal pain after meals or activity (median arcuate ligament syndrome [MALS]).

Nerve Supply of the Gut and Pelvic Organs

Sympathetic innervation (from the thorax to the abdomen, through the diaphragm):

- The intermediolateral part of spinal segments **T1–12 and L1–L2** is responsible for the sympathetic innervation.
- They run as white (myelinated) pre-ganglionic *rami communicantes* with the ventral rami of the spinal nerves and, **without synapsing**, to the paravertebral sympathetic ganglia.

Three splanchnic nerves emerge and pass through the crura of the diaphragm and synapse as follows:

- The **greater splanchnic nerve** (T5–T9) to the coeliac ganglion
- The **lesser splanchnic nerve** (T9–T10 or T10–T11) to the aorticorenal ganglion
- The **least** (lowest) splanchnic nerve, often absent (T11–T12 or T12–L2), to synapse with the renal ganglion

The thoracic sympathetic trunk continues downwards as the lumbar and then sacral sympathetic trunk and upwards as the cervical sympathetic trunk.

The sympathetic visceral nerves contain both afferent (pain fibres) and efferent fibres.

In the abdomen:

- The **lumbar sympathetic trunk** consists of four interconnecting ganglia, which give rise to grey *rami communicantes* to the ventral rami of the lumbar nerves. These **vascular and cutaneous** post-ganglionic fibres supply the branches of the abdominal aorta in addition to the skin.

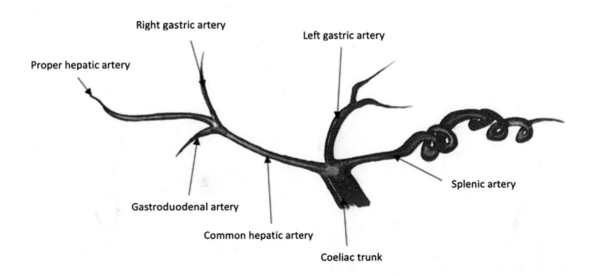

FIGURE 5.14 The branches of the coeliac trunk which supply the foregut. (Courtesy of Calum Harrington-Vogt.)

- The **lumbar splanchnic nerves** are four lumbar splanchnic nerves arising from L1–L2 spinal segments that innervate the smooth muscles and glands by joining the coeliac, inferior mesenteric (hindgut), and hypogastric plexuses (pelvic viscera, including the neck of the bladder and the prostate gland).

Parasympathetic innervation

- The **two vagi** (anterior and posterior) arise on the lower oesophagus from the oesophageal plexus and supply the foregut and midgut (down to the distal part of the transverse colon) (see **Section 6**).

Enteric Nervous System

The GI tract (GIT) from the upper oesophagus to the anus is controlled by the enteric nervous system (ENS), which is independent of the central nervous system. The autonomic nervous system (ANS) has a modulatory function. The ENS is mainly found within the myenteric plexus (Auerbach's plexus, between the longitudinal and circular muscle layers) from the upper oesophagus to the anus, and the submucous plexus (Meissner's plexus, although this can be either absent or minimal in the oesophagus and stomach).

The ENS is an autonomously operating system composed of afferent, interneurons, and efferent neurons and a huge number of small ganglia that regulate both the longitudinal and circular smooth muscle activity, bowel absorption, transmucosal fluid fluxes, and blood flow. Some scientists have nicknamed this extensive network our "second brain".

Coeliac Plexus

It is also known as the solar plexus, due to its appearance being likened to the radiation of light from the sun. This plexus is formed by the communications between the greater (T5–T9) and lesser (T10–11) splanchnic nerves and the anterior and posterior vagal trunks. It consists of ganglia and intercommunicating fibres and is located anterior to the upper abdominal aorta, behind the stomach and the lesser sac. Its branches supply the liver, pancreas, spleen, stomach, kidneys, suprarenal glands, genital organs, and midgut. Afferent nerve stimuli pass within the coeliac plexus (see "Pancreatic Cancer").

The **superior hypogastric plexus** lies over the bifurcation of the aorta in the pre-sacral space. It receives post-ganglionic sympathetic fibres from the thoracic and lumbar splanchnic nerves and parasympathetic fibres from S2 to S4 (*nervi erigentes*). It is connected to the **inferior hypogastric plexus** via two nerves (the hypogastric nerves), which pass along the internal iliac vessels. For information on the **inferior hypogastric plexus**, see **Section 6**.

Distal End of the Oesophagus

The oesophagus is a muscular tube, approximately 25 cm long, connecting the pharynx at the level of C6 to the stomach. It is formed by the diverticulum appearing in the ventral wall of the pharynx, with the tracheo-oesophageal septum splitting the pharynx into ventral and dorsal portions. The thoracic part of the oesophagus finally passes through the oesophageal hiatus, with both anterior and posterior vagi, at the level of T10 (tip: "oesophagus" has 10 letters).

The intra-abdominal segment (below the diaphragm) is short in length (1 to 2.5 cm). The oesophagogastric junction is at the level of T10–T11.

There are two high-pressure zones: at the junction of the laryngopharynx and oesophagus and at the lower oesophageal sphincter (LOS).

Gross Anatomy of the Distal End of the Oesophagus
Four layers

- *Mucosa (inner layer):* lined by non-keratinised squamous epithelium.
- *Submucosa:* contains the mucous glands, which produce mucus from goblet cells to moisturise the oesophagus, in addition to the extensive vascular (arterial and venous) networks and nerve cells (Meissner's plexus).
- *Muscularis (muscular layer):* composed of outer longitudinal and inner circular smooth muscle. Helps in peristaltic movements to push the food bolus toward the stomach. The muscularis of the upper part is skeletal (striated) and that of the middle part is mixed.
- *Adventitia (outer layer):* a fibrous layer which attaches the oesophagus to adjacent structures. The phreno-oesophageal ligament connects the lower oesophagus to the oesophageal diaphragmatic hiatus.

The **lower oesophageal sphincter (LOS)** is a physiological, rather than an anatomical, sphincter. The LOS relaxes to allow food to enter the stomach and constricts to prevent reflux of acid and stomach contents up the oesophagus. There are at least two components: the first is intrinsic, from the circular muscle of the lower oesophagus, and the second is extrinsic, due to the encircling right crus of the diaphragm. The LOS represents a high-pressure zone between the negative intrathoracic pressure transmitted to the thoracic part of the oesophagus and the positive pressure of the short intra-abdominal oesophagus.

The LOS is supplied by the ANS (vagi and sympathetic fibres from the greater and lesser splanchnic nerves T5–T12) in addition to its intrinsic nervous system.

The anterior vagus is closely related to the outer surface of the outer longitudinal muscle, but the posterior vagus lies loose behind and to the right of the oesophagus (see the later discussion on truncal vagotomy).

On oesophagogastroduodenoscopy (OGD), the transition from the oesophageal mucosa to gastric mucosa is manifested by a colour change from pale pink mucosa to deeper-coloured gastric mucosa (the zigzag or Z-line).

Blood Supply

The abdominal part of the oesophagus is supplied by the oesophageal branches of the left gastric artery, which arises from the coeliac trunk, as well as branches from the short gastric arteries. There is also some contribution from the left phrenic artery.

Venous drainage of the abdominal portion occurs through the left gastric vein draining into the hepatic portal vein and to the azygos and hemiazygos venous system. The connection with the oesophageal tributaries that drain into the azygos/hemiazygos venous system forms part of the portosystemic connection, which opens up in **portal hypertension** (oesophageal varices) and can cause vomiting of blood (haematemesis).

Nerve Supply and Lymph Drainage

The oesophagus is innervated by both parasympathetic (vagus) and sympathetic (afferent and efferent) fibres (greater and lesser splanchnic nerves). The vagi are the predominate motor innervation to the oesophagus.

The lymph drainage of the lower third of the oesophagus is to the left gastric and coeliac nodes. In lower oesophageal cancer, the mediastinal lymph nodes may also be involved.

CLINICAL NOTES

GASTRO-OESOPHAGEAL REFLUX DISEASE (GORD)

Stomach contents, including gastric acid, flow back into the oesophagus.

BARRETT'S OESOPHAGUS

The cells lining the oesophagus switch from normal stratified squamous to simple columnar epithelium and goblet cells (metaplasia), due to chronic reflux of gastric acid up the oesophagus, which can accompany sliding hiatus hernia (see next). This is a pre-cancerous condition. Patients with this condition need a regular upper endoscopy and biopsy to detect malignant changes.

HIATUS HERNIA

There are two main types:

Sliding hiatus hernia

- The most common form
- LOS slides upwards, resulting in reflux oesophagitis

Rolling hiatus hernia

- Para-oesophageal hernia
- Part of the stomach squeezes through the oesophageal hiatus of the diaphragm, which can result in serious complications due to the blood supply being cut off, causing ischaemia of that part of the stomach. This is a surgical emergency (**Figure 5.15**)

CANCER OF THE OESOPHAGUS

The cardia is a common site for the development of oesophageal cancer (**Figure 5.16**) (see also **Section 2**). The main symptom is an increasing dysphagia to both solids and liquids and weight loss.

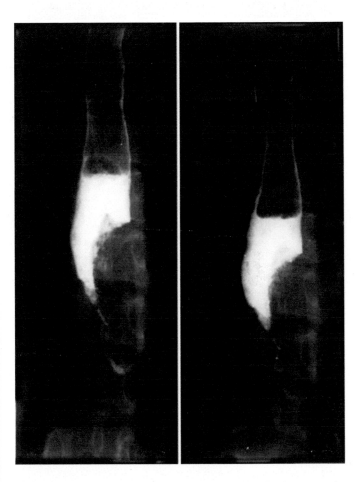

FIGURE 5.16   Contrast X-ray (barium swallow) of an oesophageal cancer, showing filling defect and rat-tail appearance. (Courtesy of Qassim F. Baker.)

ACHALASIA

This is failure of the LOS to relax. It is due to absent or a low number of ganglion cells of the myenteric plexus at the LOS, resulting in difficulty in swallowing (dysphagia) and regurgitation of undigested food and even aspiration to the respiratory passages (**Figure 5.17**).

Investigation of patients who present with persistent dysphagia include endoscopic examination of the oesophagus, stomach, and duodenum. This is performed by inserting a flexible fibreoptic endoscope through the mouth down to the pharynx and the oesophagus to check for abnormalities like growths and also to take samples for histopathological examination (biopsy). Depending on the extent of oesophageal blockage, the examination is extended down to the stomach and duodenum.

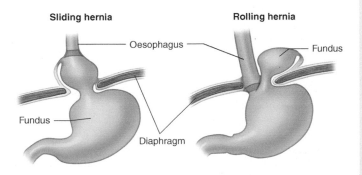

FIGURE 5.15   Types of hiatus hernias. (Courtesy of Calum Harrington-Vogt.)

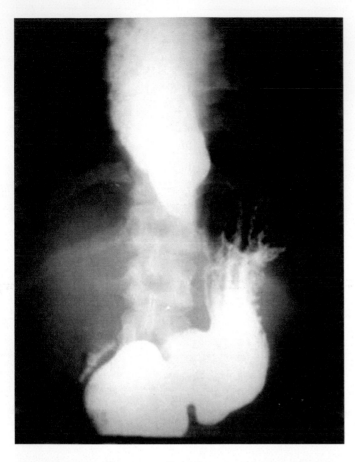

FIGURE 5.17 Barium swallow showing dilated oesophagus due to achalasia. (Courtesy of Qassim F. Baker.)

Stomach

The stomach is a hollow muscular organ located in the upper abdomen towards the left hypochondrium. It is the part of the foregut which extends from the distal oesophagus to the duodenum. Its functions include:

- Mechanical degradation of food
- Production of mucus, protecting the mucosa from the noxious action of hydrochloric acid (HCl)
- HCl production from parietal cells
- Pepsin production from the chief cells as an inactive form (to change to an active form of pepsinogen in the acidic environment created by HCl and start protein digestion to smaller peptides and amino acids)
- Endocrine secretions, e.g., gastrin, hormone secretion from G cells at the pyloric antrum (to stimulate HCl secretion)
- Secretion of intrinsic factor for vitamin B_{12} absorption

The stomach is related posteriorly mainly to the lesser sac and the pancreas and is divided into four regions: cardia, fundus, body, and pylorus.

- The **cardia** is the region adjacent to the oesophageal opening, where the stratified squamous epithelium of the oesophagus changes to simple columnar epithelium.

- The **fundus** is the most superior, dome-shaped part of the stomach to the left of the cardia and related to the left dome of the diaphragm.
- The **greater curvature** extends from the left of the gastro-esophageal junction over the fundus to the pylorus.
- The **body** is the largest region of the stomach and extends to the *incisura angularis* at the lesser curvature. The body of the stomach is involved in the digestion of food through the action of acid, enzymes, and mechanical degradation.
- The **lesser curvature** starts at the cardia down to the pylorus and is shorter than the greater curvature.
- The **pyloric region** is a continuation of the distal part of the body of the stomach from the *incisura angularis* to the pylorus. It starts with the **pyloric antrum**, moves to the **pyloric canal** (1 to 2 cm), and ends at the **pyloric sphincter or pylorus** (anatomical and physiological sphincter between the stomach and the duodenum composed of smooth muscle controlling the release of chyme from the stomach). The pyloric sphincter is under neural (vagal and sympathetic) and hormonal control.

The gastric wall consists of four layers (Figure 5.18).

The **mucosa** is the thick innermost layer. It consists of simple columnar epithelium and goblet cells (mucus production is important in mucosal protection by neutralising acid). In addition, there is a deeper lamina propria, which is loosely adherent to the mucosa and to a thin layer of smooth muscle called the muscularis mucosa. Folds of the inner surface of the stomach are known as **rugae**, and these can expand to accommodate large volumes of food intake.

The second layer is the **submucosa**, and it consists of fibrous connective tissue and the submucosal nerve plexus, or **Meissner's plexus** (part of the ENS).

The **muscular layer** is composed of inner oblique smooth muscle and is responsible for mechanical degradation of the solid luminal bolus. The middle layer is circular, and at the pylorus it forms the pyloric sphincter. The outermost layer is longitudinal and is responsible for peristaltic contraction.

Auerbach's or myenteric plexus is part of the ENS.

The **serosa (visceral peritoneum)** is the outermost layer. The stomach is completely covered by the visceral peritoneum, except for a very small area near the cardiac orifice posteriorly. The peritoneum leaves the greater curvature as the greater omentum, which hangs down like an apron to roll back and attach to the transverse colon and the gastrosplenic omentum (see above).

The visceral peritoneum leaves the lesser curvature as the lesser omentum.

The main anatomical relations of the stomach are:

- *Anteriorly:* the left lobe of the liver and the anterior abdominal wall
- *Superiorly:* oesophagus and left dome of the diaphragm
- *Inferiorly:* head and neck of the pancreas (within the curve of the duodenum)
- *Posteriorly:* the lesser sac separates the stomach from the anterior surface of the pancreas, splenic artery, visceral surface of the spleen, left suprarenal gland, and upper pole of the left kidney (stomach bed)

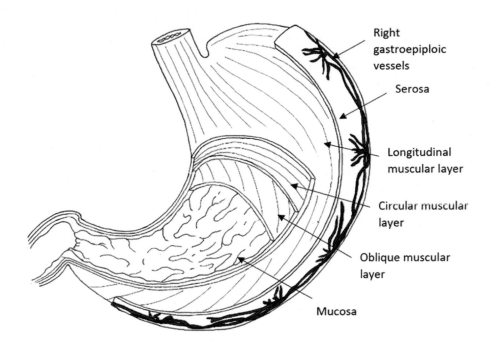

FIGURE 5.18   Layers of the stomach. (Courtesy of Calum Harrington-Vogt.)

Arterial Blood Supply and Venous Drainage

The stomach has a generous blood supply derived from the branches of the coeliac trunk. The arteries freely anastomose (**Figure 5.19**).

The lesser curvature of the stomach receives blood from the anastomoses of the **left and right gastric arteries** (within the layers of the lesser omentum).

The greater curvature of the stomach receives blood from the anastomoses of the **left and right gastro-epiploic arteries**. The **gastroduodenal artery** supplies the pyloric part of the stomach.

Origin of arteries:

- Coeliac trunk → left gastric artery
- Splenic artery → left gastro-epiploic artery and the short gastric arteries
- Common hepatic artery → right gastric artery and gastro-duodenal artery → right gastro-epiploic artery

Venous drainage is via the accompanying veins, which finally drain to the hepatic portal vein. The short gastric veins drain the fundus and upper part of the stomach and drain into the splenic vein.

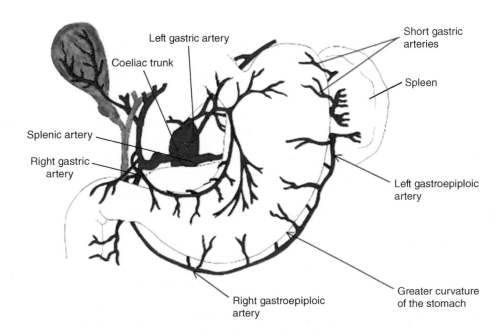

FIGURE 5.19   Arterial blood supply of the stomach. (Courtesy of Calum Harrington-Vogt.)

Nerve Supply

From both the parasympathetic fibres (vagus) and sympathetic fibres (greater and lesser splanchnic nerves via the coeliac plexus). The vagi are responsible for the motility and acid/pepsin secretion in the stomach. Truncal vagotomy, an operation to cut both vagi above the cardia, although now rarely performed, is used to treat patients with peptic ulcers, to decrease HCl secretion, and to help heal gastric and duodenal ulcerations. This operation has largely been superseded by the use of proton pump inhibitors (PPIs).

The sympathetic supply is inhibitory to the muscles of the stomach and constricts the pylorus. It also transmits the afferent pain fibres from the stomach.

Lymph Drainage

Lymphatic drainage is to the nodes found on the greater and lesser curvatures. These then drain to the coeliac lymph nodes, important when radical gastrectomy is considered for gastric cancers.

CLINICAL NOTES

Gastric cancers are mainly epithelial (carcinoma). They can cause a variety of presentations, such as iron deficiency anaemia (due to chronic blood loss), obstruction of the gastric outflow (gastric outlet obstruction), or GI bleeding (haematemesis/melaena). They are often diagnosed at a late stage and carry a poor prognosis. In countries with a high incidence of gastric carcinoma such as Japan, endoscopic screening is utilised to detect the cancer at an early stage. Endoscopic mucosal resection (EMR) is one of the options for treating early gastric and oesophageal cancers. Other malignant tumours include gastric lymphoma (the stomach is the most common site for extranodal non-Hodgkin's lymphoma).

Pyloric stenosis (gastric outlet obstruction) is a blockage to the flow of partially digested food to the duodenum. This can be an acquired condition, due to scarring from chronic duodenal ulcer, or cancer of the distal part of the stomach (**Figure 5.20**).

Congenital pyloric stenosis (**Figure 5.21**) results in projectile **bile-free vomiting**, usually within the first 4 weeks after birth. This is due to idiopathic hypertrophy of the circular muscle of the pylorus. Pyloromyotomy (division of the thickened pylorus) is the surgical procedure used following correction of water and electrolyte abnormalities, as the result of repeated vomiting.

GASTROSTOMY FEEDING

This is one of the forms of enteral nutrition used when it is not possible to take food by mouth, for example, in patients with stroke and dysphagia.

Percutaneous endoscopic gastrostomy (PEG) is performed with the help of a gastroscope to insert a feeding tube through the anterior abdominal wall into the stomach. Further tubes may be extended through the pylorus and the duodenum into the jejunum (PEG-J tube).

Rarely, the gastrostomy is done as an open procedure.

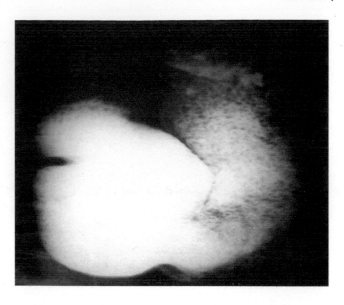

FIGURE 5.20 Barium meal of a 50-year-old adult with repeated vomiting showing dilated stomach and cut-off at the gastroduodenal junction. Gastroscopy and biopsy revealed antral cancer. (Courtesy of Qassim F. Baker.)

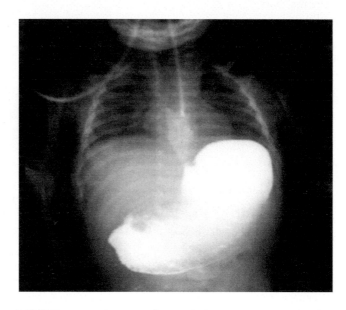

FIGURE 5.21 Gastrografin meal showing congenital pyloric stenosis in a 4-week-old child. (Courtesy of Qassim F. Baker.)

Duodenum

The duodenum (from Latin, with its length being equivalent to the breadth of approximately 12 fingers) is the first segment of the small intestine which originates from both the foregut and midgut. It is a C-shaped tube about 25 cm in length which starts from the pylorus of the stomach and ends at the duodenojejunal junction (DJJ), connecting the stomach to the jejunum of the small intestine. It consists of a proximal and distal part, in which the proximal part starts at the pylorus and ends at the major duodenal papilla.

Gross Anatomy of the Duodenum

By convention, the duodenum is divided into four parts, D1 to D4 (superior, descending, horizontal, and ascending) (**Figure 5.22**).

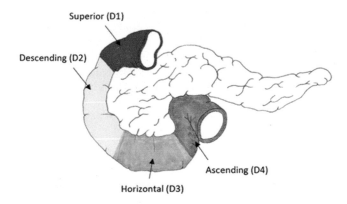

FIGURE 5.22 Parts of the duodenum. (Courtesy of Calum Harrington-Vogt.)

D1: superior Part (L1 Level)

Starts from the end of the pylorus of the stomach and ends at the superior duodenal flexure.

It passes superiorly, and the first inch (the duodenal cap) attaches to the liver by the hepatoduodenal ligament (part of the lesser omentum) and is intraperitoneal.

The first part of the duodenum is the most common site for duodenal ulceration (DU) and its complications such as bleeding, perforation, and gastric outlet obstruction.

Peptic Ulcer

An ulcer is a discontinuity in the epithelial lining (skin or mucosa). The current theory for the cause of gastric and duodenal ulcers is due to the presence of *Helicobacter pylori*, a type of gram-negative bacteria. Other causes include disruption between the balance of the amount of acid produced and the production of the mucus barrier (which offers protection) caused by the ingestion of medications like non-steroidal anti-inflammatory drugs (NSAIDs) such as aspirin, which damage the mucosa.

The gastroduodenal artery passes behind this part, which can bleed profusely with a penetrating posteriorly sited duodenal ulcer, resulting in vomiting of blood (**haematemesis**) and the passage of black tarry stool (**melaena**), due to the digestion of haemoglobin by the gastric and intestinal secretions (*vide infra*, upper and lower GI bleeding). Also, a peptic ulcer sited anteriorly in the first inch of D1 may perforate into the peritoneal cavity causing peritonitis (**Figures 5.23–5.25**).

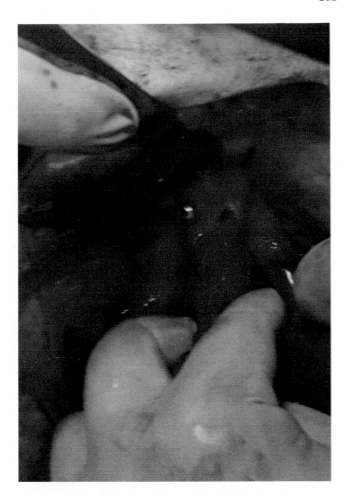

FIGURE 5.24 Operative view of perforated ulcer in the anterior part of the first part of the duodenum. (Courtesy of Ali M. Hassan.)

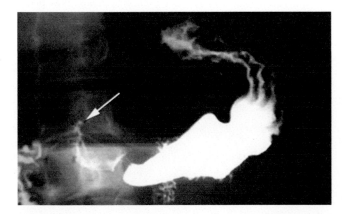

FIGURE 5.23 Barium meal showing ulcer crater *(arrow)* in the first part of the duodenum. (Courtesy of Qassim F. Baker.)

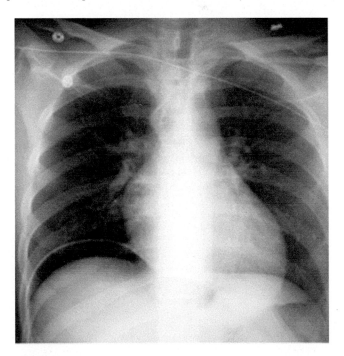

FIGURE 5.25 Chest X-ray showing air under the right dome of the diaphragm due to perforated duodenal ulcer. (Courtesy of Qassim F. Baker.)

D2: Descending Part (Extends from L1 to L3)

Starts at the superior duodenal flexure and ends at the inferior duodenal flexure. Passes inferiorly, lateral to the head of the pancreas, and overlies the hilum of the right kidney and IVC.

Contains the **major duodenal papilla**, which demarcates the opening of the CBD and the main pancreatic duct (ampulla of Vater) and the beginning of the midgut.

The peritoneum covers its anterior aspect. This part can be mobilised by incising the peritoneum on its lateral aspect and reflecting the duodenum medially (this procedure is called **Kocher's manoeuvre** which helps in surgical exposure of the lower end of the CBD).

Carcinoma of the head of the pancreas can compress the duodenum (duodenal obstruction), and it is an important cause of obstructive jaundice.

D3: Inferior Part (At the Level of L3)

Starts at the inferior duodenal flexure. Passes to the left and anteriorly to the IVC and aorta. The SMA, originating from the anterior aspect of the abdominal aorta, can compress this part of the duodenum and cause partial or complete duodenal obstruction (superior mesenteric syndrome).

D4: ascending Part (Extends from L3 to L2)

Ascends anteriorly towards the duodenojejunal junction, where it ends. The DJJ is the demarcation point between upper and lower GI bleeding.

The **ligament of Treitz** (or suspensory ligament of the duodenum) is formed of double folds of the peritoneum; it suspends the fourth part of the duodenum to form the DJJ and marks the origin of the jejunum.

Blood Supply and Venous Drainage

The proximal part of the duodenum (ending at the major duodenal papilla) receives its blood supply from the superior pancreaticoduodenal artery, which is a branch of the gastroduodenal artery, arising from the common hepatic artery.

The proximal part of the duodenum's venous drainage occurs at the prepyloric vein and the superior pancreaticoduodenal vein, which both drain into the hepatic portal vein.

The part of the duodenum which originates from the midgut receives arterial supply from the inferior pancreaticoduodenal (from the SMA). Its venous drainage is to the portal vein.

Nerve Supply and Lymphatic Drainage

The duodenum is innervated by both sympathetic (greater and lesser splanchnic nerves) and parasympathetic fibres from the vagus (via the coeliac plexus).

Lymphatic drainage is to the pancreaticoduodenal lymph nodes.

Learning Point

The major duodenal papilla is the line of demarcation between the foregut and midgut.

CLINICAL NOTES

UPPER GI BLEEDING

Refers to gut bleeding proximal to the DJJ. Common causes include bleeding peptic ulcers, variceal bleeding due to portal hypertension, gastric tumours, and Mallory-Weiss syndrome (tear at the gastro-oesophageal junction, usually following severe vomiting and retching).

LOWER GI BLEEDING

Refers to bleeding distal to the DJJ (common causes are diverticular disease, colonic polyps and cancer, angiodysplasia, and bleeding from a Meckel's diverticulum). The presentation can be acute with passing fresh blood per rectum (haematochezia) or as chronic loss (which results in iron deficiency anaemia; a common example is right colonic cancer). Note that severe upper GI bleeding may present as bleeding per rectum.

Duodenal atresia is a congenital condition due to failure of canalisation of the duodenum, usually distal to the major duodenal papilla. The new-born baby is presented with bile-stained vomiting (compare with congenital pyloric stenosis, see above).

The Pancreas

The pancreas is a long organ that develops from both the dorsal and ventral mesogastria as dorsal and ventral buds. It lies deeply seated on the posterior abdominal wall in the upper abdomen, behind the stomach. It is a secondarily retroperitoneal organ which has both endocrine (secretion of insulin and glucagon by the islet cells of Langerhans to regulate blood sugar level) and exocrine (release of enzymes for the digestion of lipids, proteins, and carbohydrates) functions.

Gross Anatomy of the Pancreas

The pancreas can be divided into the following parts (**Figure 5.26**):

- *Head:* embraced by the C-shaped duodenum.
- *Neck:* the junction between the head and the body of the pancreas; it overlies the origin of the portal vein.

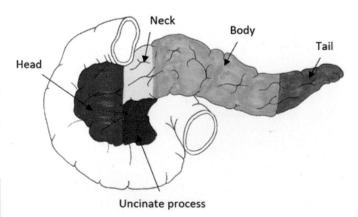

FIGURE 5.26 Parts of the pancreas. (Courtesy of Calum Harrington-Vogt.)

- *Body:* the largest part, which lies behind the stomach, anterior to the aorta and the emerging SMA. The transverse mesocolon attaches to the anterior surface of the pancreas. The splenic artery runs a tortuous course along the superior border of the body, and the splenic vein runs posteriorly and indents the body.
- *Tail:* it is related to the hilum of the spleen, so it needs to be protected during splenectomy to avoid postoperative pancreatic fistula.

The uncinate (*Latin:* "hook") process is that part of the head which lies posterior to the superior mesenteric vessels.

Blood Supply and Lymphatic Drainage

The pancreas receives its blood supply mainly from the pancreatic branches of the splenic artery. The head receives an additional blood supply from the anterior and posterior superior pancreaticoduodenal and inferior pancreaticoduodenal arteries, which arise from the gastroduodenal and superior mesenteric arteries, respectively.

Venous drainage of the pancreas is via the splenic vein, which drains into the hepatic portal vein.

The lymphatic drainage of the pancreas is to the pancreaticosplenic nodes and pyloric nodes. Both drain into the coeliac and superior mesenteric lymph nodes.

Nerve Supply

The pancreas's nerve supply comes from the parasympathetic fibres (vagus) and sympathetic fibres (thoracic splanchnic nerves and then coeliac plexus).

Duct System

Due to the double embryological origin of the pancreas, there are two pancreatic ducts.

The **main pancreatic duct** (MPD) (of Wirsung) unites with the lower CBD in a common channel arrangement (ampulla of Vater) to open in the second part of the duodenum at the major duodenal papilla. The entrance is surrounded by smooth muscle (sphincter of Oddi).

The current view is that common channel obstruction, most commonly by gallstones, explains the pathogenesis of acute pancreatitis through reflux of bile and pancreatic juice into the main pancreatic duct.

The **accessory pancreatic duct** (of Santorini) is variably present. It drains part of the head of the pancreas and opens in the duodenum at the minor duodenal papilla, 2 cm proximal to the opening of the common channel of the CBD and MPD.

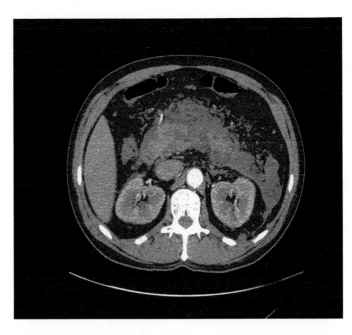

FIGURE 5.27 CT scan of the abdomen showing necrosis of the pancreas and extensive peri-pancreatic inflammatory change in a patient with acute pancreatitis. (Courtesy of Qassim F. Baker.)

PANCREATIC PSEUDOCYST

This is a collection of fluid in the lesser sac, commonly following acute pancreatitis or pancreatic trauma. Perforated posterior gastric ulcer is another rare cause. It is clinically manifested as a mass in the epigastric region a few weeks after the onset of the acute pancreatitis.

Imaging (ultrasound or CT scan) is required to establish the diagnosis.

Due to the position of the cyst posterior to the stomach, open surgical drainage may be performed via the posterior gastric wall (cystogastrostomy) if the cyst has not resolved. The pseudocyst may be dealt with laparoscopically, depending on the availability of the expertise and resources.

PANCREATIC CANCER

This is an aggressive type of cancer with a poor prognosis. The clinical presentation depends on the location of the cancer:

- Cancer of the head of the pancreas (the most common site) usually presents as obstructive jaundice due to obstruction of the lower part of the CBD.
- Carcinoma of the body of the pancreas has a poor prognosis, as it is usually diagnosed at an advanced stage, where the tumour invades the great vessels and makes resection impossible. Cancer of the body and tail presents as severe upper abdominal pain, which radiates to the back.
- Weight and appetite loss are important clinical features (the same applies to gastric cancer).

(Continued)

CLINICAL NOTES

Acute pancreatitis is autodigestion of the pancreatic tissue, mostly caused by gallstones or high alcohol consumption. Most cases are treated conservatively and rarely need urgent surgical intervention. An abdominal CT scan (**Figure 5.27**) helps in reaching a diagnosis in addition to raised serum amylase level. There are many scoring systems in clinical practice that assess the severity of acute pancreatitis.

Rarely, curative surgery is possible (**Figure 5.28**); usually, only palliative treatment is possible.

Due to the location of the pancreas on the posterior abdominal wall and its proximity to the coeliac plexus, intractable pain can result from widespread local metastasis. Coeliac plexus block is one of the options to alleviate the pain.

WHIPPLE'S PROCEDURE (PANCREATICODUODENOECTOMY)

This procedure entails removal of the head of the pancreas, duodenum, gallbladder and lower part of the CBD and sometimes the distal part of the stomach. It is indicated for operable cancer with no invasion of the portal vein or the superior mesenteric vessels. The stomach, bile duct, and MPD are then joined to the bowel. This operation is performed either as an open or laparoscopic procedure.

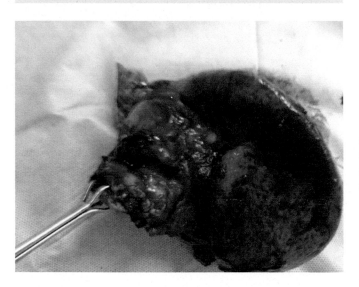

FIGURE 5.28 Distal pancreatectomy and splenectomy for cancer of the pancreatic tail. (Courtesy of Aqeel S. Mahmood.)

The Spleen

The spleen is an intraperitoneal organ and the largest of the lymphoid organs. It is surrounded by a thin capsule. It develops from the dorsal mesogastrium during the fifth week of gestation. It is located in the upper left quadrant of the abdominal cavity, between the fundus of the stomach and the left dome of the diaphragm. The spleen has immunological and haematological functions (see the discussion on post-splenectomy sepsis).

1, 3, 5, 7, 9, and 11 Rule of the Spleen:

- *1, 3, 5:* the dimensions of the spleen are $1 \times 3 \times 5$ inches.
- *7:* the spleen weighs around 7 ounces on average (although this is variable).
- *9, 11:* the spleen underlies ribs 9, 10, and 11 and is related to them at the midaxillary line.

Surface Anatomy of the Spleen

The main anatomical relations of the spleen are:

- *Anteriorly:* greater curve of the stomach, tail of the pancreas, and splenic flexure of the colon (the three structures to be safeguarded while ligating the splenic vessels during splenectomy)
- *Inferiorly:* left kidney and left suprarenal gland
- *Superiorly and laterally:* left dome of the diaphragm, separating the spleen from the left pleural cavity and left lung

Gross Anatomy of the Spleen

Can be regarded as having two surfaces: diaphragmatic and visceral (**Figure 5.29**). The diaphragmatic surface is in contact with rib cage and diaphragm.

The visceral surface contains the following impressions:

- Gastric (for the fundus of the stomach)
- Colic (in contact with the splenic flexure of the colon)
- Renal (in contact with the anterior surface of the left kidney)

The **splenic notch** is situated on the anterior border, which is clinically important when the spleen extends inferomedially, towards the right iliac fossa, and the notch can be palpated to

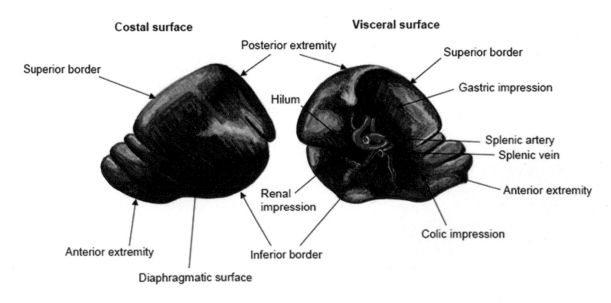

FIGURE 5.29 The costal and visceral surfaces of the spleen. (Courtesy of Calum Harrington-Vogt.)

diagnose splenomegaly (enlarged at approximately 2 to 3 times its normal size).

Peritoneal ligaments (parts of the greater omentum) are made up of two peritoneal layers. These ligaments are incised to mobilise the spleen during open or laparoscopic splenectomy.

Gastrosplenic ligament connects the spleen to the greater curvature of the stomach.

The short gastric arteries and the left gastroepiploic, arising from the splenic artery, run in it. It also contains the terminal part of the splenic artery and vein and the tail of the pancreas.

Lienorenal (or splenorenal) ligament connects the lower pole of the spleen to the left kidney.

Blood Supply and Drainage

Arterial supply to the spleen is from the **splenic artery**, the largest of the three branches of the coeliac trunk, which runs a tortuous course related to the superior border of the pancreas. Once the splenic artery enters the spleen, it usually divides into two to three branches to the upper, middle, and lower parts of the spleen. These branches divide the spleen into separate vascular segments, important in partial splenectomy where one segment can be removed without affecting others.

The splenic artery supplies the pancreas as well. The *arteria pancreatica magna* (greater pancreatic artery) is one of the largest branches of the splenic artery to the pancreas. The splenic artery is next to the aorta and iliac arteries to develop aneurysm, often clinically asymptomatic.

The splenic vein and the superior mesenteric vein (SMV) unite behind the neck of the pancreas to form the hepatic portal vein. The inferior mesenteric vein has a variable drainage between the SMV and the splenic vein, but it usually drains into the splenic vein.

Nerve Supply and Lymph Drainage

Nerve supply to the spleen is from the splenic plexus, which is derived from the coeliac plexus supplying the spleen with both sympathetic and parasympathetic nerve fibres.

The lymphatic drainage of the spleen is to the lymph nodes at the splenic hilum and to the coeliac lymph nodes.

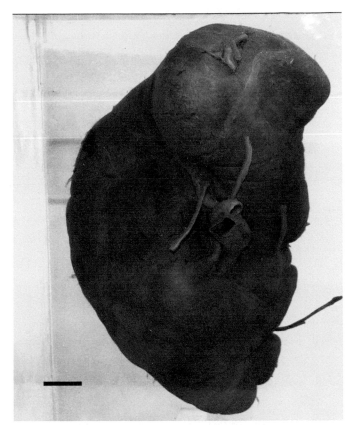

FIGURE 5.30 Splenectomy specimen in a patient with splenomegaly, bar = 2 cm. (Courtesy of Department of Anatomical Sciences, SGUL.)

Hypersplenism is the clinical term for a hyperactive spleen with excessive destruction of one or more of the blood cells (red cells, white cells, and platelets).

A common clinical question is **how to differentiate splenomegaly from an enlarged retroperitoneal organ in the left flank (e.g., an enlarged kidney)**. The answer includes:

- Direction of splenic enlargement is towards the right iliac fossa
- Palpation of splenic notch
- The enlarged left retroperitoneal mass is bimanually palpable

A **ruptured spleen** is the cause of a common surgical emergency because it can lead to life-threatening severe bleeding. The spleen is liable to injury and is the most common intra-abdominal organ injured following blunt abdominal trauma.

SPLENECTOMY

The surgical operation to remove the spleen, commonly for a badly injured spleen following trauma (**Figure 5.31**) or iatrogenic injury during the course of another operation, for example, injury to the lower pole of the spleen whilst mobilising the splenic colon flexure.

(Continued)

CLINICAL NOTES

Splenomegaly (enlarged spleen) (**Figure 5.30**) can be caused by a variety of medical conditions, which include:

- **Haematological** pathologies, e.g., haemolytic anaemia (spherocytosis, sickle cell, thalassemia), Hodgkin's and non-Hodgkin's lymphoma, leukaemia, and immune thrombocytopenic purpura (ITP).
- **Congestive causes such as portal hypertension** (mostly due to liver cirrhosis), splenic vein thrombosis, and congestive heart failure.
- **Infections** such as malaria, Epstein-Barr virus (EBV), and typhoid fever.
- **Systemic diseases** such as Felty's syndrome (rheumatoid arthritis, leucopoenia, and splenomegaly) and systemic lupus erythematosus (SLE)
- In tropical areas the most common causes of massive splenomegaly are malaria, kala-azar, and bilharziasis. Myeloproliferative disease is another cause for massive spleen.

Splenorraphy is a relatively new option in the treatment of splenic injury, and it involves suturing of the injured spleen, following certain operative criteria.

Other indications for splenectomy include ITP, spherocytosis (sometimes combined with cholecystectomy to treat gallstones due to excessive haemolysis of the red cells), hypersplenism, and for radical excision of gastric cancer.

OVERWHELMING POST-SPLENECTOMY SEPSIS (OPSS)

Splenectomy can affect the body's immunity, and serious infections with capsulated bacteria may follow. Vaccination against these bacteria is indicated either preoperatively, for elective patients undergoing splenectomy, or following emergency splenectomy, in addition to antibiotic coverage.

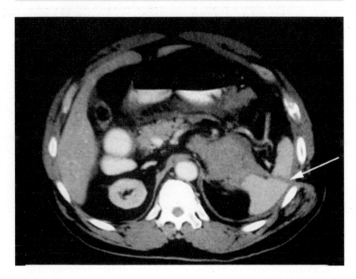

FIGURE 5.31   CT scan showing linear laceration of the spleen *(arrow)* and haemorrhage around the splenic hilum, following stab injury to the left loin. (Courtesy of Wan Khamizar.)

Liver

The liver **develops in the ventral mesogastrium**, splitting the ventral mesentery into two derivatives: anterior (falciform ligament) and posterior (lesser omentum). The falciform ligament attaches the liver to the anterior abdominal wall.

Facts about the liver

- The liver is the largest gland and the second largest organ in the body, after the skin.
- Weighing about 1.5 kg, this heavy organ is mainly supported by the attachment of the hepatic veins, usually three in number, to the IVC.
- The liver receives around 1.5 litres per minute of blood supply, 25% from the proper hepatic artery and 75% from the hepatic portal vein. It drains into the IVC via three hepatic veins. Consequently, liver trauma can be a life-threatening condition due to severe bleeding leading to hypovolaemic shock.
- The liver is located in the right upper quadrant of the abdomen, extending from the fifth intercostal space to the costal margin. This fact is essential during liver examination where palpation and percussion are required.
- Penetrating injuries to the thorax may involve the liver and other anatomically related structures, as the liver is protected by the lower right ribs.

Liver function includes

- Production of bile (essential for lipid digestion) and clotting factors
- Detoxication of harmful substances brought to the liver by the portal vein, like alcohol
- Amino acids formation and changing the toxic by-product ammonia into urea to be excreted by the kidneys
- Carbohydrate metabolism through the formation of glucose from glycogen and vice versa by storing excess glucose as glycogen
- Storage of fat-soluble vitamins like vitamin K and minerals like iron and copper
- The liver has an immunological function

Surface Anatomy of the Liver

The main anatomical relations of the liver are:

- *Superiorly:* diaphragm
- *Anteriorly:* rib cage and abdominal wall
- *Posteriorly (visceral or the posterior surface):* lower oesophagus, stomach, superior part of duodenum, and gallbladder

Gross Anatomy of the Liver

Glisson's capsule is the fibrous layer covering the liver and has somatic innervation from the lower intercostal nerves (hepatomegaly can be painful due to stretching of the capsule).

Two main anatomical lobes (split by the falciform ligament anatomically) (**Figure 5.32**):

- **Left lobe** (smaller in size)
- **Right lobe** (larger in size)

There are two accessory lobes:

- **Caudate lobe** or segment I (located superiorly on the posterior surface of the liver), found between the IVC (right) and the fissure of the ligamentum venosum (left)
- **Quadrate lobe** (located inferiorly on the posterior surface of the liver), found between the gallbladder (left) and the fissure of the ligamentum teres (right)

The liver has diaphragmatic (collective of the anterior, superior, and right surfaces) and visceral (posteroinferior) surfaces.

The **porta hepatis** is an H-shaped transverse slit (about 4 cm in length) on the posterior surface of the liver, located between the caudate and quadrate lobes, which transmits:

- Right and left branches of the hepatic artery
- Right and left branches of the common hepatic duct
- Hepatic portal vein
- Autonomic fibres (vagal and sympathetic)
- Some lymph vessels that emerge from the liver

The lesser omentum splits to embrace the porta hepatis.

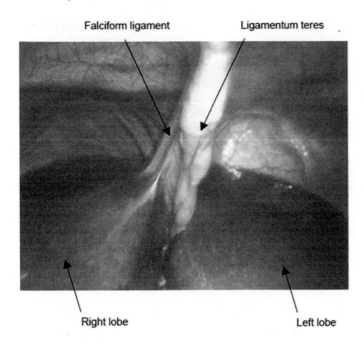

FIGURE 5.32 Laparoscopic view of the anterior view of the liver lobes and the attachment of the falciform ligament. (Courtesy of Paul Carter.)

Surgical liver segments

- The Cantlie line extends from the midpoint of the gallbladder fossa to the midpoint of the IVC and divides the liver into left and right lobes.
- The liver is divided into eight segments according to Couinaud's classification, with each segment having its own blood supply and biliary drainage. This is important in planning interventional radiology procedures such as

therapeutic embolization and specific surgical segmental or lobe resection; so, for example, we talk about resection of segment I or II, left or right lobectomy, and so on (**Figures 5.33** and **5.34**).

Peritoneal recesses

- Subhepatic space is found between the liver and the transverse colon.
- Subphrenic space is located between the diaphragm and the liver. The falciform ligament divides this into left and right spaces.
- Morison's pouch is the space between the right kidney and the visceral surface of the liver.

Fluid such as pus can collect in these spaces, e.g., following perforation of a hollow viscus. Image-guided aspiration of abscesses, where possible, avoids an open surgical procedure.

Blood Supply of the Liver

The **common hepatic artery**, originating from the coeliac trunk, gives rise to the right gastric and the gastroduodenal arteries before it passes within the free margin of the lesser omentum. It divides into the right and left hepatic arteries. The hepatic artery proper starts after the origin of the gastroduodenal artery and supplies oxygen-rich blood to the liver sinusoids.

The **hepatic portal vein** is formed by the union of the splenic and superior mesenteric veins behind the neck of the pancreas. It then passes posteriorly to the first part of the duodenum to join the hepatic artery proper and the CBD within the free margin of the lesser omentum, to divide into two branches at the porta hepatis. This vein supplies nutrient-rich, deoxygenated blood to the liver. Finally, once both oxygenated and deoxygenated blood have entered the liver and have been stripped of their essentials, blood drains into the IVC via the three hepatic veins.

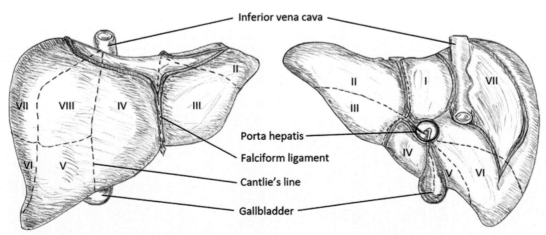

The segments are usually referred to by number (name): I (caudate); II (left lateral superior); III (left medial inferior); IV (left medial superior) (sometimes subdivided into superior and inferior parts); V (right medial inferior); VI (right lateral inferior); VII (right lateral superior); VIII (right medial superior).

FIGURE 5.33 Anterior and posterior views of the liver showing the eight liver segments. (Courtesy of Alina Humadani.)

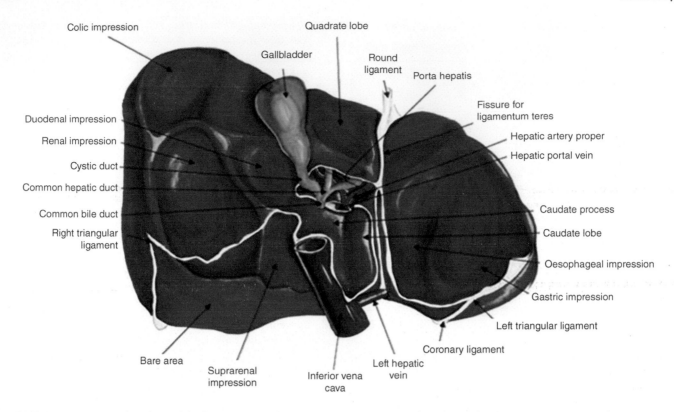

FIGURE 5.34   Visceral surface of the liver. Note the liver is tilted upside down. (Courtesy of Calum Harrington-Vogt.)

Nerve Supply

The liver, except its capsule, is innervated by the **hepatic plexus**, which contains both sympathetic (from the coeliac plexus) and parasympathetic fibres from the vagus, passing through the porta hepatis. The capsule is innervated by somatic nerves (lower intercostal nerves supply the parietal peritoneum). Pain from stretching the liver capsule by inflammatory or neoplastic conditions is well localised to the right upper quadrant of the abdomen. However, pathologies which involve the diaphragmatic surface may be felt as referred pain in the right shoulder (see the phrenic nerve, **Section 4**).

Lymphatic Drainage

The lymphatic vessels of the liver drain into the hepatic lymph nodes, which are found close to the hepatic vessels, before entering the coeliac lymph nodes. Other lymphatic vessels in the liver pass from the bare area to the mediastinal lymph nodes, found posteriorly.

CLINICAL NOTES

EXAMINATION OF THE LIVER

The lower edge of the liver extends to the right costal margin. Hepatomegaly is clinically detected by percussion from above (*chest:* resonant compared to the dullness of the liver) and by palpation starting from the lower right quadrant upwards to feel for the lower edge.

HEPATOMEGALY

An enlarged liver is caused by a variety of conditions, including viral hepatitis (mostly hepatitis A, B, and C), alcoholic liver disease due to excessive alcohol consumption, congestive heart failure, and primary and secondary liver tumours. In tropical countries, hydatid cyst (helminthic infestation with *Echinococcus granulosus*) is a common cause of hepatomegaly, as the liver is the most common body organ to harbour the disease (**Figure 5.35**).

Physical examination (see earlier) is required to give a rough estimate of the liver size, in addition to general signs like jaundice and palmar erythema. Other tests include liver function test (LFT), USS, CT, and magnetic resonance imaging (MRI).

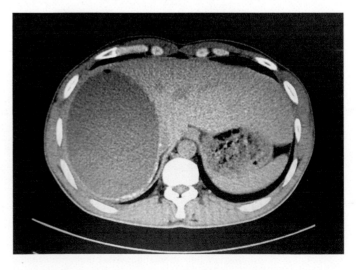

FIGURE 5.35   Twenty-five-year-old male who presented with hepatomegaly. CT image shows a thin-walled fluid collection in the right hepatic lobe, due to hydatid cyst. (Courtesy of Ahmed Alsagban.)

PORTAL HYPERTENSION

This term refers to the rise of the portal venous pressure above the normal range of 5 to 10 mm Hg. Commonly caused by liver cirrhosis through either excessive alcohol consumption or following infection with hepatitis B or C. In some countries such as Egypt, bilharziasis is an important cause of portal hypertension. The liver becomes damaged, resulting in pressure build-up within the tributaries of the portal vein. The portosystemic communications, which are normally closed, open up. Varices form in the lower oesophagus, stomach, rectum, and radiating veins from the umbilical region (caput medusa, Latin for the head of the Medusa). If the oesophageal varices rupture, severe blood loss can occur in the form of haematemesis and melaena.

LIVER METASTASIS

The liver is the most common site for metastasis from GI malignancies, often from colorectal cancer and malignant tumours from other sites like the breast, malignant melanoma, and lung cancer. Percutaneous image-guided liver biopsy is used to take small pieces of liver tissue by inserting a special needle in the midaxillary line at the level of the eighth or ninth intercostal space into the liver. The clotting screen should be within normal limits; otherwise, this procedure may risk bleeding from the liver.

The other methods to take a liver biopsy are laparoscopic and transvenous. For patients with abnormal clotting, a procedure via a small neck incision is used, cannulating the internal jugular vein and passing the catheter down the hepatic veins into the liver. This procedure needs the injection of IV contrast to delineate the veins and guide the cannula and the biopsy needle into the liver. Transjugular liver biopsy may be combined with transjugular intrahepatic portosystemic shunt (TIPSS) to treat portal hypertension.

LIVER TRANSPLANT

The liver has a peculiar ability to regenerate within a few months following injury or infections like hepatitis. However, the liver can fail acutely (acute liver necrosis) or in the long term (end-stage liver disease) and will necessitate liver transplant, which is a major surgical procedure.

In the majority of cases, the transplanted liver comes from a deceased registered donor (cadaveric), which will replace the recipient's damaged liver, or from a section of a living donor (**orthotopic transplantation**). In **heterotopic liver transplant**, an auxiliary liver graft is provided without removal of the diseased liver in the hope that the native liver recovers function (see the NICE Guidelines on liver transplantation, which can be found online).

The Gallbladder and Biliary System

The biliary system develops as an outgrowth of the foregut. It is responsible for draining bile (about 700 to 1000 mL/day, important for lipid digestion) from the liver into the duodenum. The gallbladder is a pear-shaped sac, covered by visceral peritoneum, for storage and concentration of bile secreted by the liver. It is found on the posterior side of the liver (right lobe) with a storage capacity of around 50 mL (**Figure 5.36**).

Gross Anatomy of the Gallbladder and Biliary System
The gallbladder can be divided into:

- **Fundus** (end part of the gallbladder and most dependent)
- **Body** (largest part of the gallbladder)
- **Neck** connects with the **cystic duct**

A dilatation from the neck to the body in the presence of gallstones is termed **Hartmann's pouch** (**Figure 5.37**).

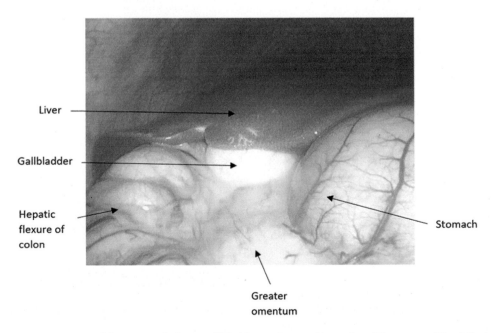

FIGURE 5.36 Laparoscopic view of the stomach, liver, gallbladder, and ascending colon. (Courtesy of Paul Carter.)

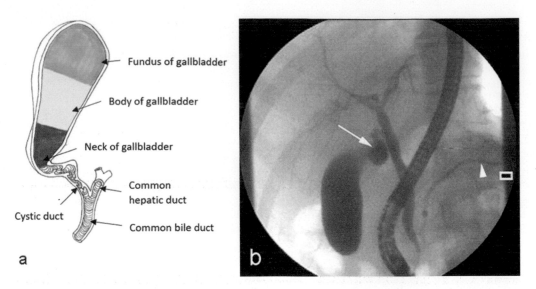

FIGURE 5.37 (a) Parts of the gallbladder and biliary system. (Courtesy of Calum Harrington-Vogt); (b) endoscopic retrograde cholangiopancreatography (ERCP) showing the biliary system, including Hartmann's pouch *(arrow)*. The main pancreatic duct (MPD) is also visible *(arrowhead)*. (Courtesy of Department of Anatomical Sciences, SGUL.)

Biliary Tree

The bile is secreted through numerous ducts from the liver; bile canaliculi lie between hepatocytes.

Extra Hepatic Biliary System

The right and left hepatic ducts at the porta hepatis form the common hepatic duct (CHD).

The common hepatic duct is joined by the cystic duct to form the CBD.

The CBD is about 3 inches in length. It divides into three parts:

- Supraduodenal, in the free border of the lesser omentum
- Retroduodenal (behind the first part of the duodenum)
- Paraduodenal or pancreatic segment (indents the posterior aspect of the head of the pancreas)

The CBD usually joins the main pancreatic duct to form the ampulla of Vater, which empties the bile into the second part of the duodenum via the major duodenal papilla, which is regulated by the sphincter of Oddi (muscular valve).

Blood Supply

The arterial supply comes from the **cystic artery**, usually originating from the right hepatic artery and passing through the hepatobiliary triangle, *vide infra*. Venous drainage of the gallbladder occurs through the cystic vein, which drains into the hepatic portal vein.

Lymphatic Drainage

Lymphatic drainage is to the cystic node found close to the neck of the gallbladder. The cystic node drains into the coeliac nodes via the hepatic lymph nodes.

Nerve Supply

The gallbladder receives innervation from the coeliac plexus (sympathetic fibres) and the vagus nerve (parasympathetic fibres). Parasympathetic innervation causes the gallbladder to contract, releasing bile into the cystic duct towards the duodenum, in addition to the cholecystokinin (CCK) hormone secreted from the duodenal mucosa.

The **hepatobiliary triangle (Calot's triangle)** is bounded by the CHD, the cystic duct, and the inferior surface of the liver. It is bridged by a double layer of peritoneum. Its main content is the cystic artery.

Identification of this triangle is of high surgical importance in both open and laparoscopic cholecystectomy.

Biliary anomalies, such as an accessory bile duct or short or long cystic duct, are common and should always be kept in mind while dissecting the hepatobiliary triangle to avoid unnecessary complications.

Endoscopic retrograde cholangiopancreatography (ERCP):

- Entails locating the major duodenal papilla and cannulation of the CBD (**Figures 5.37b** and **5.38a**). It is done by passing a side-view endoscope through the stomach and into the duodenum. ERCP is used both for diagnostic and therapeutic

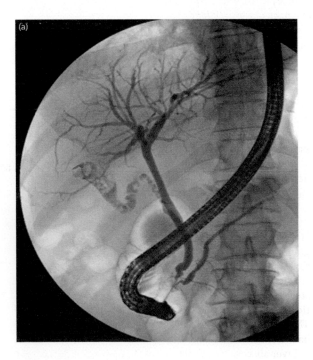

FIGURE 5.38a ERCP showing biliary system and main pancreatic duct (MPD).

purposes, such as extraction of residual stones in the CBD following cholecystectomy, splitting the sphincter of Oddi (endoscopic sphincterotomy) to assist free drainage, passing of small stones (**Figure 5.38b**), and relief of jaundice by stenting the CBD, for example, as a palliative measure in patients with inoperable pancreatic cancer.

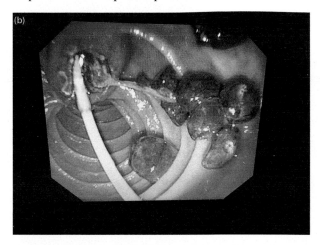

FIGURE 5.38b Intraduodenal view of ERCP sphincterotomy of the ampulla of Vater and extraction of CBD stones. (Courtesy of Akram A. Najeeb.)

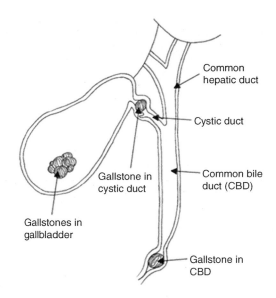

FIGURE 5.39 Expected sites of gallstones. (Courtesy of Calum Harrington-Vogt.)

CLINICAL NOTES

Gallstones (cholelithiasis) are a common condition and can be silent (asymptomatic) or symptomatic (**Figures 5.39** and **5.40**). They can cause severe pain in the upper abdomen, mainly on the right side (biliary colic).

Acute cholecystitis (inflammation of the gallbladder) usually follows obstruction of the cystic duct. However, cholecystitis can occur without the presence of gallstones (acalculous cholecystitis). Rarely, impacted gallstones in the cystic duct or the neck of the gallbladder may compress the CHD and cause obstructive jaundice, and may even cause fistula formation between the gallbladder and the CHD (Mirizzi's syndrome).

The obstructed infected gallbladder may turn into a bag of pus (empyema of the gallbladder), which necessitates urgent percutaneous pus aspiration (interventional radiology procedure) or sometimes surgical evacuation and drainage of the gallbladder (cholecystostomy).

Cholelithiasis is the most common cause of acute pancreatitis.

A big gallstone can fistulate from the gallbladder to the duodenum and move down the small bowel to its narrowest part, the ileum, and cause small bowel obstruction (gallstone ileus).

Murphy's sign: this physical examination involves the patient breathing in deeply with the examiner's hand placed at the location of the gallbladder, under the right costal margin. An inflamed gallbladder feels tender to palpation, and this sign is positive.

Post-hepatic (obstructive) jaundice occurs when gallstones pass into the CBD. Septicaemia is a serious complication which can follow infection of the bile ducts (cholangitis). The most common causative organisms are gram-negative bacilli like *Escherichia coli*.

Liver abscess (pus formation) can also follow biliary tract infections.

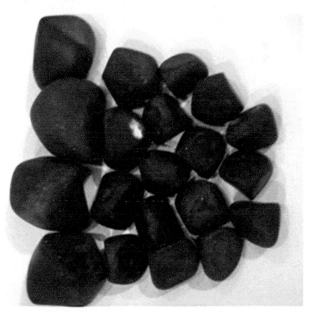

FIGURE 5.40 Gallstones removed from a cholecystectomy specimen from a patient with empyema of the gallbladder. (Courtesy of Qassim F. Baker.)

Biliary obstruction can be:

- *Intramural (lumen):* commonly by gallstones (**Figures 5.41** and **5.42**) or, rarely, by parasitic worms such as *Ascaris* or a ruptured liver hydatid cyst
- *Mural (wall):* cholangiocarcinoma (cancer of the epithelial lining of the bile duct), sclerosing cholangitis, and stricture formation following previous cholecystectomy
- Extramural (pressure from outside, commonly due to cancer in the head of the pancreas or periampullary carcinoma)

(Continued)

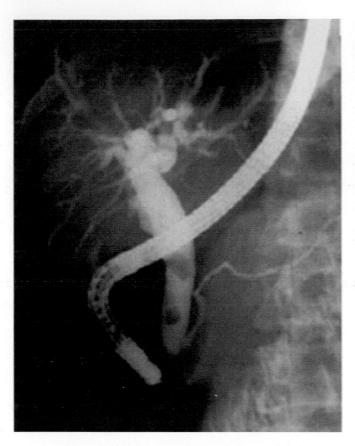

FIGURE 5.41 ERCP showing residual stones in a dilated CBD. (Courtesy of Qassim F. Baker.)

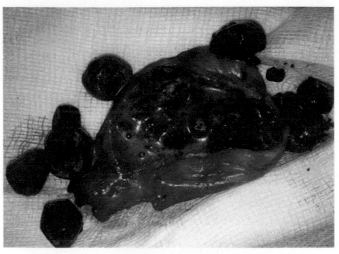

FIGURE 5.42 Surgical specimen showing gallbladder containing multiple gallstones. (Courtesy of Mohammed M. Habash.)

There are three main types of **jaundice** (yellow discolouration of the skin and sclera due to high bilirubin level in the blood) (**Figure 5.43**):

- *Pre-hepatic* (excessive red cell destruction, i.e., haemolysis, with the release of unconjugated bilirubin). Common examples are haemolytic anaemia (spherocytosis, sickle cell anaemia, thalassaemia) and malaria.
- *Intrahepatic (cholestatic):* the disruption happens in the liver, e.g., in patients with viral hepatitis.
- *Post-hepatic (obstructive):* characterised by passing dark-coloured urine, pale-coloured faeces, and sometimes itching of the skin.

In both intrahepatic and post-hepatic jaundice there is an increased level of serum conjugated bilirubin, which is water-soluble and can pass through the filtration mechanism of the kidneys and results in passing dark-coloured urine.

Learning Point

Laparoscopic cholecystectomy is one of the most common surgical procedures. Keeping in mind the presence of anomalies of the biliary system and blood supply to the gallbladder will avoid serious complications, such as perioperative severe bleeding and postoperative biliary fistulas.

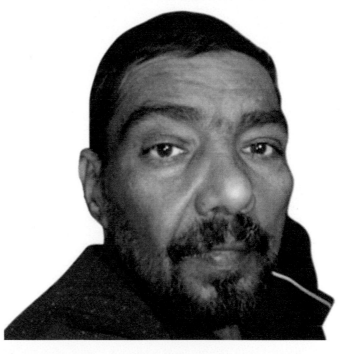

FIGURE 5.43 Patient with obstructive jaundice due to pancreatic cancer. (Courtesy of Aqeel S. Mahmood.)

QUIZ QUESTION

Q. *Why does pain from an inflamed gallbladder refer to the tip of the right shoulder?*

The Ileum and Jejunum

The jejunum and the ileum are the next parts of the small intestine. They extend from the DJJ to the ileocaecal valve. There is no clear boundary for differentiating between the jejunum and the ileum, as they both form a continuous tube which gradually changes along its length. As there is no distinct boundary between the jejunum and the ileum, they are often spoken of together as the jejuno-ileum (**Table 5.2** and **Figure 5.44**).

The wall consists of the mucosa, submucosa, muscularis, and serosa.

- The **mucosa** is designed for absorption of products of digestion, aided by the huge surface area formed by the villi. The epithelial cells renew every 3 to 5 days.
- The **submucosa** consists of a layer of connective tissue that contains the blood vessels, nerves, and lymphatics.
- The **muscular layer** is formed of outer longitudinal and inner circular layers.
- The **serosa** is formed by the visceral peritoneum.

The secretion and motility of the small bowel are controlled by its autonomic innervation and its ENS.

The **jejunum and ileum are suspended from the posterior abdominal wall by the mesentery** (see earlier), which transmits branches and tributaries of the superior mesenteric vessels, lymphatics, and autonomic nerves. The jejunum and ileum measure about 6 metres in length, while its mesentery attaches to a small strip of the posterior abdominal wall from the level of the L2 vertebra on the left to the right iliac fossa (the "root" of the mesentery).

The Superior Mesenteric Artery (SMA) (Figure 5.45)
The SMA is the artery of the midgut and supplies the bowel from the level of the major duodenal papilla (second part of the duodenum) to the splenic flexure of the colon. It arises from the abdominal aorta at the level of the L2 vertebra.

Branches

- **Inferior pancreaticoduodenal**, supplies part of the head of the pancreas and duodenum from the second part.
- **Middle colic** divides into right and left branches within the transverse mesocolon to supply the transverse colon. The left branch anastomoses with branches of the left colic artery (from the IMA) at the splenic flexure (watershed area) to form the marginal artery (of Drummond).
- **Jejunal and ileal branches** arise from the left side of the artery and connect with each other via a series of arcades (important to recognize if small bowel resection is attempted, e.g., for small bowel gangrene, injuries, tumours, or Crohn's disease).
- **Ileocolic artery** supplies the terminal ileum, caecum, vermiform appendix (appendicular artery), and ascending colon. This is the reason to resect the terminal ileum in the operation of right hemicolectomy, commonly performed for right-sided colon cancer.
- **Right colic artery** to the ascending colon up to the hepatic flexure and anastomoses with the right branch of the middle colic artery.

Corresponding tributaries join the SMV, which runs with the artery within the mesentery and which joins the splenic vein to form the hepatic portal vein behind the neck of the pancreas.

After resection of a segment of the small bowel, the two ends can be joined together (end-to-end anastomosis) in the majority of cases because of the rich blood supply of the small bowel and less contaminated contents. In comparison, immediate large bowel anastomosis is less feasible.

SMA Occlusion
The SMA can get blocked by thrombosis or emboli (for example, in patients with uncontrolled atrial fibrillation [AF]). This results in widespread bowel ischaemia, and, if not diagnosed early, bowel gangrene follows, which is usually fatal.

Nerve Supply
Visceral afferent fibres (sympathetic) pass to thoracic segments of the spinal cord via the greater and lesser splanchnic nerves. Visceral pain from small bowel obstruction is felt first in the dermatome T9–T11 (central abdominal pain). Efferent pre-ganglionic sympathetic axons travel down the greater and lesser splanchnic nerves to the coeliac plexus and to the superior mesenteric plexus to accompany the arteries arising from the SMA. They act as vasoconstrictors and inhibitors to the smooth muscles of the jejunum and ileum.

Parasympathetic innervation comes from the vagus, increasing secretomotor activity and bowel motility.

Lymphatic Drainage
The lymphatic vessels of the jejunum and ileum not only have an immune function but also help in absorption of fat and fat-soluble vitamins via lacteals in the villi. The lymphatic vessels join mesenteric lymph nodes (within the mesentery) and finally join the lymph nodes at the origin of the SMA.

Inflammation of these lymph nodes is called **mesenteric adenitis**, sometimes clinically indistinguishable from acute appendicitis, especially in children.

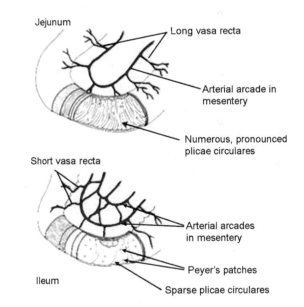

FIGURE 5.44 How to differentiate the jejunum and ileum. (Courtesy of Calum Harrington-Vogt.)

Small Bowel Obstruction
The small bowel can get obstructed and may become ischaemic (cut off of blood supply), commonly from outside causes (adhesions following previous bowel surgery or a segment of bowel being pinched off and pushed through an orifice in the body wall – obstructed inguinal, paraumbilical, umbilical, incisional, and femoral hernias), or rarely, small bowel loops are trapped into, for example, a mesenteric hole (internal hernia). In comparison to the large bowel, the small bowel is rarely obstructed by tumours (benign, like submucous lipoma, or malignant, like carcinoid tumour, lymphoma, and adenocarcinoma). If

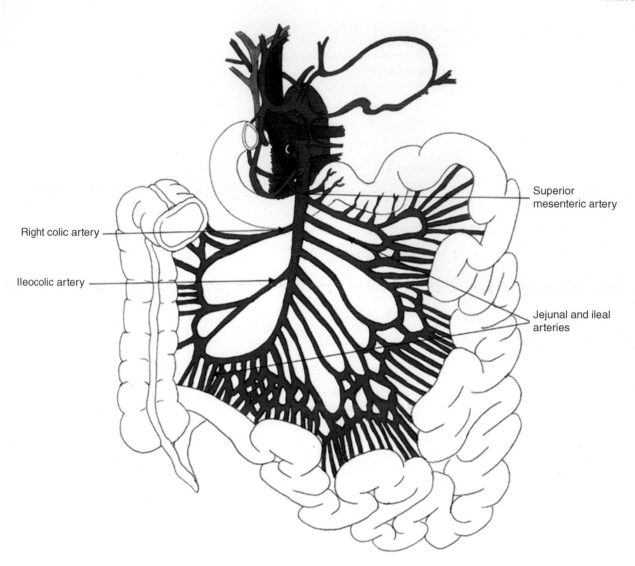

Right colic artery

Ileocolic artery

Superior
mesenteric artery

Jejunal and ileal
arteries

FIGURE 5.45 Blood supply of the small bowel and right colon. (Courtesy of Calum Harrington-Vogt.)

TABLE 5.2: Differences between the jejunum and the ileum

Jejunum	Ileum
Thicker walled, with a wider lumen relative to the ileum	Thinner-walled, with a narrower lumen relative to the jejunum
More vascularised relative to the ileum; the mesentery has fewer arterial arcades, with a longer vasa recta	Less vascularised relative to the jejunum; its mesentery has more arterial arcades compared to the jejunum, with a short vasa recta
The main site of absorption for carbohydrates, proteins, and most other nutrients extracted from food.	The ileum is the main site for lipid (and other lipid-soluble molecules), vitamin B_{12}, and bile salt absorption.
Has a much more richly folded luminal mucosal lining, which forms a dense microvilli surface, ideal for quick and efficient absorption of nutrients	The luminal mucosa is much less projected into microvilli, giving the ileum much less absorptive capacity relative to the jejunum
The jejunum has little mucosal-associated lymphoid tissue (MALT)	The ileum has MALT present facing into the lumen. These patches of lymphoid tissue are known as **Peyer's patches** and have an immunological function in the gastrointestinal tract
The jejunum has numerous pronounced plicae circulares (circular folds) projecting into its lumen	Less obvious plicae circulares. The distal ileum has barely any plicae circulares

the circulation is not restored, the bowel becomes gangrenous (black in colour, no pulsation in the branches of the SMA, and not contractile), which will necessitate resection of the gangrenous segment (**Figure 5.46**).

The classical symptoms of patients with small bowel obstruction include central colicky abdominal pain, vomiting, abdominal distension, and constipation.

Plain X-ray of the abdomen in the erect position reveals multiple air–fluid levels (**Figure 5.47**).

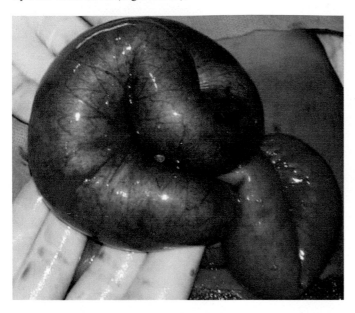

FIGURE 5.46 Ischaemic loop of small bowel (which may be still salvageable); compare this to the pink colour of healthy bowel. (Courtesy of Maan Aldoori.)

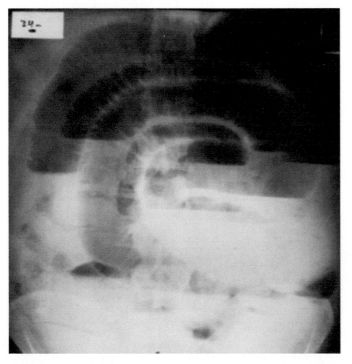

FIGURE 5.47 Plain X-ray (erect position) of a patient with small bowel obstruction showing multiple air–fluid levels in a ladder pattern appearance. (Courtesy of Qassim F. Baker.)

Learning Point

The two most common causes of small bowel obstruction are postoperative adhesions and obstructed hernias.

Crohn's Disease

This inflammatory condition of unknown aetiology can affect the whole GIT, but has a preference for the terminal ileum. It can cause small bowel obstruction, bleeding, and fistula formation into the GIT and rarely perforates into the peritoneal cavity.

Notes on Inflammatory Bowel Disease

Both Crohn's disease and ulcerative colitis (UC) are forms of inflammatory bowel disease (IBD). In medical school exams, the features in **Table 5.3** are often used to distinguish between the two.

TABLE 5.3: Comparison between the main two types of inflammatory bowel disease

Crohn's Disease	Ulcerative Colitis
Occurs anywhere within the GIT (commonly the terminal ileum, often rectal sparing)	Confined to the colon, always affects the rectum
Skip lesions possible	Continuous lesions, extending proximally from the rectum; sharp transition from normal to inflamed colon
Transmural inflammation – strictures and fistulae therefore more common than UC	Mucosal inflammation

Note: Some patients have overlapping features of UC and Crohn's disease. IBS can therefore be considered a spectrum between the two. Care is often shared between medical and surgical teams.

Meckel's Diverticulum

A Meckel's diverticulum is an outpouching of a segment of bowel from the anti-mesenteric border, commonly in the terminal ileum (**Figure 5.48**). It represents a patent remnant of the proximal part of the vitelline duct (omphalomesenteric duct) arising from the distal ileum (see the discussion on the umbilicus for more information).

Meckel's diverticulum is classified as a **true diverticulum**, as it involves all the layers of the gut (including the muscular layer, not just the mucosa), in contrast to false diverticuli of the colon. There may be some heterotopic epithelium of gastric, pancreatic, or colonic type. The gastric epithelium may undergo ulceration and bleed, causing bleeding per rectum.

Most patients who have a Meckel's diverticulum are asymptomatic and do not need to have bowel resection surgery.

Meckel's diverticulum has a 2, 2, 2, 2 record; with 2% of the population possessing a Meckel's diverticulum, it being located approximately 2 feet from the ileocaecal junction proximally, usually 2 inches in length, and typically presenting before the age of 2.

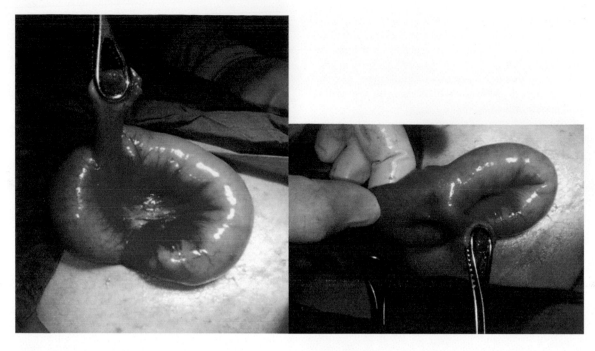

FIGURE 5.48   Meckel's diverticulum. (Courtesy of Mohammed H. Aldabbagh.)

Meckel's diverticulum, if symptomatic, usually produces symptoms early on in life. Inflamed diverticulum usually produces symptoms similar to acute appendicitis and is often misdiagnosed for acute appendicitis; only at operation is Meckel's diverticulum usually diagnosed. Other complications include bleeding per rectum and invagination of the bowel segment containing the

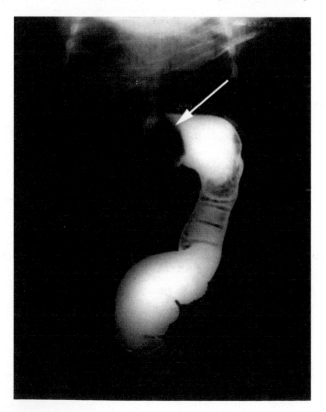

FIGURE 5.49   Barium enema of a child with ileocolic intussusception showing the meniscus sign *(arrow)*. (Courtesy of Qassim F. Baker.)

diverticulum into another adjacent bowel segment (intussusception), causing bowel obstruction (*vide infra*).

Intussusception

Intussusception is the invagination of a proximal bowel segment into another one, causing bowel obstruction. The most common type is ileocolic (the distal ileum telescopes into the proximal colon but may go farther down the colon). It mostly affects children in their first year, with the peak age at 9 months. The diagnosis can be achieved by USS of the abdomen. Contrast barium enema is more diagnostic (**Figure 5.49**) and can be used as a therapeutic measure as well to undo the bowel invagination under fluoroscopic screening. If radiological reduction fails, a laparotomy is indicated before bowel gangrene establishes, in which case it will need a bowel resection. In adults, intussusception may have an underlying bowel condition such as small bowel tumours, e.g., submucous lipoma or lymphoma.

Large Bowel or Large Intestine

Extends from the ileocaecal valve to the anus and is derived from the distal midgut (caecum, ascending colon, proximal two-thirds of transverse colon), hindgut (distal one-third of the transverse colon, descending and sigmoid colon, and rectum), and the proctodeum. The division between the midgut and the hindgut is at the splenic flexure (watershed area between the SMA and IMA). The large bowel's main function is storage and transmission of the intestinal contents, absorption of water and electrolytes, vitamin production (by the commensal bowel bacteria), and absorption of vitamins such as B and K.

Layers of the colon

- Mucosa, lined by columnar epithelium
- Submucosa, connective tissue that contains the blood vessels, lymphatics, and nerves
- Inner circular muscle
- Outer longitudinal muscle

• Serosa, complete peritoneal covering on the caecum, transverse colon, and sigmoid colon; the ascending and descending colon are covered only anteriorly by the peritoneum

The colon does not have a continuous covering of longitudinal smooth muscle; the longitudinal smooth muscle takes the form of three thin whitish bands known as the ***taeniae coli*** (*taenia:* latin, "ribbon") which aid in the peristalsis of bowel contents. As the colon does not have a continuous covering of longitudinal smooth muscle, it can form diverticuli (protrusions of the mucosa) in high-pressure areas of the colon, such as the sigmoid colon.

The **rectum** is retroperitoneal and **has a continuous covering of longitudinal smooth muscle**, so it is immune to the formation of diverticuli (see **Section 6**, Pelvis and Perineum).

The small intestine is separated from the large intestine by the ileocaecal valve. This valve is usually competent, allowing the passage of bowel contents in one direction and preventing backflow to the small bowel.

If there is an obstructing lesion distally along the large intestine or the rectum, there will be a build-up of bowel contents proximally causing dilation of the colon, and especially of the wide-lumened caecum, which may end up with caecal perforation and faecal peritonitis (a very serious type of bacterial peritonitis).

The transverse and sigmoid colon have a mesentery, while the rest of the colon is secondarily retroperitoneal, and therefore partially covered by peritoneum. The caecum, however, is frequently intraperitoneal, but usually has no mesentery. The sigmoid colon can twist around its mesentery (volvulus), which results in huge abdominal distension.

The colon has a dual arterial supply:
• From the SMA (see earlier)

The IMA gives rise to the following branches:
• Left colic
• Sigmoidal arteries, running through the sigmoid mesocolon
• IMA continues as the superior rectal artery

See **Section 6** for more information.

The **marginal artery of Drummond** runs on the mesenteric margin of the colon and is formed by the anastomosis of ileocolic, right colic, middle colic, and left colic arteries. The most susceptible part is at the splenic flexure (watershed area; this explains ischaemic colitis at this site) (**Figure 5.50**).

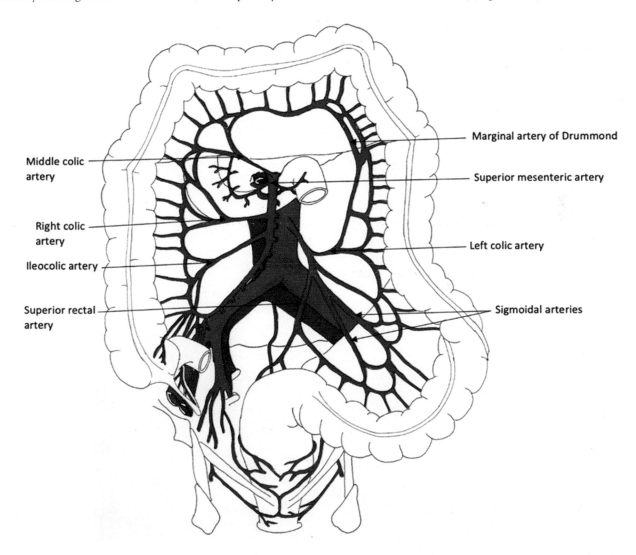

FIGURE 5.50 The arterial supply of the colon. (Courtesy of Calum Harrington-Vogt.)

Lymphatic drainage of the colon follows the arterial blood supply. The colic lymph nodes can be divided into epicolic, paracolic, intermediate, and pre-terminal (near to the origins of the SMA and IMA).

Radical colonic resection aims at removal of the colic lymph nodes, draining the excised part of the colon (right, left, or total colectomy).

How to differentiate the large from the small bowel:

- The presence of taeniae coli
- Appendices epiploicae, small fatty projections on the free surface of the colon
- Wider calibre of the large bowel
- Sacculations (haustrations) seen on radiological examination of the colon

Parts of the Colon

Caecum

This part of the colon is a blind sac, lying below the ileocaecal junction (ileocaecal valve). It has a large diameter which makes it susceptible to distension and perforation with increased intracolonic pressure (see earlier). Rarely, the appendix and the caecum fail to descend to the RIF and stay in a subhepatic position. In this case, pain from an inflamed appendix may be mistaken for acute cholecystitis.

The vermiform appendix (*vermiform*: latin, "worm-like") is a narrow blind tube which is attached to the caecum on its posteromedial aspect. It has a mesentery (the mesoappendix) and is frequently completely covered by peritoneum. Traditionally, McBurney's point is the surface marking on the anterior abdominal wall to indicate the site of the base of the appendix (see **Figure 5.10**).

The taeniae coli of the caecum converge and surround the vermiform appendix (a practical way to locate the appendix at operation is by following the taeniae coli). The appendix is supplied by the appendicular artery, which usually arises from the ileocolic artery (from the SMA) (**Figure 5.51**). The tip of the appendix varies in position and can lie behind the caecum (retrocaecal), down in the pelvis (pelvic), anterior or posterior to the ileocaecal junction, and rarely, ascending behind the visceral surface of the liver (subhepatic); appendicectomy in this case will necessitate ligation and division of the base of the appendix and the appendicular vessels first and continuing the dissection upwards, behind the caecum and ascending colon, until complete excision of the appendix.

Acute appendicitis is the most common cause for acute abdomen needing surgical intervention and is mostly due to obstruction of its lumen, e.g., by faecolith (solid particle of faeces). The appendicular artery is an end artery, so thrombosis of this artery due to acute appendicitis can lead to gangrene and perforation of the appendix, causing localised or generalised peritonitis, a serious surgical emergency (**Figure 5.52**). The appendix can be removed via an open approach or laparoscopically (**Figure 5.53**).

The greater omentum and loops of small bowel may surround the inflamed appendix and form an inflammatory mass (**appendicular mass**), which can be felt as a tender mass in the right iliac fossa. Most cases are treated conservatively (non-operatively) with IV antibiotics and close clinical observation.

As part of the midgut, the pain of acute appendicitis is usually first felt around the umbilicus (**visceral pain**). The pain sensation is conducted via afferent sympathetic nerves to the T10 segment of the spinal cord, and this is the same spinal segment that supplies the skin at the level of the umbilicus. When the inflammation reaches the parietal peritoneum, it will be more localised and sharper (**somatic pain**). Older patients can develop acute appendicitis, but consideration must be given to an obstructing lesion on the right side of the colon, such as carcinoma. Usually, a preoperative CT scan is arranged to rule out right colon cancer. Psoas sign is due to inflammation of the parietal peritoneum overlying the iliopsoas muscles (flexors of the hip joint) due to, for example, a retrocaecal appendicitis and is manifested clinically by pain on extension of the hip joint.

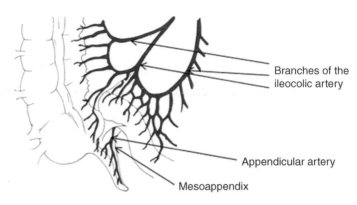

Branches of the ileocolic artery

Appendicular artery

Mesoappendix

FIGURE 5.51 Blood supply of the appendix and right side of the colon. (Courtesy of Calum Harrington-Vogt.)

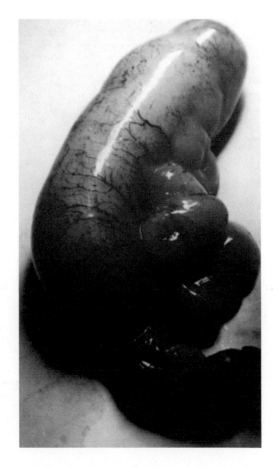

FIGURE 5.52 Specimen of inflamed distended appendix. (Courtesy of Qassim F. Baker.)

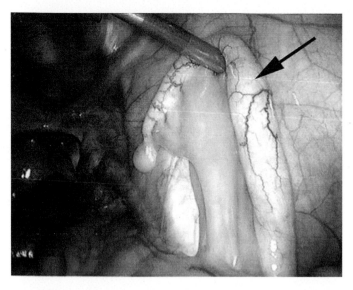

FIGURE 5.53 Laparoscopic view showing the vermiform appendix *(arrow)*. (Courtesy of Paul Carter.)

Differential diagnosis of pain in the RIF, in addition to acute appendicitis, should include:

- Other bowel pathologies such as Crohn's disease, mesenteric adenitis, and caecal and ascending colon cancer
- *Gynaecological causes:* complicated ovarian cysts, acute salpingitis, mittelschmerz (midcycle bleeding), and ectopic pregnancy
- Urological causes such as ureteric colic and urinary tract infection (UTI)

Ascending Colon

The ascending colon runs from the ileocaecal junction to the **hepatic flexure**, where the colon bends to the right to form the transverse colon.

The hepatic flexure is related to the visceral surface of the liver. Lesions of the hepatic flexure, such as cancer, should be part of the differential diagnosis of pain in the right upper quadrant of the abdomen (common causes include biliary and hepatic problems).

The blood supply of the ascending colon comes from the ileocolic and right colic arteries.

Transverse Colon

The transverse colon runs across the upper abdomen, starting at the hepatic flexure and ending at the splenic flexure, and is suspended from the transverse mesocolon. The splenic flexure is higher than the hepatic flexure. The gastrocolic omentum from the greater curve of the stomach fuses with the anterior part of the transverse colon and continues inferiorly as the **greater omentum**.

The transverse colon is rarely interposed between the diaphragm and the liver, and on imaging, the air within the colon may be mistaken as hollow viscus perforation (Chilaiditi's syndrome).

The blood supply is from the middle colic artery, which runs within the transverse mesocolon.

Descending Colon

Starts at the splenic flexure and ends at the pelvic brim, where it becomes the sigmoid colon.

The blood supply is from the left colic artery and upper sigmoidal arteries (branches of the IMA).

The **white lines of Toldt** are zones of avascular peritoneum originally described **along the lateral edges of the ascending colon and descending colon** at the meeting point of the visceral peritoneum and the peritoneum of the posterior abdominal wall. They are important in open, laparoscopic, or robotic mesocolic excision (excision of the tumour-bearing segment and its mesocolon).

In the operation of right or left colectomy, the colon should be mobilised first by cutting through the bloodless line of parietal peritoneum along the paracolic gutter; the blood supply is then secured with clips or ligatures.

On the right side the following structures need to be identified and safeguarded:

- Right ureter, which is retroperitoneal but **frequently adherent to the parietal peritoneum**
- Right gonadal vessels
- The second part of the duodenum; unnoticed injury may result in the development of duodenal fistula, which can be missed

On the left side, the left ureter and gonadal vessels need to be identified.

Sigmoid Colon

This starts as a continuation of the descending colon and ends at the level of the third sacral vertebra to become the rectum. It is suspended by an inverted V-shaped structure: the sigmoid mesocolon.

CLINICAL NOTES

Stomas are openings in the small or large bowel delivered to the skin surface of the abdomen to divert bowel contents to a bag, which is fixed to the abdominal wall, mostly necessary during surgery for large bowel obstruction.

Colostomy is an opening in the colon to divert contents after relieving obstruction or to protect anastomosis following large bowel resection. The sigmoid and transverse colon are the most suitable to be brought to the skin in view of their mesenteries (sigmoid and transverse mesocolon, respectively). Colostomy can be temporary (with bowel continuity restored after a while) or can be permanent, for example, following excision of the rectum in abdominoperineal resection.

Ileostomy is an opening in the ileum (usually in the last part) which is brought to the skin surface, for example, following total removal of the colon (total colectomy) or to protect a distal colonic anastomosis.

Colorectal carcinoma (CRC) is one of the most common surgical cancers and starts in the mucosa. Certain pathological conditions can predispose to CRC; among these are IBD (UC and Crohn's disease) and familial adenomatous polyposis (FAP, **Figure 5.54**).

The extent of colorectal cancer can be staged according to the degree of bowel wall invasion, involvement of the regional lymph nodes, and presence of liver metastasis (common site for cancer spread). See **Section 6**.

In minimal access surgery (laparoscopic surgery), the transverse colon is at risk of injury while inserting the trocar, prior to insufflation of the peritoneal cavity.

(Continued)

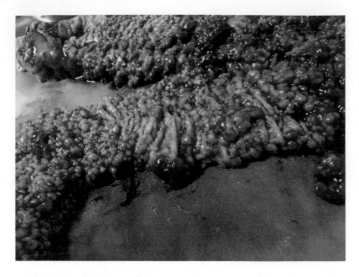

FIGURE 5.54 Colectomy specimen showing the colon riddled with extensive polyps due to familial adenomatous polyposis (FAP). (Courtesy of Rashide Yaacob.)

Diverticulosis of the colon (**Figure 5.55**) refers to the protrusion of the colonic mucosa, usually in the sigmoid colon. It is a common finding, which is usually asymptomatic, but can become complicated in the form of inflammation (acute diverticulitis), localised or generalised peritonitis due to bowel perforation, bleeding per rectum (which can be profuse), and fistula formation (tracking to another organ, e.g., the urinary bladder).

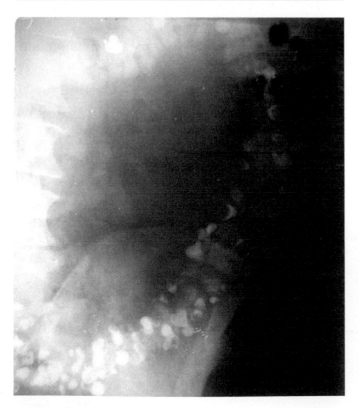

FIGURE 5.55 Barium enema showing extensive diverticulosis of the descending and sigmoid colon. (Courtesy of Qassim F. Baker.)

COMMON CAUSES OF LARGE BOWEL OBSTRUCTION

The large bowel is commonly obstructed by cancer, especially on the left side of the colon (**Figure 5.56**) and rectum. Other causes include volvulus, faecal impaction, and foreign bodies inserted into the rectum.

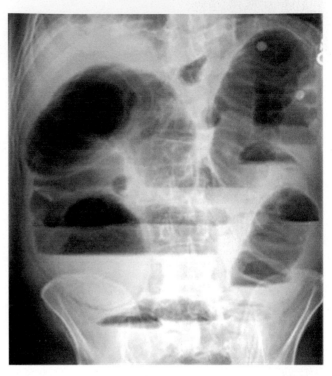

FIGURE 5.56 Plain X-ray of the abdomen showing colonic distension due to obstructing distal colon cancer. The ileocaecal valve is competent, so the small bowel is not distended

SIGMOID VOLVULUS

Sigmoid volvulus is a condition where a loop of bowel, commonly the sigmoid colon, twists around its mesentery, which results in cutting off of its blood supply and bowel gangrene. Patients with this condition present with a sudden onset of abdominal pain, vomiting, constipation, and massive abdominal distension (**Figures 5.57** and **5.58**).

Hirschsprung's disease is a congenital disease due to a lack of nerve cells (aganglionosis) of usually a short segment of the distal colon and rectum, which impairs peristalsis and causes constipation and large bowel obstruction in affected neonates (**Figure 5.59**).

ISCHAEMIC COLITIS

This term refers to the pathological changes which follow lack of blood supply (ischaemia) to the colon, specifically to the mucosa. It typically affects the watershed area at the junction of the territories of the SMA and IMA (splenic flexure). The main cause is atherosclerosis, and ischaemic colitis is a disease of older patients. The main clinical presentation is abdominal pain and rectal bleeding.

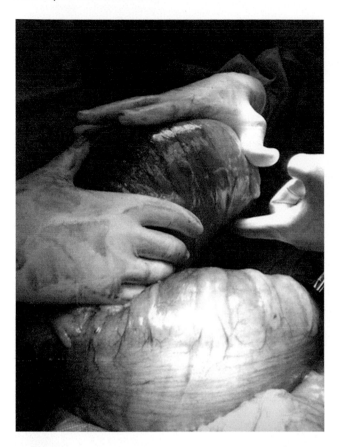

FIGURE 5.57 Volvulus of sigmoid colon. (Courtesy of Maan Aldoori.)

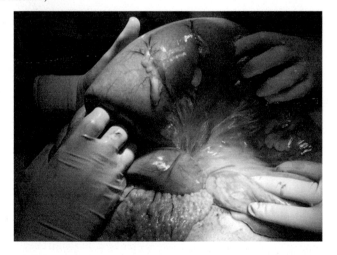

FIGURE 5.58 Ischaemic sigmoid colon in a 52-year-old man who presented with sudden lower abdominal pain and distension due to sigmoid volvulus. (Courtesy of Walid M.G. El-Haroni.)

Posterior Abdominal Wall

What are the structures that form the posterior abdominal wall?

- Lumbar vertebrae and the intervening intervertebral discs and connecting ligaments
- Muscles
- Diaphragm (see **Section 4**)
- Lumbar plexus

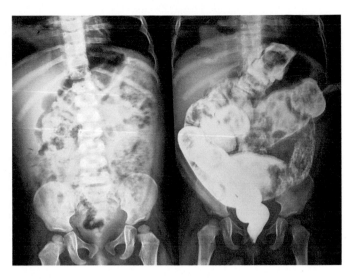

FIGURE 5.59 Plain X-ray and barium enema of a 3-year-old child with chronic constipation, faecal impaction, soiling, and abdominal distention, diagnosed with Hirschsprung's disease. (Courtesy of Mohammed H. Aldabbagh.)

There are five **lumbar vertebrae**:

- The lumbar vertebrae have a large kidney bean–shaped body with a triangular vertebral foramen (**Figures 5.60a** and **5.60b**).
- They have short, thick, and broad spinous processes and long, slender transverse processes. The pedicles are relatively strong, whilst the laminae are broad and short.
- The superior articular facets are concave and face postero-medially, whilst the inferior articular facets are convex facing anterolaterally. This reciprocity means that the lumbar spine is the most flexible region of the vertebral column, allowing flexion, extension, lateral flexion, and axial rotational movement.
- L5 has the largest body and is significantly deeper anteriorly, contributing to the lumbosacral angle.

The vertebral lamina extends from the base of the spinous process to the junction of the upper and lower articular facets. It has an anterior surface towards the vertebral canal and a posterior surface that gives attachment to the erector spinae muscles.

The **ligamenta flava** (*singular:* ligamentum flavum), yellow in colour because of their elastin content, are paired structures which run between adjacent vertebral laminae (**Figure 5.61**).

The intervertebral disc is composed of the peripheral annulus fibrosus (fibrocartilage) surrounding a gel-like centre, the nucleus pulposus (**Figure 5.62**).

Intervertebral discs contribute 25% of the total length of the vertebral column. They separate the vertebrae, which aids movement of the column. In addition, they act as a shock absorber to any mechanical force exerted on the column.

Sacralisation of L5 and lumbarization of S1 are congenital abnormalities – S1 takes lumbar characteristics, and L5 takes sacral characteristics.

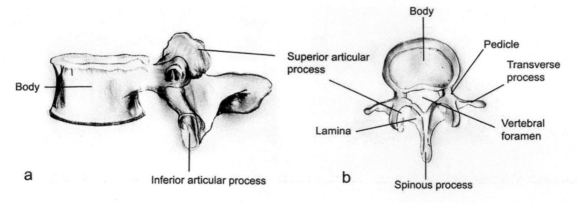

FIGURE 5.60   Lateral (a) and superior (b) view of a lumbar vertebra. (Courtesy of Aditya Mavinkurve.)

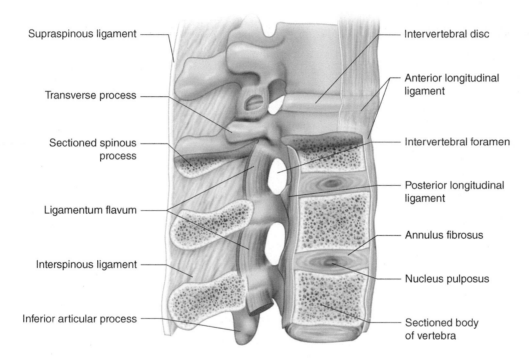

FIGURE 5.61   Diagram showing the ligaments of the vertebral column. (Courtesy of Gabriela Barzyk.)

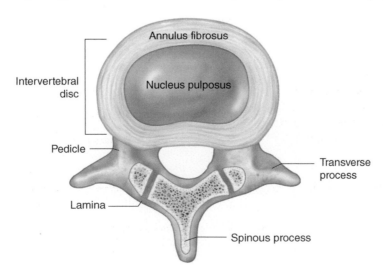

FIGURE 5.62   Diagram of a vertebra and intervertebral disc. (Courtesy of Gabriela Barzyk.)

Anatomical Planes

The lumbar vertebrae are important for identifying specific planes of the abdomen and pelvis:

- The adult spinal cord typically terminates at L1 (L3 in children) and continues as the conus medullaris.
- *L1:* transpyloric plane.
- *L3:* subcostal plane.
- Body of L4 is usually at the middle point of the horizontal line, joining the highest points of the iliac crests (intercristal line).
- *L5:* trans-tubercular plane; see the discussion on the division of the anterior abdominal wall.

CLINICAL NOTES

Degenerative disc disease results from alterations in the collagen composition of the nucleus pulposus and annulus fibrosus, which occur with age. Ossification and thickening of the endplates alter the shear and tensile force distribution across the disc. Annular tears develop, resulting in extrusion (fragmentation of the nucleus pulposus) or prolapse (escape of nuclear fluid – **posterolateral is the most common route**). Symptoms include localised back pain and muscular and radicular pain in the lower limbs from nerve root compression (sciatica). The main sites for slipped disc are L5–S1 and L4–L5.

Laminectomy is one of the most common orthopaedic operations performed to gain access to the spinal canal to relieve pressure on the spinal cord or cauda equina. Spinal stenosis is the most common indication for laminectomy (see **Section 1B**). Other indications include intervertebral disc herniation and primary or secondary tumours (metastatic spread to the vertebrae).

Changes in the height or curvature of the column can lead to compression of spinal nerve roots, resulting in radicular pain and loss of function.

Spondylosis is a form of osteoarthritis in the vertebral column and leads to the formation of osteophytes. Symptoms result from localised osteophyte compression of the nerve root, leading to unilateral lower limb radiculopathy, muscle spasm, and back pain.

The first symptoms of **osteoporosis** may result from wedge compression fractures of the lumbar vertebrae. Reduced bone mineral density leads to fragility fractures from minimal trauma. Fractures result in localised vertebral tenderness, a kyphotic spinal curvature, and reduced vertical height.

L5 is a common site for **spondylolysis** (a stress fracture of the vertebral arches) and **spondylolisthesis** (anterior dislocation of vertebrae).

Flexion-distraction fractures (seatbelt injury, for example) are common in the lumbar region, and spinal stenosis occurs from vigorous flexion, resulting in compression of the anterior portion of the vertebral body and a transverse fracture in the posterior element.

SPINAL METASTASIS

Metastases of cancer to the vertebral column are common, due to its extensive blood supply, and it is believed to be related to the extensive valveless veins of the paravertebral plexus, often referred to as Batson's plexus, which connects the thoracic veins and the pelvic veins, draining the prostate, bladder, and rectum. In descending order, the most common cancers which metastasise to the spine are prostate, breast, lung, thyroid, and renal.

Muscles of the Posterior Abdominal Wall

The following muscles lie on each side of the vertebral column:

- Psoas major and iliacus
- Quadratus lumborum
- Transversus abdominis (see discussion on the abdominal wall muscles)
- The posterior part of the diaphragm

Psoas Major

Origin

The name psoas comes from Greek ("of the loin"). This muscle lies along the lumbar spine and originates from the tips of the transverse processes and sides of the vertebral bodies of T12–L5 and the intervening intervertebral discs. It unites with the iliacus muscle, which originates from the upper part of the iliac fossa, to form the **iliopsoas**, and passes deep to the inguinal ligament to be inserted into the lesser trochanter of the femur. **The lumbar plexus runs within the muscle (Figure 5.63)**. It is covered by the psoas fascia, part of the lumbar fascia.

The nerve supply is from branches from L1 to L3 of the lumbar plexus. The iliacus is supplied by the femoral nerve (*vide infra*, "Lumbar Plexus").

In terms of action, both the iliacus and the psoas major are flexors of the hip joint.

Psoas abscess refers to a collection of pus within the psoas fascia. The causes include TB of the spine and spreading infection from infective focus in the GIT or the urinary system. The pus collection may track down the upper thigh, posterior to the inguinal ligament, and present as a mass in the groin (see **Section 6**).

Quadratus Lumborum

This quadrangular sheet of muscle lies lateral to the psoas major and originates from the inner lip of the iliac crest and the iliolumbar ligament, to be inserted into the 12th rib and transverse processes of the upper four lumbar vertebrae.

The nerve supply is from the lumbar plexus. See the anatomy of diaphragm, **Section 4**, for more information.

In terms of action, it helps in respiration by fixing the 12th rib and also acts as an extensor and lateral flexor of the spine.

Lumbar Plexus

The lumbar plexus is formed from the **ventral rami of spinal nerves L1–L5 and T12 (Figures 5.63** and **5.64)**. The plexus forms lateral to the intervertebral foramina on either side of the vertebrae. The course of the branches is described in relation to the psoas major, as well as the quadratus lumborum and iliacus (**Table 5.4**).

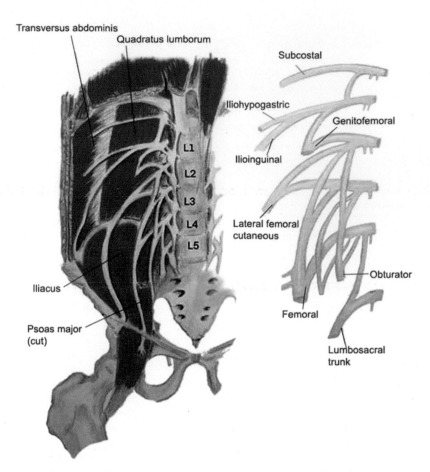

FIGURE 5.63   Nerves of the lumbar plexus and their relations with the psoas major and quadratus lumborum. (Courtesy of Kathryn DeMarre.)

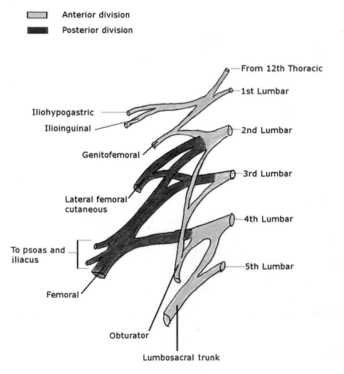

FIGURE 5.64   The branches of the lumbar plexus. (Courtesy of Gabriela Barzyk.)

CLINICAL NOTES

The **ilioinguinal nerve** may be blocked with local anaesthetic during inguinal hernia operations, 2 cm medial and 2 cm superior to the ASIS. It can also be damaged in open appendicectomy and inguinal hernia repair, causing loss of innervation to the conjoint tendon, predisposing to postoperative direct inguinal hernia. The nerve might also suffer entrapment during open hernia repair (herniorraphy), which results in postoperative chronic groin pain.

The **genitofemoral nerve** is important in eliciting the cremasteric reflex (L1, L2), which is used in neurological examination of the lumbar plexus; the reflex is particularly noticeable in new-born males. (See Further Reading: role of the genitofemoral nerve in testicular descent.)

The **obturator nerve** can be irritated by ovarian pathology, due to its close association with the ovary, passing just lateral to it in its descent. Irritation results in referred pain to the knee and inner thigh.

Femoral nerve (L2–L4) block: 2 cm below the inguinal ligament, 1 cm lateral to the femoral artery. When accessing the femoral vein for taking a blood sample, it is important to find the femoral pulse and go medially, as the femoral nerve can be damaged if you go lateral to the pulse.

The **saphenous nerve** is a sensory branch of the femoral nerve and the longest cutaneous nerve in the body. It can be damaged in varicose vein surgery, e.g., stripping of the great saphenous vein; see **Section 7**.

TABLE 5.4: The nerves of the lumbar plexus

Nerve	Spinal Segment	Course	Innervates
Iliohypogastric	T12 and L1	Lateral to psoas major and runs inferolateral across quadratus lumborum, posterior to kidneys. Passes between the transversus abdominis and internal oblique muscles	Sensory to skin of suprapubic and the posterolateral gluteal skin. Motor to internal oblique and transversus abdominis
Ilioinguinal	L1	Lateral to psoas major, inferior to iliohypogastric, runs inferolateral across quadratus lumborum and iliacus. **Pierces posterior wall of inguinal canal** and accompanies spermatic cord through superficial inguinal ring	Sensory to skin of upper medial aspect of thigh and anterior one-third of scrotum/labia majora. Motor branches to internal oblique and transversus abdominis (conjoint tendon)
Genitofemoral	L1 and L2	**The only nerve that pierces anterior surface of psoas major**. Splits into genital and femoral branches, which course separately through the deep inguinal ring and femoral sheath, respectively	Genital branch sensory to anterior genitalia and motor to cremasteric muscle. Femoral branch sensory to upper anterior aspect of thigh
Lateral femoral cutaneous (lateral cutaneous nerve of the thigh)	L2 and L3	Lateral to psoas major, runs inferolateral across iliacus, 1–2 cm medial to ASIS and inferior to inguinal ligament	Sensory to skin on anterolateral aspect of thigh
Obturator	L2–L4 (Ventral divisions)	• Descends **at medial border of psoas major** • Runs along lateral pelvic wall, lateral to the internal iliac vessels and the ovary on medial surface of obturator internus • Passes through obturator foramen	• Sensory to medial aspect of the thigh down to knee • Motor to adductor muscles of thigh (adductor longus, brevis, and part of magnus), as well as gracilis and obturator externus • Somatic branches to the pelvic peritoneum
Femoral	L2–L4 (Dorsal divisions)	• Emerges **in groove between iliacus and psoas major** at lateral border of psoas major • Passes inferior to inguinal ligament lateral to femoral artery and **outside femoral sheath** • Splits into anterior and posterior divisions	• Sensory to anterior aspect of thigh and medial aspect of leg and foot via saphenous nerve • Motor branches to quadriceps femoris (knee extensors) and iliacus, pectineus and sartorius (hip flexors) • *Knee jerk:* L3–L4

The Retroperitoneal Space

The retroperitoneal space is an anatomical space posterior to the parietal peritoneum of the posterior abdominal wall, which is superiorly closed by the diaphragm (**Figure 5.65**).

Contents of the retroperitoneal space

- Suprarenal glands (adrenal glands)
- Urinary organs (kidneys, ureters)
- *Bowel:* most of the duodenum, ascending and descending colon

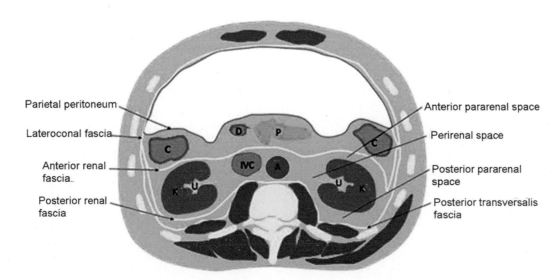

FIGURE 5.65 Cross-section of lumbar region showing the retroperitoneal organs. C: Colon, P: Pancreas, D: Duodenum, K: Kidney, U: Ureters, IVC: Inferior vena cava, A: Aorta. (Courtesy of Adam Lebby.)

- Pancreas
- Major vessels (abdominal aorta; common, internal, and external iliac arteries and their branches; IVC and corresponding iliac veins; origins of the azygos and hemiazygos veins – see **Section 4**).
- Lumbar plexus and abdominal autonomic plexuses
- Gonadal vessels
- Pre-aortic and para-aortic lymph nodes, cisterna chyli, and the origin of the thoracic duct (see **Section 4**)
- Connective tissue, including fat (retroperitoneal lipoma or liposarcoma can develop here and reach a huge size)

Suprarenal Glands

Each caps the upper pole of the kidney. There are two parts to each adrenal gland, of different embryological origins.

The **cortex (mesodermal origin)** has three layers: the zona glomerulosa, zona fasciculata, and zona reticularis (*mnemonic:* GFR).

This part is hormone-secreting as follows:

- *Zona glomerulosa:* mineralocorticoids such as aldosterone
- *Zona fasciculata:* corticosteroids such as hydrocortisone
- *Zona reticularis:* sex hormones (androgen, progesterone, and oestrogen)

Hormonal secretion is regulated by adrenocorticotropic hormone (ACTH) from the anterior pituitary gland.

Medulla (neural crest origin) is part of the sympathetic system (chromaffin cells) and secrets the catecholamines adrenaline and noradrenaline. The sympathetic pre-ganglionic fibres (via the greater splanchnic nerves) bypass the coeliac plexus to supply the chromaffin cells of the adrenal medulla, which can be considered post-ganglionic neurons.

Blood Supply

The adrenal glands have one of the richest blood supplies in the body relative to their weight.

The arteries are the superior suprarenal, middle suprarenal, and inferior suprarenal arteries from the inferior phrenic, abdominal aorta, and renal artery, respectively.

The venous drainage is via the adrenal vein to the IVC on the right side and to the renal vein on the left side (note that the right adrenal vein is quite short – an important operative consideration during removal of adrenal gland tumours).

Common clinical problems include Cushing's syndrome (due to excessive secretion of corticosteroids) and phaeochromocytoma (usually presents as intermittent or constant hypertension due to excessive catecholamine secretion from the adrenal medulla).

Removal of the adrenal gland/glands (adrenalectomy) can be performed via an open procedure, laparoscopic intraperitoneal/posterior extraperitoneal, or robotic surgery.

The Kidneys

Each kidney is a bean-shaped structure which lies on each side of the vertebral column from the level of T12–L3. The normal adult kidney measures about $12 \times 6 \times 3$ cm and weighs about 130 to 150 g. The right kidney lies at a slightly lower level, due to the position of the right lobe of the liver. Above each kidney is the suprarenal (adrenal) gland. Each has anterior and posterior surfaces, two borders: lateral convex and medial concave, which contains a vertical slit, the hilum of the kidney, for the passage of the renal vein, renal artery, ureter, branches of the renal plexus (sympathetic from the lower thoracic segments and parasympathetic from the vagus), and lymphatics.

Each kidney consists of an outer area (cortex) and an inner area (medulla); the nephron is the functional unit.

The embryology is as follows (**Figure 5.66**):

- The kidneys are derived from intermediate mesoderm.
- A **urogenital ridge** forms on either side of the aorta, from which the kidneys develop cranially to caudally through three sequential stages:
  - *Pronephros:* this is non-functional, and forms the nephrotomes, paired tubules draining into the pronephric duct, which regress by the end of week 4 of gestation.
  - *Mesonephros:* develops caudally to the pronephros and drains into the mesonephric ducts (Wolffian ducts). These carry out rudimentary kidney functioning, until many regress around 2 months of gestation. Some of these persist, opening into the cloaca of the embryo. The ureteric bud is also derived from the caudal end of the mesonephric ducts and later forms the collecting system of the mature kidney.

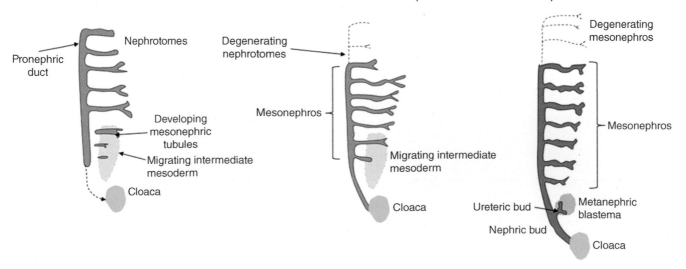

FIGURE 5.66 Embryological development of the kidneys. (Courtesy of Adam Lebby.)

- *Metanephros:* develops between the 5th and 12th weeks of gestation at the sacral level. Derived from the mesonephric duct (ureteric bud) and metanephric blastema (caudal intermediate mesoderm). Ultimately, this forms the mature kidney.
  - *Collecting system:* (**From the ureteric bud**) Ureter, renal pelvis, major and minor calyces, collecting ducts
  - *Excretory system:* (**From metanephric blastema**) Nephrons (Bowman's capsule enclosing the glomerulus, proximal convoluted tubule, loop of Henle, distal convoluted tubule)

The kidneys begin caudally in the embryo (initially sacral), and so the initial vascular supply is from the common iliac and middle sacral arteries. However, as the embryo grows and elongates, the kidneys come to sit in the lumbar region (ascension). Instead of pulling their blood supply with them (as seen in the testicular arteries), the kidneys send out new arterial branches to the aorta, thus forming the mature renal arteries. The caudal arteries then regress. This process of ascending can be deranged, leading to a number of **malformations (Figures 5.67** and **5.69**).

Posteriorly

Posterior abdominal wall (the diaphragm, psoas major, quadratus lumborum, and transversus abdominis). The diaphragm separates the upper pole from the pleura. Also related to the 11th and 12th ribs and upper nerves of the lumbar plexus (iliohypogastric, ilioinguinal in addition to the subcostal nerve) (see **Section 4** for information on the relationship of the pleura to the lower ribs).

The kidney is surrounded by a **fibrous capsule**, then the **perinephric fat**, which is surrounded by the **perinephric fascia** (of Gerota), which encloses the adrenal gland as well. This is of surgical importance when embarking on radical nephrectomy for renal cancer. The perinephric fat and fascia must be removed en bloc, including the suprarenal gland. The kidney hilum lies at the transpyloric plane. **The renal vein is the most anterior, and the ureter is the most posterior.** This explains the posterior approach to dealing with the removal of renal stones, while the anterior approach is more appropriate to secure the pedicle while removing tumours, such as renal cell carcinoma (RCC). However, more stone operations are performed by the interventional radiologists (percutaneous nephrolithotomy) than by open surgery.

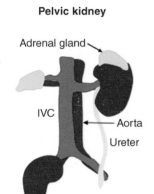 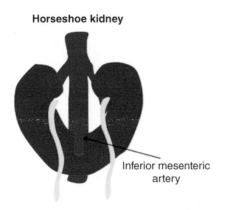 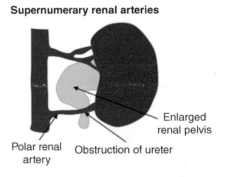

Pelvic kidney

Adrenal gland
IVC
Aorta
Ureter

Horseshoe kidney

Inferior mesenteric artery

Supernumerary renal arteries

Enlarged renal pelvis
Polar renal artery
Obstruction of ureter

FIGURE 5.67 Developmental anomalies of the kidneys. (Courtesy of Adam Lebby.)

Main functions of the kidneys include:

- Excretory function
- Maintenance of water, acid–base balance, and blood pressure
- Hormonal function (secretion of erythropoietin, renin–angiotensin system to control blood pressure, secretion of vitamin D active metabolite 1,25-dihydroxycholecalciferol)

Anatomical Relations

Anteriorly

Right kidney: second part of duodenum and hepatic flexure of the colon. The hepatorenal pouch of Morison separates the upper pole of the right kidney from the visceral surface of the right lobe of the liver and is one of the sites of peritoneal fluid collection due to its connection to the right paracolic gutter and the right subphrenic space.

Left kidney: pancreatic body and tail medially, with spleen laterally and splenic flexure of the colon related to the lower pole.

Arterial blood supply is through the renal arteries. These arise at a right angle from the abdominal aorta, below the origin of the SMA at the level of intervertebral discs between L1 and L2. The right renal artery passes posteriorly to the IVC. However, some 30% of people have accessory renal arteries. These mostly arise from the abdominal aorta. Accessory arteries may compress the pelviureteric junction (PUJ) and cause hydronephrosis. Extrarenal branches include the inferior suprarenal artery, branches to the upper ureter, renal capsule, and perinephric fascia (**Figure 5.68**).

- Each renal artery divides into an anterior and a posterior division.
- Five segmental arteries (understanding this is especially important when planning partial nephrectomy for cancer of the upper or the lower pole).
- Lobar, interlobar, arcuate, and interlobular arteries.
- Afferent arterioles to the glomeruli.
- Efferent arterioles to peritubular capillary plexus.
- Venous ends of capillaries to the interlobular veins, arcuate, and interlobar veins, and then to the renal vein.

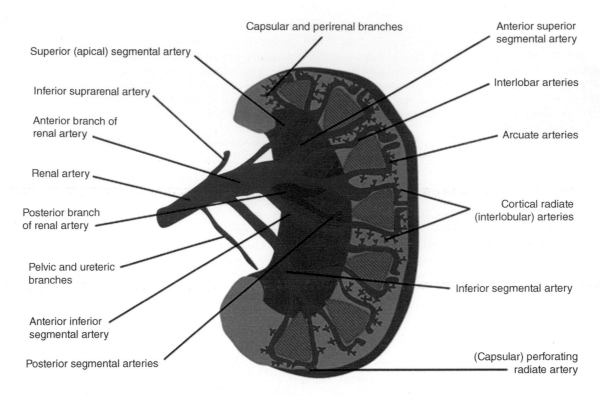

FIGURE 5.68   Diagram of renal blood supply with the renal pelvis removed. (Courtesy of Adam Lebby and Alina Humdani.)

The kidneys have a high contribution of blood flow through the renal arteries (about 20% of cardiac output per minute), so renal trauma can result in severe blood loss and hypovolaemic shock. The left renal vein passes anterior to the aorta, where it receives the left gonadal vein; see **Section 6**. Each renal vein drains into the IVC.

Lymphatic drainage is through four to five lymphatic trunks to the lateral aortic lymph nodes.

Nerve supply is via autonomic nerves: sympathetic pre-ganglionic fibres that run with T12–L1 (least splanchnic nerve) to the renal and coeliac plexuses. Renal pain from stretching of the renal capsule, due to inflammation (e.g., glomerulonephritis) or obstruction of the PUJ, is felt in the back and flanks (T12 and L1 nerve distribution; see information on ureteric colic, later).

Parasympathetic is from the vagus nerve.

CLINICAL NOTES

- Ureteric colic (see **Section 6**, Pelvis and Perineum).
- Renal artery stenosis is one of the causes of secondary hypertension, which can be correctable (other causes include phaeochromocytoma and coarctation of the aorta).
- Kidney tumours, commonly RCC, which may be manifested as haematuria and unilateral loin pain.

- The right renal vein is shorter than the left. Malignant kidney tumours may extend down the renal vein into the IVC, making removal of the malignant emboli more difficult on the right side.
- Kidney infections (pyelonephritis), inflammation (glomerulonephritis), and nephrotic syndrome are common clinical conditions.
- Acute kidney injury and CKD (for more details see Baker & Aldoori, 2009).
- Kidney injuries, which can be part of injuries to other abdominal organs. Most renal injuries are treated conservatively, and nephrectomy (surgical removal of the kidney) is kept as the last resort for severely shattered or avulsed kidneys.
- Pelvic kidney results from failure of ascent. It forms one of the differential diagnoses of masses in the RIF or left iliac fossa (LIF).
- Horseshoe kidney (**Figure 5.69**) is a congenital anomaly where the lower poles of each kidney are united. The IMA prevents the ascent of the isthmus that bridges the lower poles of the kidneys. This anomaly predisposes the kidneys to stone formation and repeated UTI.
- *Supernumerary arteries:* non-regression of caudal arteries can lead to multiple renal arteries. This increases the risk of pressure on the ureter, leading to back-up of urine into the kidney and hydronephrosis.

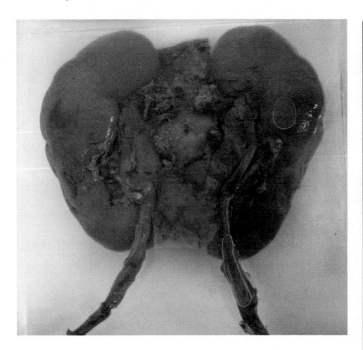

FIGURE 5.69 Horseshoe kidney. (Courtesy Dept. of Anatomical Sciences, SGUL.)

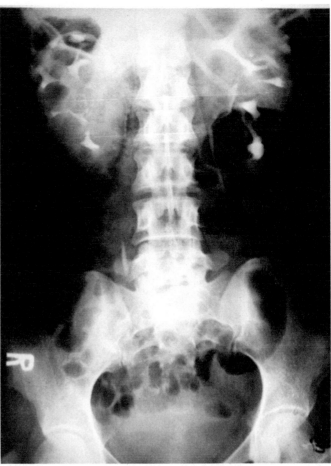

FIGURE 5.70 IVU examination showing spider leg configuration of bilateral polycystic kidneys. (Courtesy of Qassim F. Baker.)

- Polycystic kidney disease is an autosomal dominant disorder, characterised by the formation of multiple cysts within the kidneys in adult life. The end stage is chronic renal failure (**Figure 5.70**).
- Agenesis of one or both kidneys (failure of the kidney to develop) is rare but important to note when embarking on nephrectomy during explorative laparotomy for trauma.

KIDNEY TRANSPLANTATION

Because of its longer renal vein, the left kidney is the preferred side for live donor nephrectomy. The donor kidney is positioned retroperitoneally in one of the iliac fossae, and the renal artery and vein are anastomosed to the corresponding external iliac vessels, while the ureter is attached to the bladder.

CLINICAL EXAMINATION

Palpation of the kidneys should be done as part of any abdominal examination. In a healthy adult with no anatomical malformation, it is unlikely that you will be able to palpate any more than the inferior pole of the kidney, when the patient is supine and in full inhalation. Even this may not be possible in all patients.

Note: The right kidney is sometimes more palpable in very thin patients or children, as it sits lower due to the liver.

To examine a kidney, one should use both hands, in a technique known as balloting: the lower hand pushes up from the back in the costophrenic angle, whereas the upper hand pushes into the abdomen from the upper quadrant, lateral to the rectus abdominis muscle.

An easily palpable or tender kidney is abnormal and should raise clinical suspicion of renal pathology, including but not limited to neoplasia, infection, obstruction, or trauma. The clinical history should be thorough to help elucidate potential pathology. Back examination should be part of a proper abdominal exam to check the spine and for swelling and tenderness at renal angles, e.g., perinephric abscess.

Revision Questions

Q1.

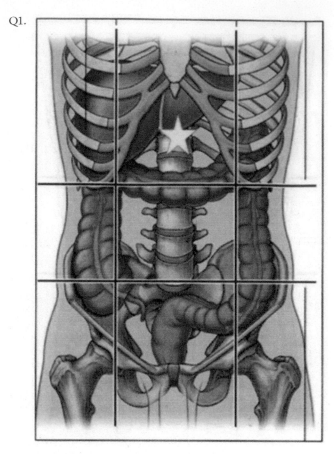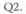

(Courtesy of Dept. of Anatomical Sciences, SGUL.)

Q1A. Which of the following best describes the region indicated by the star?
a. Epigastric
b. Left hypochondrium
c. Right hypochondrium
d. Suprapubic
e. Umbilical

Q1B. Which of the following best describes the region of the gut from which pain may be referred to this region?
a. Appendix
b. Ileum
c. Jejunum
d. Pylorus
e. Sigmoid colon

Q2.

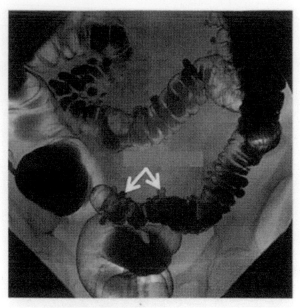

(Courtesy of the Dept. of Anatomical Sciences, SGUL.)

Q2A. Which of the following best describes the features indicated by the arrow?
a. Appendices epiploicae
b. Colonic diverticula
c. Haustra
d. Mesenteric lymph nodes
e. Taeniae coli

Q2B. Which of the following best describes the abdominal region where pain emanating from these features would be felt most?
a. Epigastric
b. Lower left quadrant
c. Umbilical
d. Upper right quadrant
e. Upper left quadrant

Q3. Embryologically, what does the parietal peritoneum arise from?
a. Ectoderm
b. Endoderm
c. Neuroectoderm
d. Somatic mesoderm
e. Splanchnic mesoderm

Q4. Which of the following is a secondarily retroperitoneal organ?
a. Ascending colon
b. Kidney
c. Liver
d. Stomach
e. Ureter

Q5. What is the anterior relation of the epiploic foramen?
   a. Hepatoduodenal ligament
   b. Hepatogastric ligament
   c. Parietal peritoneum covering the IVC
   d. Visceral peritoneum covering the caudate lobe of the liver
   e. Visceral peritoneum covering the superior aspect of the duodenum

What is Pringle's manoeuvre?

Q6. Which structure helps to divide the infracolic compartment into its right and left components?
   a. Ligament of Treitz
   b. Mesentery proper
   c. Mesoappendix
   d. Sigmoidal mesocolon
   e. Transverse mesocolon

Q7. Which structure runs posterior to the apex of the sigmoid mesocolon?
   a. Common iliac artery
   b. Common iliac vein
   c. Inferior vena cava
   d. Left ureter
   e. Right ureter

Q8. The ligamentum teres (round ligament) is a remnant of which embryological structure?

Q9. The ligamentum venosum is a remnant of which embryological structure?

Q10. Which of the following structures is contained within the lateral umbilical folds?
   a. Inferior epigastric artery
   b. Superior epigastric artery
   c. Umbilical artery
   d. Umbilical vein
   e. Urachus

Q11. Why do patients with pelvic peritonitis flex their knee and hip?

Q12.

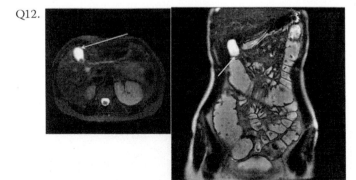

(Courtesy of the Dept. of Anatomical Sciences, SGUL.)

Q12A. Which term best describes the structure indicated by the arrows?
   a. Common bile duct
   b. Cystic duct
   c. Fundus of gallbladder
   d. Neck of gallbladder
   e. Quadrate lobe

Q12B. Inflammation of the structure indicated by arrows may be perceived as pain arising in which of the following regions?
   a. Epigastric region
   b. Left hypochondrium
   c. Right hypochondrium
   d. Suprapubic region
   e. Umbilical region

Q13.

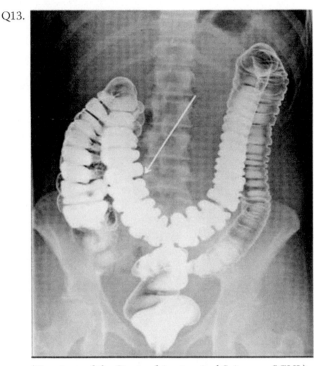

(Courtesy of the Dept. of Anatomical Sciences, SGUL)

Q13A. Which of the following best describes the structure indicated by the arrow?
   a. Ascending colon
   b. Caecum
   c. Descending colon
   d. Sigmoid colon
   e. Transverse colon

Q13B. Which of the following best describes the arterial supply of the region of the gut marked by the arrow?
   a. Ileocolic
   b. Jejunal
   c. Left colic
   d. Middle colic
   e. Right colic

Q14.

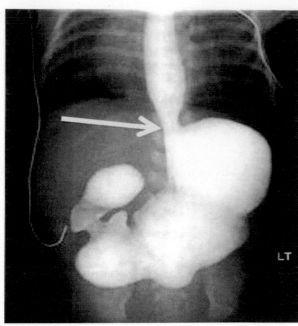

(Courtesy of the Dept. of Anatomical Sciences, SGUL.)

Q14A. Which of the following best describes the region of the stomach indicated by the arrow?
   a. Body
   b. Cardia
   c. Fundus
   d. Pylorus
   e. Pyloric antrum

Q14B. What is the usual vertebral level of the region indicated by the arrow?
   a. T6
   b. T8
   c. T10-T11
   d. T12
   e. L2

Q15.

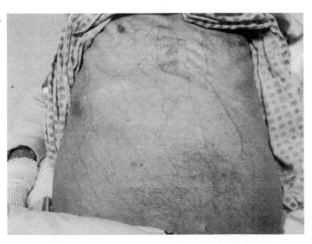

(Courtesy of the Dept. of Anatomical Sciences, SGUL.)

Q15. What is the azygos system? What can cause engorgement of the anterior abdominal wall veins? What are the sites of portosystemic anastomosis?

Answers

A1A. a
A1B. d
A2A. b
A2B. b
A3.   d
A4.   a
A5A. a
A5B. Applying pressure to the free border of the lesser omentum through the epiploic foramen to control bleeding during surgery
A6.   b
A7.   d
A8.   Left umbilical vein
A9.   Ductus venosus
A10. a
A11. Patients with peritonitis lie still on one side or the other, with the knees and hips flexed to relax the anterolateral abdominal muscles (the psoas sign).
A12A. c
A12B. c
A13A. e
A13B. d
A14A. b
A14B. c
A15. The azygos system connects the IVC and SVC outside the right atrium, giving a path for blood to return to the right atrium if either vena cava is blocked. Its main function is to drain the intercostal spaces and the posterior thoracic wall. See **Figure 4.8** and **Table 4.2** in **Section 4**.

Engorgement of the veins of the anterior abdominal wall can be caused by portal hypertension and IVC obstruction.

Sites of portosystemic anastomosis include the lower oesophagus, inferior and superior rectal veins, and veins on the anterior abdominal wall; some are radiating from the umbilicus (caput medusa).

Further Reading

Baker Q and Aldoori M. 2009. Clinical Surgery: A Practical Guide. CRC Press.

Blake PG and Daugirdas JT. Peritoneal Dialysis: https://abdominalkey.com/physiology-of-peritoneal-dialysis. June 2016.

Fraumeni D. Splenectomy and Subsequent Mortality in Veterans of the 1939-45 War. *Lancet* 1977;310(8029):127–129.

McLatchie, et al. 2013. Oxford Clinical Handbook of Clinical Surgery. Oxford Press. 4e. Pages: 554–555.

Newland et al. Overwhelming Post-Splenectomy Infection (OPSI). *BMJ* 2005; 331:417–418.

The Operation of Lumbar Sympathectomy. https://www.sciencedirect.com/topics/medicine-and-dentistry/lumbar-sympathectomy

Raine, et al. 2018. Oxford Handbook for the Foundation Programme. Oxford Press. 5e. Page 440.Swerdlow NJ, Wu WW, & Schermerhorn ML. Open and Endovascular Management of Aortic Aneurysms. https://www.ahajournals.org/doi/full/10.1161/CIRCRESAHA.118.313186 Feb. 2019.

6

ANATOMY OF THE PELVIS AND PERINEUM

Reviewed by Paul Carter, Qassim F. Baker, and Philip J. Adds

Learning Objectives

- Understand the overall anatomy of the pelvis
- Understand the blood supply and innervation of the pelvic organs
- Describe the function and components of the pelvic floor
- Know the pelvic organs and understand the clinical implications of their location
- Understand the overall anatomy of the rectum and anal canal
- The perineum
- The male genital organs
- The female genital organs
- Revision questions

The Pelvic Girdle

Consists of the two innominate (coxal) bones, the sacrum, and the coccyx, which enclose the pelvic cavity (**Figures 6.1** and **6.2**). **The main functions of the pelvic girdle are**:

- Transmission of body weight from the spine to the femurs, via the sacroiliac joints
- Protection and support of pelvic organs, including the bladder, rectum, and the internal reproductive organs
- Provide attachment for the muscles of the anterior and posterior abdominal walls, buttocks, and thighs

Components of the Pelvic Girdle

The pelvic brim divides the **true (lesser) pelvis**, below the brim, from the **false (greater) pelvis**, above the brim (which can be considered part of the abdominal cavity). The true pelvis has an inlet (pelvic brim), cavity, and outlet. The pelvic cavity projects posteriorly from the abdominal cavity towards the buttocks.

What Is Meant by the Pelvic Brim?

The pelvic brim extends from the sacral promontory (the anterior lip of the superior surface of S1) to the upper part of the pubic symphysis and includes the ala of the sacrum, the arcuate line of the ilium, the ilio-pubic eminence, and the pectineal line of the pubis.

The Pelvic Outlet

The pelvic outlet is diamond-shaped and consists anteriorly of the lower border of the pubic symphysis and the two ischiopubic rami (forming the pubic arch); posteriorly it consists of the ischial tuberosities, sacrotuberous ligaments, and coccyx.

The Innominate Bone

- The innominate or coxal bone (*os coxa*) consists of three bones (ischium, ilium, and pubis) which fuse at the "Y-shaped" cartilage in the acetabulum ("vinegar cup" in Latin); this is where the head of the femur articulates with the pelvis to form the hip joint.
- During puberty the cartilage ossifies and the three bones fuse.
- The ilium is the largest and most superior portion of the innominate bone. Superior to the acetabulum, the ilium expands to form the **ala**, the winged portion of the ilium, which articulates with the alar surface of the sacrum at the synovial sacroiliac joint and transmits all the forces of the upper body downwards.
- The ilium is composed of three surfaces: gluteal (on the outside), iliac (forming the iliac fossa, above the pelvic brim), and a sacropelvic surface. The gluteal surface has the anterior, inferior, and posterior gluteal lines, which provide attachment points for the gluteal muscles (see **Section 7**, Lower Limb).
- The iliac crest extends between the posterior superior iliac spine (PSIS) and the anterior superior iliac spine (ASIS), which is the most anterior part; it has inner and outer lips.

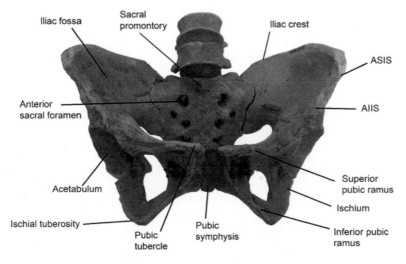

FIGURE 6.1 Pelvic girdle. (Courtesy of Qassim F. Baker.)

DOI: 10.1201/9781003312895-7

The external lip of the iliac crest has four muscle attachments:

- External oblique
- Latissimus dorsi (LD; this attachment is detached when creating an LD flap, commonly for breast reconstruction)
- Tensor fasciae latae
- Internal oblique

The internal lip of the iliac crest has four muscle attachments:

- Transversus abdominis
- Quadratus lumborum
- Sacrospinalis (erector spinae)
- Iliacus (mainly originates from the iliac fossa)

See **Section 5** for more information on the muscles of the anterior abdominal wall.

The horizontal **intercristal line** is between the highest points of the iliac crests and corresponds to the level of L4-L5. It is used for lumbar puncture positioning and insertion of epidural catheters.

The pectineal line (Latin *pecten*, "comb") is a ridge on the superior ramus of the pubic bone, which joins the arcuate line to form the iliopectineal line. The **pectineus muscle** arises from the superior pubic ramus (pectineal line) and inserts onto the pectineal line of the femur. It forms a quadrangular sheet of muscle in the upper and medial thigh and part of the floor of the femoral triangle. It is mainly an adductor of the thigh and is supplied by the femoral and obturator nerves.

The **pubic tubercle** is a projection lateral to the pubic symphysis that gives attachment to the adductor longus and the medial end of the **inguinal ligament**, which originates on the ASIS.

The **spermatic cord** passes down to the scrotum, superior to the pubic tubercle. The pubic tubercle is an important landmark in differentiating between inguinal and femoral hernias. Inguinal hernias are above and medial to the pubic tubercle, whereas femoral hernias are below and lateral.

The **pubic arch** is formed by the pubic symphysis in the middle and the bodies of the inferior pubic rami at the sides.

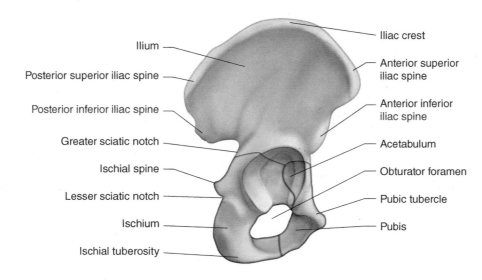

FIGURE 6.2   The lateral aspect of the innominate bone. (Courtesy of Chun Ho.)

The Arcuate Line

The **arcuate line** is a smooth, rounded border on the internal surface of the ilium. It is inferior to the iliac fossa and iliacus muscle (which attaches, with the psoas major muscle, onto the lesser trochanter of the femur) and above the medial aspect of the acetabulum. The pelvis is orientated so that the pubic symphysis and ASIS are in the same vertical plane. Therefore, the posterior aspect of the iliac fossa is superior to the arcuate line, and the anterior portion of the iliac fossa is anterosuperior. The line indicates where weight is transferred from the sacroiliac joint to the hip joint. The arcuate line is continuous with the pectineal line (*vide infra*).

The ilium provides muscle attachment to the sartorius (at the ASIS) and piriformis, from the area below the posterior inferior iliac spine (PIIS).

The Pubic Bone

- Composed of three parts: body, superior ramus, and inferior ramus.
- The pubic symphysis joins the two pubic bones at a secondary cartilaginous joint.

The angle at the lower end of the pubic symphysis is called the **subpubic angle**.

Learning Point

Typically, secondary cartilaginous joints occur in the median plane of the body and permit limited movement. Examples include the pubic symphysis, manubriosternal joint, and intervertebral discs.

The Ischium

The ischium is the lower part of the innominate bone. It is inferior to the ilium and posterior to the pubis. The superior part of the ischium forms one-third of the acetabulum.

The ischium consists of:

- The body and ramus. The deep and superficial transverse perineal muscles originate from the body of the ischium.

- The ramus of the ischium ascends to join the inferior ramus of the pubis (forming the ischiopubic ramus), and together form the lower boundary of the obturator foramen. It is the partial origin for the gracilis and adductor magnus.

The **ischial tuberosity** is a bony prominence on the posterior portion of the superior ischial ramus. It marks the lateral boundary of the pelvic outlet and carries the body weight in the sitting position.

- Structures attaching to the ischial tuberosity include extensors of the hip, (the hamstring muscles) and the sacrotuberous ligament.

The **ischial spine** is a posterior bony projection from the body of the ischium and gives attachment to the superior gemellus muscle, sacrospinous ligament, and coccygeus muscle.

The ischial spine is an important landmark between the greater and lesser sciatic notches. The pudendal nerve passes beneath the piriformis muscle and medial to the ischial spine (site for pudendal nerve anaesthesia in obstetrics).

The **greater sciatic notch** is located on the ilium, directly inferior to the PIIS. The **sacrospinous ligament** attaches from the ischial spine to the sacrum and converts the greater sciatic notch into the greater sciatic foramen, which is partly filled by the piriformis (see **Section 7**, Lower Limb, gluteal region).

The **lesser sciatic notch** is located on the ischium, directly inferior to the ischial spine. The sacrotuberous ligament attaches from the ischial tuberosity to the sacrum, posterior to the sacrospinous ligament, creating the lesser sciatic foramen from the lesser sciatic notch (which transmits the nerve to the obturator internus and its tendon, the pudendal nerve, and internal pudendal vessels).

For further details review the anatomy of the buttock in **Section 7**, Lower Limb.

Lateral Pelvic Wall

The **obturator foramen** is bounded by the pubis anteriorly and the ischium posteriorly and is covered by the **obturator membrane**, except for a small superolateral passage, the **obturator canal**, for the passage of the obturator nerve (from the lumbar plexus) and the obturator vessels to supply the medial (adductor) compartment of the thigh (see **Section 7**, Lower Limb).

The **obturator internus** muscle takes its origin from the pelvic aspect of the obturator membrane and the surrounding bone. Its tendon passes through the lesser sciatic foramen to insert onto the greater trochanter of the femur. It is a lateral rotator of the femur at the hip joint and is supplied by its own nerve from the sacral plexus.

The **obturator externus muscle** originates from the outer part of the obturator membrane and the adjacent bones of the obturator foramen and inserts into the trochanteric fossa of the femur. It is supplied by the obturator nerve and helps in stabilising the hip joint.

The Sacrum (Figure 6.3)

The sacrum consists of the union of five vertebrae. It articulates, above, with L5 vertebra and, below, with the coccyx and, laterally, with the iliac bones at the sacroiliac joint (a synovial joint with limited movement). Ossification and fusion of the sacrum are not complete until age 18 to 35 years.

The **anterior and posterior sacral foramina** (four, on both the pelvic and the dorsal surfaces of the sacrum) are the sites for exit of the ventral and dorsal rami of the sacral spinal nerves S1–S4, respectively.

The **median sacral crest**, posteriorly, represents the fused spinous processes of the sacral vertebrae and can be felt on the upper part of the cleft between the buttocks.

The lower three fused sacral vertebrae are associated with the retroperitoneal lower third of the rectum.

The **sacral hiatus** (through which the fifth sacral spinal nerves exit) is situated at the lower end of the sacral canal and is flanked by two bony prominences (sacral cornua, which form an important landmark to find the hiatus). It is located about 5 cm above the tip of the coccyx.

The **coccyx** (*Greek:* "cuckoo", from its resemblance to a cuckoo's beak) is usually composed of four fused vertebrae. It articulates at its upper end with the sacrum. The anterior surface of the coccyx can be felt by rectal digital examination.

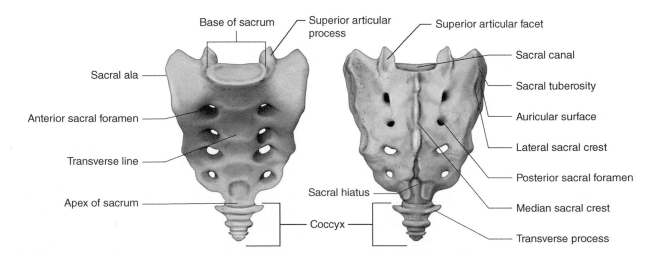

FIGURE 6.3 Anterior and posterior aspects of the sacrum and the coccyx. (Courtesy of Callum Moffitt.)

CLINICAL NOTES

- *Bone marrow transplant:* the iliac crest is easily accessible and provides a large reservoir of bone marrow cells.
- *Bone graft:* bone grafting involves the transplantation of bone tissue into bones which have been damaged from different causes, e.g., trauma. The iliac crest is the most common site for bone tissue donation.

Fractures of the sacrum and coccyx are rare; however, neurological deficit is common if they do occur.

Caudal regression syndrome is underdevelopment of the sacrum and coccyx.

Cauda equina syndrome is compression of the cauda equina. This can be a consequence of herniated disc compression at L5–S1, ruptured disc, tumour, or abscess (see **Section 1B**, Spinal Cord).

The sacrum is the most common site for development of a rare sarcoma, known as **chordoma**, from the remnants of the notochord.

PELVIC FRACTURE

This commonly follows road traffic accidents or falling from heights. The fracture can be displaced or non-displaced, depending on the integrity of the pelvic ring (**Figure 6.4**). Displaced fractures result from more than one fracture or dislocation of the sacroiliac joint or symphysis pubis. The pelvis almost always fractures in two places; therefore, if one fracture is identified, always look for another fracture.

Complications include:

- **Hypovolaemic shock**, from internal haemorrhage due to rupture of the thin pelvic veins.
- **Injuries to other organs** such as the urethra, bladder, and rectum. Therefore, it is important to perform a rectal examination on all patients with a pelvic fracture.

QUIZ QUESTION

Q. *What are the expected clinical problems in the management of the patient in* **Figure 6.4** *in an A&E department?*

Blood Supply of the Pelvic Organs

Arterial Supply

The main arterial supply is from the **internal iliac artery**, a branch of the common iliac artery at the level of the sacroiliac joint (the other division is the external iliac artery, which continues as the common femoral artery underneath the inguinal ligament).

The internal iliac artery divides into anterior and posterior divisions at the level of the upper margin of the greater sciatic notch (**Figure 6.5**).

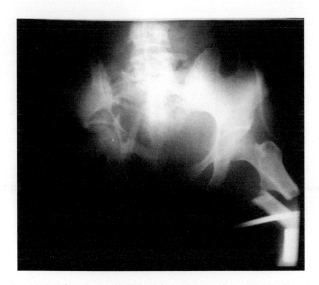

FIGURE 6.4   X-ray of the pelvis and upper femora showing severe disruption of the pelvic ring and comminuted fracture of the upper left femur. (Courtesy of Qassim F. Baker.)

Branches of the Anterior Division

The anterior division contains nine arteries: three arteries supplying the bladder, three arteries supplying the viscera, and three arteries supplying the body wall.

Arteries supplying the bladder

- *Umbilical artery:* extends from the fetus to the placenta during embryonic life; after birth, the proximal part remains as the superior vesical artery, the occluded distal part becomes the medial umbilical ligament (see **Section 5**, Abdomen)
- *Superior and inferior vesical arteries:* supply the bladder, ductus deference, seminal vesicles, and the prostate gland

Arteries supplying the viscera

- *Middle rectal (see information on the blood supply of the rectum):* supplies the lower part of the rectum; may be absent in both sexes, especially in females
- *Vaginal and uterine arteries:* in females, the vaginal artery may replace the inferior vesical artery; see later discussion on the blood supply of the vagina

Arteries supplying the body wall

- *Internal pudendal artery:* follows the course of the pudendal nerve (leaving through the greater sciatic foramen to enter the gluteal region, then enters the ischiorectal fossa through the lesser sciatic foramen within the Alcock's canal, giving off the inferior rectal artery through its course in the fossa)
- *Obturator artery:* passes with the obturator nerve to the adductor compartment of the thigh
- *Inferior gluteal artery:* enters the buttock through the great sciatic foramen, underneath the piriformis; supplies the gluteus maximus

Branches of the *posterior* division (supply *parietal* structures) –

Remember that the posterior division supplies the *p*arietal structures.

- *Superior gluteal artery:* the largest branch of the internal iliac artery (see anatomy of the gluteal region in **Section 7**,

Lower Limb) and runs above the piriformis and enters the buttock through the greater sciatic foramen to supply the three gluteal muscles (maximus, medius, and minimus)

- *Lateral sacral artery (or arteries):* supply the skin and muscles dorsal to the sacrum after exiting through the posterior sacral foramina
- *Iliolumbar artery:* supplies the iliacus, quadratus lumborum, and psoas major

Intraoperative ligation of the internal iliac artery can be lifesaving in cases of uncontrollable bleeding during pelvic surgery, for example, after pelvic trauma and during hysterectomy.

of the pubic symphysis and is about 10 cm in the adult male compared to 11.2 cm in the female; the **transverse diameter** is measured between the furthest points of the inlet (13.1 cm in the female to 12.5 in the male).

For the pelvic outlet, the following diameters can be elicited:

- **The transverse diameter** of the outlet, the distance between the ischial tuberosities, measures approximately 11.8 cm in the female compared to 8.5 cm in the male.
- **The AP diameter** of the outlet, the distance between the tip of the coccyx and the inferior border of the pubic symphysis, is approximately 12.5 cm in the female, 8.0 cm in the male.

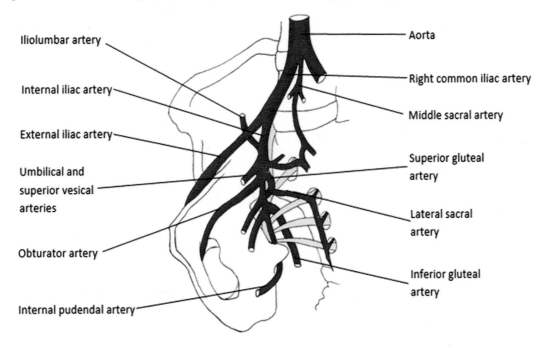

FIGURE 6.5   Arterial blood supply of the pelvis. (Courtesy of Calum Harrington-Vogt.)

Venous Return

The veins correspond to the branches of the internal iliac artery. They converge to form the internal iliac vein. The internal iliac vein unites with the external iliac vein to form the common iliac vein. The union of the right and left common iliac veins forms the inferior vena cava (IVC) at the level of L5. The only exception is the iliolumbar vein, which drains into the common iliac vein.

Lymphatics of the Pelvis

These accompany the blood vessels and, therefore, the lymph nodes are named accordingly (internal iliac, common iliac lymph nodes).

Sexual Dimorphism

Male and female pelvises have evolved differently, as a result of the female pelvis being adapted for childbirth. These differences are useful in differentiating between male and female skeletons (**Table 6.1**).

Diameters of the Female Pelvis

The diameter of the female pelvis is very important in relation to the diameter of the skull of the fetus. Measurement of this is known as pelvimetry and nowadays uses plain radiographs or magnetic resonance imaging (MRI) scanning of the pelvis. The pelvic diameters are as follows.

Of the inlet (superior pelvic aperture):

- The **anterior-posterior (AP) diameter** is measured from the midpoint of the sacral promontory to the upper border

- The **diagonal conjugate diameter**, the distance between the sacral promontory and the lower border of the pubic symphysis, is approximately 12.5 cm in the adult female
- The **interspinous distance**, the distance between the ischial spines, is approximately 9.5 cm in the adult female

It is important to note that the widest point of the pelvic *inlet* is the transverse diameter, whereas the widest point of the pelvic *outlet* is the AP diameter. This is the reason the fetal head must rotate 90 degrees during labour to pass through the pelvic cavity.

TABLE 6.1: The differences between male and female pelvises

Male	Female
Smaller and less wide (optimised for bipedal locomotion)	Larger, wider, and rounder (to aid in childbirth)
Iliac crest is higher	Iliac crest is lower
Sacrum is longer, narrower, and straighter	Sacrum is shorter, wider, and rounder
Subpubic angle is acute	Subpubic angle is obtuse
Greater sciatic notch is narrow	Greater sciatic notch is wider
Acetabula are closer together	Acetabula are wide apart
Pelvic inlet is slightly heart shaped	Pelvic inlet is oval
Pelvic outlet is narrow and oval	Pelvic outlet is more circular

Types of pelvises (Figure 6.6)

- *Gynaecoid (Female type):* the most suitable pelvis shape and dimensions for childbirth, as the inlet is ovoid in shape and its transverse diameter is greater than the AP diameter.
- *Platypelloid (Flat pelvis):* there is a flat inlet and a prominent sacrum, with the transverse diameter being greater than the AP diameter; the subpubic arch is wide, and the ischial spines are prominent
- *Android (Male type):* this pelvis has a wedge- or a heart-shaped inlet, with a prominent sacrum, and consequently narrow AP diameter; the reduced pelvic outlet leads to increased risk of complications during childbirth.
- *Anthropoid (Ape-like):* the pelvic inlet is oval, and the AP diameter of the pelvic inlet is greater than the transverse diameter with a narrow subpubic angle.

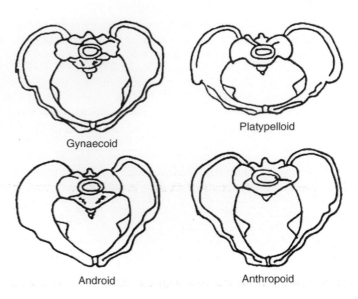

FIGURE 6.6 Pelvis types. (Courtesy of Chun Ho.)

Innervation of the Pelvis

Sacral Plexus

The sacral plexus is formed from the ventral rami of spinal nerves L4–S4. There is a contribution from the lumbar plexus by the **lumbosacral trunk** (L4, L5), which connects the two plexuses. The nerves are on the anterior surface of the piriformis muscle on the posterior pelvic wall. Ultimately, they converge towards the greater sciatic foramen and unite to form a flattened band, which continues as the sciatic nerve. There are numerous branches arising from the sacral plexus, as shown in **Figure 6.7** and **Table 6.2** (see also **Figure 7.3** in **Section 7**, Lower Limb).

The plexus lies on the posterior surface of the pelvis between the piriformis muscle and pelvic fascia. It is posterior to the internal iliac vessels, ureter, and sigmoid colon, on the left side.

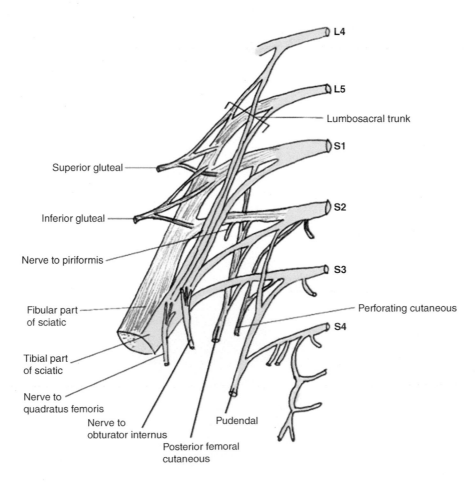

FIGURE 6.7 The branches of the sacral plexus. (Courtesy of Gabriela Barzyk.)

TABLE 6.2: Branches of the sacral plexus

Nerve	Spinal Segment	Course	Innervates
Sciatic (main lateral nerve)	L4–L5 to S1–S3	Passes inferior to piriformis, through greater sciatic foramen and descends in the posterior thigh to the popliteal fossa, where it divides	Provides sensory and motor innervation via its two branches; it also innervates the hamstring muscles
Common peroneal (common fibular)	L4–L5 to S1–S2	Winds around the neck of the fibula and then divides into superficial and deep branches, which descend on the lateral and anterior aspects of the leg, respectively, towards the foot	Provides sensory and motor innervation to the anterior and lateral compartments of the leg
Tibial	L4–L5 to S1–S3	Continues down the posterior aspect of the leg towards the foot	Provides sensory and motor innervation to the posterior compartment of leg (see **Section 7**, Lower Limb)
Superior gluteal nerve	L4–L5 to S1	Travels through the greater sciatic foramen superior to piriformis	Motor innervation to gluteus medius, gluteus minimus, and tensor fasciae latae
Inferior gluteal nerve	L5 to S1–S2	Travels through the greater sciatic foramen inferior to piriformis	Motor innervation to gluteus maximus
Nerve to piriformis	S1 and S2	Enters along the anterior surface of piriformis	Motor innervation to piriformis
Nerve to quadratus femoris and inferior gemellus	L4–L5 to S1	Exits via greater sciatic foramen and passes anterior to sciatic nerve and the anterior surfaces of innervated muscles	Motor innervation to quadratus femoris and inferior gemellus Articular branches to the hip joint
Nerve to obturator internus and superior gemellus	L5 to S1–S2	Exits pelvis via the greater sciatic foramen, inferior to piriformis, and gives a branch to the superior gemellus; it then crosses the ischial spine and re-enters the pelvis through lesser sciatic foramen to give rise to the obturator internus branch	Motor innervation to obturator internus and superior gemellus
Posterior cutaneous femoral nerve (posterior cutaneous nerve of the thigh)	S1–S3	Exits through the greater sciatic foramen inferior to piriformis	Gluteal branch (inferior cluneal nerve) provides skin sensation to the skin of the inferior part of the buttock Perineal branch supplies the posterior part of the scrotum or the labia majora Cutaneous branch supplies the posterior thigh, down to the popliteal fossa
Nerve to levator ani	S4		Motor innervation to levator ani
Pudendal nerve	S2–S4	Initially leaves through greater sciatic foramen, crosses sacrospinous ligament laterally, then wraps around the ischial spine and re-enters pelvis through lesser sciatic foramen, where it joins the internal pudendal vessels and accompanies these through the pudendal canal (Alcock's canal), which is formed by the fascia over the obturator internus muscle	Splits into three branches: inferior rectal nerve, perineal nerve, and dorsal nerve of penis/clitoris Inferior rectal nerve is the first branch, gives sensory supply to area below the pectinate line (in lower part of anal canal) and perianal skin, as well as motor supply to the external anal sphincter The perineal branch supplies sensation to the posterior two-thirds of the scrotum/labia majora and minora and perineum Motor function to perineal muscles, including bulbospongiosus, ischiocavernosus, external urethral sphincter, and levator ani Dorsal nerve of penis/clitoris provides sensation to (skin) of penis/clitoris
Perforating cutaneous nerve	S2–S3		Supplies skin on the lower medial aspect of the buttock
*Pelvic splanchnic nerves (nervi erigentes)	S2–S4	Travel from the sacral plexus to corresponding inferior hypogastric plexuses bilaterally	Provide parasympathetic innervation to pelvic and genital organs, as well as the hindgut

* The **pelvic splanchnic nerves**, or *nervi erigentes*, arise from the ventral rami of S2–S4, which carry **parasympathetic fibres**. They join the superior hypogastric plexus before travelling to the inferior hypogastric plexus, where they synapse and supply the pelvic and genital organs.

The **superior hypogastric plexus** lies at the bifurcation of the aorta and consists of sympathetic and visceral afferent fibres. It is connected to the inferior hypogastric plexus via the hypogastric nerves, which lie on the medial aspect of the descending ureters.

The **inferior hypogastric plexus (pelvic plexus)** lies extraperitoneally along the pelvic sidewall towards the base of the bladder and, in the male, to the prostate gland and on each side of the seminal vesicles; in the female, it lies on each side of the cervix and vaginal fornix. The inferior hypogastric plexus is mainly composed of sacral sympathetic splanchnic nerves and the parasympathetic splanchnic pelvic nerves.

The parasympathetic supply of the large bowel, from the splenic flexure to the upper half of the anal canal, arises from branches of the hypogastric plexuses, containing fibres from the pelvic splanchnic nerves, which accompany the branches of the artery of the hindgut, i.e., the inferior mesenteric artery (see the discussion on the hindgut in **Section 5**, Abdomen). The pelvic splanchnic nerves also form some of the afferent pain sensation pathway from the sigmoid colon and rectum, as well as from the cervix in females.

The *nervi erigentes* can be damaged in pelvic surgery, e.g., excision of rectal cancer or radiotherapy.

Pelvic Part of the Sympathetic Innervation

There are two sacral sympathetic trunks, which are continuations of the lumbar sympathetic trunks. They pass medial to the anterior sacral foramina of the sacrum. These trunks contain four to five ganglia and send post-ganglionic grey *rami communicantes* that accompany the sacral and coccygeal nerves to supply pelvic organs, e.g., male internal reproductive organs (vas deferens, seminal vesicles, and prostate gland), perineum, and the lower limb. Note that the sympathetic nerves relax organs and tighten sphincters, whereas the parasympathetic nerves do the opposite. The sympathetic trunk ends as a structure called the ganglion impar.

CLINICAL NOTES

- The sacral plexus is formed from the ventral rami of spinal nerves L4–S4 and lies on the anterior surface of the piriformis. The acronym SIPPS helps to remember the important nerves of the plexus: S (superior gluteal), I (inferior gluteal), P (posterior femoral cutaneous), P (pudendal), and S (sciatic).
- *Anal tone:* S2–S4 (anal tone and the anal reflex can be lost in spinal cord injuries).
- *Ankle jerk:* S1.

- The **sciatic nerve** is the thickest nerve in the human body; it innervates most of the muscles in the lower limb (see the distribution of the femoral and obturator nerves in **Section 7**, Lower Limb). It emerges deep to the piriformis in the posterior compartment of the thigh. Lower back problems such as intervertebral disc herniation, degenerative disc disease, lumbar spinal stenosis, and piriformis hypertrophy can result in compression and irritation of the fibres destined for the sciatic nerve; this is known as sciatica and results in pain extending from the lower back down the leg to the foot, depending on the affected nerve roots.
- Superior and inferior gluteal nerves supply the main abductors of the lower limb. The inferior gluteal nerve can be damaged during hip replacement. **These nerves have no cutaneous innervation** (see the anatomy of the buttock in **Section 7**, Lower Limb).
- A **pudendal nerve block** is used to anaesthetise the perineum in order to perform instrumental deliveries or repair an episiotomy. To perform a pudendal nerve block, it is first necessary to palpate the ischial spine per vagina before guiding the needle, as the nerve passes medial to the tip of the ischial spine (**Figure 6.8**). Damage to the pudendal nerve can lead to inability to differentiate between faeces and flatus, leading to faecal incontinence. The pudendal nerve is responsible for both faecal and urinary continence (the inferior rectal branch supplies the external anal sphincter, and the perineal branch supplies the external urinary sphincter). Calling the pudendal nerve, the "social nerve" helps students to understand part of its function (personal communication, Prof. Richard Tunstall).

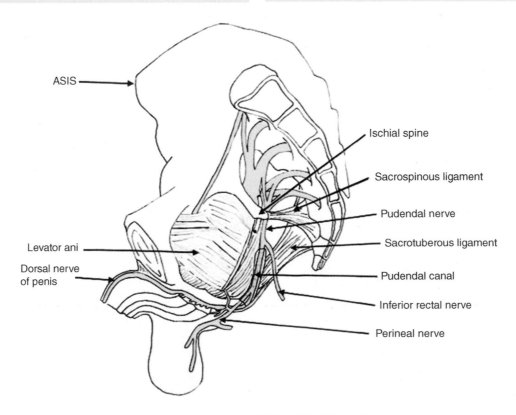

FIGURE 6.8   The pudendal nerve and its branches. (Courtesy of Fallon O'Neill.)

Pelvic Floor (Pelvic Diaphragm) (Figure 6.9)

The levator ani

- Separates the pelvic cavity from the perineum
- Forms slings around the rectum, vagina, and urethra to assist in urinary and anal continence
- Provides support for pelvic organs such as the bladder, rectum, and uterus
- Plays an important part in labour by rotating the fetal head from its transverse position upon entering the pelvic cavity to the AP position required to safely exit the pelvic outlet

The pelvic floor muscles contract in response to increased intra-abdominal pressure, such as coughing or lifting heavy objects.

The levator ani is a flat sheet of muscle which originates from the posterior aspect of the pubis, the lateral wall of the pelvis (tendinous arch on the obturator internus fascia), and the ischial spine. The paired levators form a gutter-like arrangement which slopes downwards and forwards and which constitutes the pelvic floor.

The **nerve supply** to the levator ani is from the sacral plexus: nerve to levator ani (S3–S4) on the pelvic surface and both the perineal and inferior rectal branches of the pudendal nerve on the perineal surface.

The levator ani receives its blood supply from the inferior gluteal, inferior vesical, and pudendal arteries.

The **ischiococcygeus** (also known as the coccygeus) is not part of the levator ani, but together they form the pelvic diaphragm. This triangular, rather fibrous muscle, at the posterior aspect of the levator ani, originates from the ischial spine and inserts into the lower end of the sacrum and the coccyx. The coccygeus lies on the pelvic surface of the sacrospinous ligament and may fuse with it.

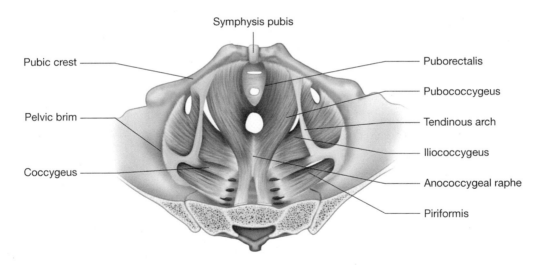

FIGURE 6.9   Superior view of the male pelvic diaphragm. (Courtesy of Xi Ming Zhu.)

The muscle can be divided into three parts: **pubococcygeus** (further subdivided into pubourethralis, pubovaginalis in the female, or puboprostaticus in the male), **iliococcygeus** (from the tendinous arch of the obturator internus), and **puborectalis**. These muscles all insert into a fibrous midline raphe (the **anococcygeal raphe**). The pubococcygeus also inserts into the perineal body.

These three muscles constitute the main part of the pelvic diaphragm.

Medial to the pubococcygeus is the **puborectalis**, which arises from the posterior aspect of the ischiopubic rami. Its fibres decussate behind the rectum to form a sling around the anorectal junction and fuse with the external anal sphincter.

Pelvic Organs

Embryology

The cloaca is divided by the urorectal septum into the urogenital sinus and the anorectal canal. The urogenital sinus develops into the urinary bladder and its neck and the phallic segment. The phallic segment forms the penile urethra in the male and the vestibule of the vagina in the female.

Ureter

For its embryology, see the embryology of the ureter in Section 5, Abdomen.

The ureter is a retroperitoneal muscular tube that connects the renal pelvis to the bladder. It is about 25 to 30 cm in length. It leaves the renal pelvis (ureteropelvic junction [UPJ]) posterior to the renal vessels. The ureter runs lateral to the tips of the transverse processes of the lumbar vertebrae.

Note how the tips of the transverse processes of the lumbar vertebrae, the sacroiliac joints, and the ischial spines form a useful guide to identify radio-opaque stones within the course of the ureter on a kidney, ureter, and bladder (KUB) X-ray.

The ureter is divided into three parts:

1. *Abdominal ureter:* from the UPJ to the pelvic brim, anterior to the sacroiliac joint, at the bifurcation of the common iliac artery. It is crossed anteriorly by the gonadal vessels ("bridge over water"). On the left side, the apex of the sigmoid mesocolon, containing the sigmoidal vessels, runs anterior to the ureter. In a sigmoid colectomy, the ureter should be clearly identified, as it may be densely adherent to the diseased colon (bowel cancer or complicated diverticular disease). The same applies on the right side when removing right colon cancer (right hemicolectomy). The ureter is usually adherent to the posterior peritoneum.
2. *Pelvic ureter:* passes from lateral to medial, towards the bladder wall, and is about half of its total length, i.e., 12.5 cm. In the male, the vas deferens loops over it, just before it enters the bladder. The ureter travels to the bladder accompanied by inferior vesical vessels and branches of the inferior hypogastric (pelvic) plexus. In the female, the ureter courses posterior to the ovary and then reaches the base of the broad ligament of the uterus. Finally, just before entering the bladder, it passes the anterior vaginal fornix. **Note the close proximity of the ureter to the uterine vessels**. This is the site where ureteric injuries most commonly occur during gynaecological procedures.
3. *Intramural ureter:* a short segment passing obliquely through the bladder wall. The oblique course prevents reflux of urine during urinary bladder contraction. The ureters receive vascular supply from the renal arteries, abdominal aorta, gonadal arteries, common and internal iliac arteries, and the superior and inferior vesical arteries. This rich blood supply helps in mobilising the ureter during operations without compromising its vascularity.

Nerve Supply of the Ureter
Aortic plexus, superior hypogastric, and inferior hypogastric plexuses (i.e., most nerves it passes).

The ureter has three constrictions:

* At the UPJ
* Where it crosses the pelvic brim
* Ureterovesical junction (intramural part)

These constrictions are common sites for stone impaction (Figure 6.10).

How to identify the ureter at operation? The following can be of great help in identifying the ureter, especially during difficult surgery due to adhesions or local cancer spread:

* The ureter crosses the bifurcation of the common iliac vessels.
* The ureter vermiculates on gentle pinching, due to peristalsis (Kelly's sign).
* A hugely dilated ureter (hydroureter) can be aspirated with a needle and syringe.

CLINICAL NOTES
* The ureters are at risk of injury during pelvic surgery and hysterectomy. The ureter lies inferior to the uterine artery (female) or the vas deferens (male). This can be remembered as "water under the bridge".
* Stones impacted in the lower ureter can be felt during a vaginal examination through the lateral fornices. Note that this is the only location in the body where stones in the ureters can be palpated.
* The most common clinical problem is ureteric colic.

Ureteric colic is a severe intermittent pain due to contraction of ureteric smooth muscle to overcome an obstruction, usually due to a stone (calculus). The pain may radiate to the lower abdomen ("from loin to groin"), testis, or tip of the penis.

In contrast to patients with peritonitis, who lie still and avoid moving, patients with ureteric colic are restless in bed (very useful clinical observation).

The urinalysis usually shows frank or microscopic haematuria (blood in the urine) and sometimes signs of a urinary tract infection (UTI) (presence of bacteria, raised white blood cells [WBCs] and nitrates).

The main risk of a ureteric stone is obstruction of the ureter with the development of hydroureter and hydronephrosis (**Figure 6.10**).

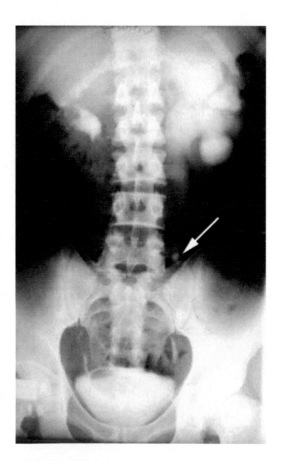

FIGURE 6.10 Intravenous urogram (IVU) showing obstructed left ureter (hydroureter) and kidney (hydronephrosis) due to stone *(arrow)* in the left ureter. (Courtesy of Qassim F. Baker.)

Non-contrast abdominal computed tomography (CT) is now the standard investigation which is requested for patients with ureteric colic (**Figure 6.11**).

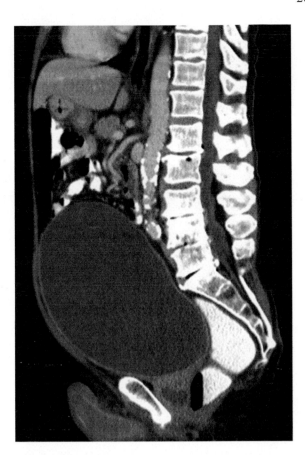

FIGURE 6.12 Sagittal CT reformat of the abdomen and pelvis showing distended urinary bladder. (Courtesy of Mudhar Hassan.)

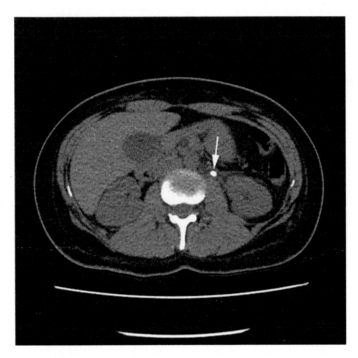

FIGURE 6.11 Non-contrast abdominal CT showing a proximal stone in the left ureter *(arrow)*. (Courtesy of Mudhar Hassan.)

The Bladder

The bladder is a distensible, three-sided, pyramidal-shaped, hollow muscular structure that can store more than 1000 mL of urine in acute urinary retention (**Figure 6.12**). It consists of an apex, base, superior surface, and two sloping inferolateral surfaces. The bladder is lined by multilayered epithelium called the urothelium (traditionally called transitional cell epithelium), which also lines the ureter and renal pelvis. It is extraperitoneal when empty but becomes increasingly intraperitoneal as it fills.

The **detrusor muscle** (smooth muscle) is the muscular layer of the urinary bladder. The bladder lies in the pelvis, but when distended, it extends into the abdominal cavity and can be clinically detected as a suprapubic swelling. When the bladder is empty, it is covered by the parietal peritoneum anteriorly. The bladder is separated from the rectum in the male by the rectovesical pouch; in the female, the vesicouterine pouch separates the uterus from the bladder.

In children up to the age of 6 years, the bladder is an abdominal organ because the pelvis is not yet large enough to accommodate the bladder.

The bladder receives blood supply from the anterior division of the internal iliac arteries, including the superior and inferior vesical arteries, with small contributions from the obturator, inferior gluteal, and uterine arteries (in the female).

See information on the urachus, in **Section 5**, Abdomen, for more information.

The urge to micturate

Stretch receptors in the bladder wall stimulate the parasympathetic nerves (pelvic splanchnic nerves S2–S4) to contract the detrusor muscle and relax the internal urinary sphincter (involuntary). The external urethral sphincter (voluntary) is controlled by the perineal branch of the pudendal nerve, S2.

CLINICAL NOTES

Cystitis is the most common clinical problem related to the bladder. It is more frequent in females because of their shorter urethra, which allows organisms to reach the bladder more easily.

Acute urinary retention is the inability to voluntarily empty the bladder and is the most common urological emergency, especially in males with urethral obstruction from prostatic enlargement. Passing a urinary catheter might be needed if other measures fail to alleviate the problem.

Bladder tumours are usually manifested by the passage of blood in the urine (haematuria) (*vide infra*).

Suprapubic cystostomy (insertion of a catheter into the bladder, just above the symphysis pubis, in the midline) is usually performed under local anaesthetic when it is not possible to empty the bladder via the urethra.

(Continued)

Cystoscopy is the visualisation of the inside of the bladder via an endoscope passed through the urethra and is a common procedure used to diagnose and treat bladder pathologies, such as tumours (by taking a biopsy, transurethral resection of bladder tumour [TURBT]), or as part of other procedures to treat prostatic hypertrophy (transurethral resection of the prostate [TURP]) (**Figure 6.13**). Also used for retrograde insertion of ureteric catheters and double J stents (pigtail) to treat ureteric obstruction and ensure free urinary drainage from the kidney.

Structures seen during cystoscopy:

- The **trigone** is a triangular-shaped area at the bladder base, which connects the internal urethral orifice, ureteric orifices, and **interureteric fold**. The trigone contains stretch receptors that signal the need to micturate. The rugae of the bladder will flatten when the bladder distends, and the bladder will become increasingly intraperitoneal.

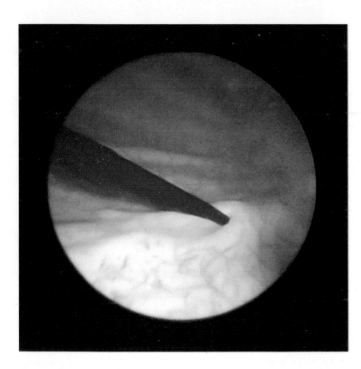

FIGURE 6.13   A blood jet through the left ureteral orifice during a cystoscopy, a sign of bleeding from the left upper urinary tract. (Courtesy of Mudhar Hassan.)

INJURIES OF THE BLADDER

The bladder can be injured in the following circumstances:

- Perioperative, such as when dissecting a pelvic tumour or during gynaecological operations,

including hysterectomy and caesarean section. This is why an indwelling urinary catheter, e.g., Foley's catheter, is routinely inserted before pelvic surgery to keep the bladder empty and less liable to injury.
- *Radiotherapy to treat pelvic cancers:* this treatment can damage the bladder (radiation cystitis) with risk of perforation/fistula formation.
- Long and difficult labour.
- Instrumentation of the bladder such as cystoscopy, TURBT, and TURP.
- *External trauma (blunt or penetrating injuries):* bladder injury should be excluded in all patients with pelvic trauma.

The injury of the bladder can be mild, such as contusion of the bladder wall, or more serious with urine extravasation extraperitoneally or intraperitoneally (especially injuries sustained with a full bladder).

HAEMATURIA

The presence of blood in the urine. Haematuria can be microscopic (blood visible only under high-powered microscopy) or frank (macroscopic), with or without clots.

There are many causes, which can be generally divided into:

- **Traumatic** (external trauma to the renal system such as renal, bladder, or urethral injuries).
- **Iatrogenic injuries** (inflicted during a surgical, therapeutic, or diagnostic procedure) form an important cause, including bladder and urethral injuries during catheterisation and endoscopic operations (TURT and TURP and cystoscopy; see "Injuries of the Bladder", above).
- **Inflammatory conditions** such as glomerulonephritis, pyelonephritis, cystitis, and prostatitis.
- **Stone formation**, which usually starts in the kidneys and then travels down the ureter causing ureteric colic and obstruction (see **Figure 6.10**) and can impede urinary function, is an important cause of haematuria. However, stones can form in the bladder and cause haematuria and UTIs. Typically, the spiky oxalate stones irritate the urothelium of the bladder (**Figure 6.14**).
- **Neoplastic conditions** such as renal cell carcinoma (RCC) and bladder and prostate tumours.

In some countries, such as Egypt (infection was diagnosed in mummies 3000, 4000, and 5000 years old) and Iraq, parasitic infection with *Schistosoma haematobium* causes bilharziasis, which presents as frank haematuria and may end up with the development of bladder cancer (usually of the squamous cell type). *Further Reading:* M.R. Barakat, Epidemiology of Schistosomiasis in Egypt: Travel through Time. Journal of Advanced Research 2013.

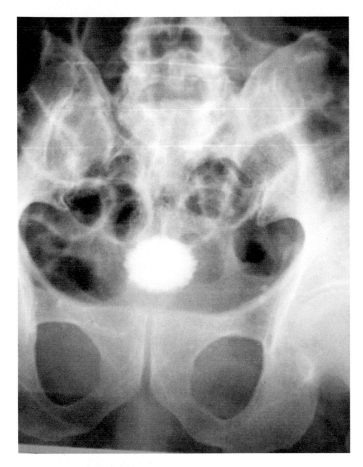

FIGURE 6.14 Plain X-ray of the pelvis showing a large vesical stone. (Courtesy of Abdel-Aziz Abdel-Ghany.)

Rectum and Anal Canal

The rectum and upper anal canal are derived from the embryological hindgut (endodermal origin).

The rectum (Latin, "straight") is a 12- to 15-cm muscular tube and is a continuation of the sigmoid colon at the rectosigmoid junction, at the level of the third sacral vertebra. Unlike many primates, which have a straight rectum, the human rectum follows the curvature of the sacrum and has lateral curves (two on the right and one on the left). The **rectum has a complete longitudinal muscle layer** (which explains the non-existence of diverticuli in the rectum), in contrast to the colon, where the longitudinal muscle layer is restricted to the three taeniae coli.

The rectosigmoid junction is a common site for cancer.

Houston's valves are mucosal shelves that correspond with the three rectal curves and can be seen on sigmoidoscopy. The lower one-third of the rectum is completely retroperitoneal, while the upper one-third is covered by peritoneum anteriorly and laterally. The middle one-third is covered on the anterior aspect only.

The rectum continues as the anal canal, at the anorectal junction, by curving backwards. The puborectalis (part of the levator ani) forms a loop at the anorectal junction, and this marks the transition from rectum to anal canal. The dilated lower part of the rectum is called the rectal ampulla.

Related Fascial Layers

Denonvillier's fascia (recto-prostatic fascia or recto-vaginal fascia in females) is a fascial layer extending superiorly from the perineal body to the floor of the recto-vesical pouch of the peritoneum in the male. It separates the prostate and base of the bladder from the rectum and covers the seminal vesicles and ductus deferens ampulla.

It is an important landmark when performing radical prostatectomy (removal of the prostate gland) for prostatic cancer.

Presacral fascia is the part of the endopelvic fascia which lines the anterior part of the sacrum.

Mesorectum (mesorectal fascia) is the connective tissue that surrounds the rectum and contains fatty tissue, the superior rectal artery and vein, and lymph nodes. Posteriorly, it connects the rectum with the pre-sacral fascia and blends anteriorly with the recto-prostatic fascia or recto-vaginal fascia. There is special emphasis on total mesorectal excision (TME) to decrease the incidence of local recurrence of cancer.

Waldeyer's fascia extends between the pre-sacral fascia and the mesorectum from the S2 to S4 level.

Blood supply

- Superior rectal artery (continuation of the inferior mesenteric artery at the pelvic brim and divides into two terminal branches)
- Middle rectal artery (from the anterior division of the internal iliac artery, or sometimes from the inferior vesical or the vaginal artery, sometimes absent)
- Inferior rectal artery (branch of the internal pudendal artery) supplies the anal canal, the external and internal sphincters, and the perianal skin, in addition to the lower rectum
- Small contribution from the middle sacral artery, which runs on the lumbosacral vertebrae within the presacral space

Venous drainage

- Tributaries of the rectal plexus drain to the superior rectal vein → inferior mesenteric vein → splenic vein (portal circulation)
- Middle rectal vein → internal iliac vein (systemic circulation)
- Inferior rectal vein → internal pudendal vein → internal iliac vein (systemic circulation)

Engorged anal and rectal veins (haemorrhoids) can be a feature of portal hypertension due to connections between the portal and caval systems in this region.

Nerve supply

- Sympathetic (lumbar splanchnic L1, L2)
- Parasympathetic (*nervi erigentes* S2–S4)

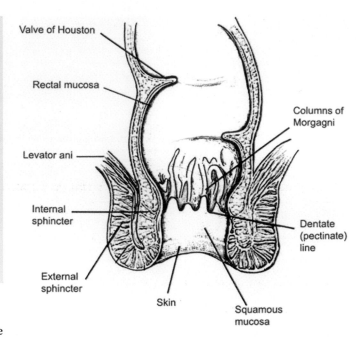

FIGURE 6.15 Lower rectum and anal canal. (Courtesy of Chun Ho.)

Lymphatic drainage of the rectum and anal canal above the dentate line

- Pararectal lymph nodes (of Gerota) in the mesorectum and then along the lymphatics accompanying the superior rectal artery to the pre-aortic lymph nodes
- Lymphatics along the middle and inferior rectal arteries to the internal iliac lymph nodes

The Anal Canal

The anal canal is a muscular tube about 3 to 4 cm long, extending posterior-inferiorly from the rectum to the anal orifice, situated within the anal triangle of the perineum, below the pelvic diaphragm. Its wall consists of the epithelium lining and internal and external sphincters, in addition to the neurovascular structures (**Figure 6.15**).

It lies between the ischioanal (ischiorectal) fossae, which allows expansion of the canal during defaecation. Posteriorly the anal canal is connected to the coccyx through the anococcygeal ligament. Anteriorly it is connected to the perineal body.

The **dentate** ("tooth-like") **or pectinate** ("like a comb") **line** delineates the upper and lower anal canals, which vary in embryological origin. The upper part arises from endodermal and mesodermal tissue, while the lower part arises from ectodermal tissue (proctodeum), where there is a change in the type of epithelium from the columnar epithelium of the embryological hindgut to the non-keratinised squamous epithelium of the anus. Below the intersphincteric groove, the epithelium becomes keratinised squamous epithelium.

The differences between the upper and lower anal canals are listed in **Table 6.3**.

Anal columns (of Morgagni) are longitudinal folds in the upper part of the anal canal separated by furrows and are joined at their lower ends by the valve-like folds called the **anal valves**. The anal glands open into the anal valves. Perianal abscesses are believed to arise from infection of the branched anal glands that may penetrate the internal sphincter.

Anal cushions are normal protrusions of vascular subepithelial tissue from the internal haemorrhoidal plexus, above the dentate line, which correspond to the terminal branches of the superior rectal vessels and play a role in anal continence by sealing the

TABLE 6.3: The differences between the upper two-thirds and lower one-third of the anal canal

Embryonic origin	Above the dentate line (endoderm)	Below the dentate line (ectoderm)
Blood supply	Superior rectal artery (continuation of inferior mesenteric artery)	Inferior rectal artery (from the internal pudendal artery)
Nerve supply	Sympathetic fibres from the inferior mesenteric plexus relax bowel and contract internal sphincter. *Parasympathetic (from the pelvic splanchnic nerves)*: contracts bowel and relaxes internal sphincter during defaecation	Inferior rectal nerve from the pudendal nerve (somatic)
Lymphatic drainage	Pararectal to pre-aortic lymph nodes	Superficial inguinal lymph nodes
Epithelial lining	Columnar epithelium	Stratified, squamous non-keratinised epithelium

anal canal. They are sited at the left lateral, right posterior, and right anterior, which corresponds to 3, 7, and 11 o'clock, respectively, when viewed through a proctoscope with the patient in the lithotomy position.

The **internal sphincter** (smooth muscle) is a continuation of the inner circular muscle of the rectum. It is tonically contracted at rest but becomes relaxed secondary to distension of the lower rectum.

It is innervated by the sympathetic and parasympathetic pelvic splanchnic nerves from the inferior hypogastric plexus.

The **external anal sphincter** (striated muscle) surrounds the anal canal, outside the internal sphincter. The old classification into subcutaneous superficial and deep components is no longer valid, and the whole muscle acts as one unit. It is superiorly blended with the puborectalis (part of the levator ani) (see **Figure 6.9**) and anteriorly attached to the perineal body and can be injured during childbirth. Posteriorly, it is attached to the coccyx via the anococcygeal ligament.

Its nerve supply is from the inferior rectal branch of the pudendal nerve. The external anal sphincter enables voluntary closure of the anus and can be voluntarily contracted for a short time to resist passing faecal matter.

The **conjoint longitudinal muscle** is a continuation of the longitudinal muscle of the large bowel which runs between the external and the internal sphincters. It is supplied by autonomic nerves and acts to shorten and widen the anal canal on defaecation.

Anal continence is enabled by sympathetically mediated contraction of the internal sphincter in addition to the contraction of the external sphincter and anal cushions (see earlier).

Common causes of faecal incontinence include injury to the anal sphincter during childbirth and iatrogenic injuries to the anal sphincters that follow anal surgery for high fistula-in-ano, haemorrhoidectomy, or internal sphincterotomy for treatment of anal fissures. Spinal injuries can also result in faecal incontinence.

CLINICAL NOTES

Internal haemorrhoids (piles) are abnormally dilated anal cushions (see earlier), which contain blood vessels called the sinusoids. They can become engorged and can bleed following repeated intra-abdominal pressure and straining in patients with constipation.

Internal haemorrhoids are **painless (above the dentate line)** but tend to bleed (fresh bright blood during or shortly after defaecation). They appear as anal bulges at the 3, 7, and 11 o'clock positions when looked at in the lithotomy position. This type is called grade I haemorrhoids.

Internal haemorrhoids can prolapse to the outside and can reduce either spontaneously (grade II) or by manual reduction (grade III). Grade IV haemorrhoids are prolapsed outside the anal verge. Prolapsing haemorrhoids (piles) may strangulate when the blood supply becomes occluded by the constricting action of the anal sphincters.

External haemorrhoids are below the dentate line (from the external haemorrhoidal plexus) and **can become painful**, especially if they become thrombosed.

Learning Point

All patients with rectal bleeding, with or without recent changes in bowel habits, should be thoroughly investigated, including a full anorectal examination, to exclude anorectal or colonic pathologies, including cancer (see NICE Guidelines, 2017: https://cks.nice.org.uk/topics/gastrointestinal-tract-lower-cancers-recognition-referral/).

Painful Perianal Conditions

Commonly seen in clinical practice and may be referred to A&E or the colorectal clinic:

- *Perianal haematoma:* a collection of blood around the anus which results from rupture of superficial blood vessels.

- *Anorectal suppuration:* pus formation commonly around the anal verge (perianal abscess) or in the ischiorectal fossa. Perianal abscess may end up with fistula formation (track between the lining of the anal canal and the skin); the most common type is intersphincteric. Rare but more complicated trans-sphincteric fistula can prove difficult to treat. Fistula-in-ano can be associated with bowel disease such as Crohn's disease.

- *Anal fissure:* a crack at the lower part of the anal canal, most commonly posteriorly, which causes pain when passing stools and can bleed. Digital examination is contraindicated in patients with acute anal fissure. If conservative measures fail to heal the fissure, day case surgery may be considered (lateral internal sphincterotomy).

- *Anal ulcerations:* can be caused by a variety of diseases such as Crohn's disease, tuberculosis (TB), squamous cell carcinoma, malignant melanoma, and sexually transmitted disease (STD; herpes, syphilis) in addition to trauma.

Digital rectal examination (DRE) or per rectum (PR) examination is an important bedside examination of the anal verge, anal canal, and lower rectum. It is usually performed with the patient lying in the left lateral position with their hips and knees flexed to their chest.

What structures can be felt on performing a PR examination?

Males: the prostate gland (size, consistency, tenderness, and presence of median sulcus between the two lateral lobes) and seminal vesicles (usually palpable only if inflamed or enlarged).

Females: the cervix can be felt as well as any masses present within the recto-uterine pouch, e.g., ovarian cysts.

Tenderness may be elicited on PR exam in patients with pelvic peritonitis (infection of the pelvic peritoneum from a septic focus such as acute appendicitis).

Palpable pathologies such as rectal polyps, tumours, and the presence of blood/mucus on the gloved finger should be noted.

Further evaluation of the anal canal, rectum, and sigmoid colon requires either a sigmoidoscopy or colonoscopy (**Figure 6.16**).

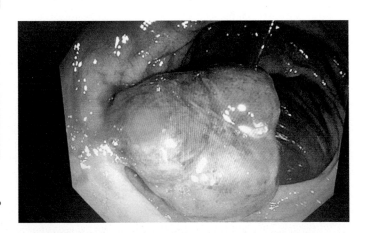

FIGURE 6.16 Endoscopic view of rectal polyp. (Courtesy of Akram A. Najeeb.)

The Perineum

Defined as a diamond-shaped region between the thighs, caudal to the pelvic diaphragm.

The perineum is divided into two triangles by an imaginary line between the ischial tuberosities:

* *Anterior:* urogenital triangle
* *Posterior:* anal triangle

The boundaries of the perineum are:

* *Anterior:* lower end of the pubic symphysis
* *Lateral:* ischiopubic rami and sacrotuberous ligaments
* *Posterior:* tip of the coccyx

* The **deep pouch** contains the compressor urethrae muscle and the sphincter urethrovaginalis, a skeletal muscle sphincter complex surrounding the urethra and vaginal orifices

The vagina and the urethra traverse the deep and superficial pouches. The urethra is surrounded by both inner circular smooth muscle (as a continuation of the detrusor muscle of the bladder, under autonomic control) and outer skeletal muscle (innervated by the pudendal nerve).

Stress incontinence (leakage of urine during actions that increase the intra-abdominal pressure such as coughing or sneezing) is the most common type of incontinence in women and is due to problems with the closing mechanism of the bladder.

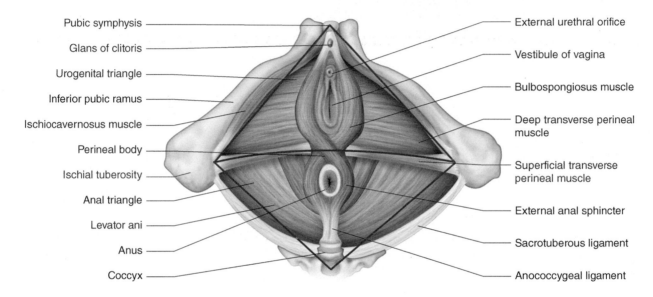

FIGURE 6.17   The triangles of the female perineum. (Courtesy of Hatidzhe Masteva.)

The **perineal body** (central tendon of the perineum) is a median, fibromuscular mass between the urogenital and anal triangles and is situated midway between the two ischial tuberosities (between the posterior commissure of the labia majora and the anus). It is an important attachment point for the perineal muscles that supports the pelvic floor.

The **anterior urogenital triangle** is further divided by the perineal membrane (a triangular sheet of connective tissue that lies between the ischiopubic rami) into superficial and deep pouches.

The **posterior (anal) triangle** contains the anal canal, internal and external anal sphincters, and ischioanal fossa (one on each side of the anal canal).

Female Perineum (Figure 6.17)

Urogenital triangle:

* The **superficial pouch**, which contains the structures that form the root of the clitoris and includes the bulbospongiosus, ischiocavernosus, and superficial transverse perineal muscles, in addition to the lesser vestibular (Skene's) glands and the greater vestibular (Bartholin's) glands.

> ### CLINICAL SIGNIFICANCE
>
> During childbirth, the perineal body can be stretched or torn, leading to the prolapse of pelvic viscera. This could be avoided by a mediolateral episiotomy (favoured), where the perineum is cut. This prevents uncontrolled tears of the perineal body (**Figure 6.18**).

Male Perineum

* The urethra pierces the urogenital diaphragm in the urogenital triangle.
* The superficial perineal pouch contains the root of the penis and the superficial perineal muscles: bulbospongiosus, ischiocavernosus, and superficial transverse perineal muscles, all supplied by the pudendal nerve.
* The deep perineal pouch contains the deep transverse perineal muscles, membranous urethra, and bulbourethral

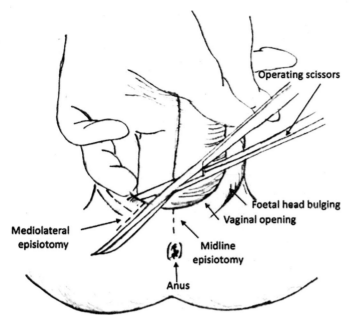

FIGURE 6.18 Diagram of mediolateral episiotomy. (Courtesy of Naomi Bartholomew.)

glands. The membranous urethra is surrounded by the circular muscle fibres of the external sphincter urethrae.

- The deep transverse perineal muscles arise from the ischial rami and are inserted into the perineal body. They are, in addition to the sphincter urethrae, supplied by the pudendal nerve.

The **ischioanal fossa (ischiorectal)**, on each side, is situated lateral to the anal canal between the obturator internus muscle and its fascia laterally and the pelvic diaphragm (levator ani) and its inferior fascia, as well as the external anal sphincter, medially. The pudendal canal (Alcock's canal), which contains the internal pudendal vessels and pudendal nerve, is a fascial compartment on the lateral wall of the ischioanal fossa. The fossa is filled with fat and contains the inferior rectal nerve and vessels. Abscess formation can occur at the ischioanal fossae and may develop a fistula to the rectum or the anal canal.

Anatomy of the Male Genital Tract and Inguinal Canal

During early development, the external genitalia of both sexes are similar in structure and appearance. This is the **indifferent stage**. Subsequently, in the male, the scrotal folds fuse, forming the scrotum (remaining as the labia majora in the female), while the urethral folds fuse in the midline to surround the penile urethra (remaining as the labia minora in the female). The genital tubercle then elongates to form the phallus. Thus, by 9 weeks, the differences between the male and female sexes are apparent. With a common origin, male and female anatomical structures are comparable (**Table 6.4**).

TABLE 6.4: Comparison of male and female genital structures

Male Structures	Female Structures
Testes	Ovaries
Penis	Clitoris
Scrotum	Labia majora
Penile skin	Labia minora
Seminal vesicles	N/A
Prostate gland	Paraurethral/lesser vestibular/Skene's gland
Bulbourethral gland	Greater vestibular/Bartholin's gland
Bulb of penis	Vestibular bulbs
Glans penis	Clitoral glans
Crura of penis	Clitoral crura
Foreskin	Clitoral prepuce
Gubernaculum testis	Round ligament of uterus and the ligament of the ovary

Note: The prostatic utricle (a depression on the urethral crest in the male) is the analogue of the uterus and vagina in females and represents the distal end of the fused paramesonephric ducts (*vide infra*, female reproductive tract).

The male external genitalia (Figure 6.19) consist of:

- Penis
- Scrotum
- Testes
- Epididymides (*singular:* epididymis)
- Vasa deferentia (*singular:* vas deferens – also known as the ductus deferens)

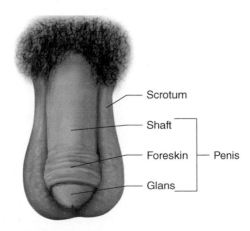

FIGURE 6.19 External male anatomy. (Courtesy of Gabriela Barzyk.)

The Penis

When describing the dorsal and ventral surfaces of the penis, note that, in the anatomical position, the penis is erect and comprises the root, penile body (shaft), and glans penis, from proximal to distal. The penis develops from the genital tubercle.

fold of skin that covers the glans and is surgically removed in circumcision.

Thus, the **shaft of the penis** is composed of the three corpora (the three cylindrical bodies of the penis). Buck's fascia, also called the investing deep fascia of the penis, surrounds these three corpora (**Figure 6.20**).

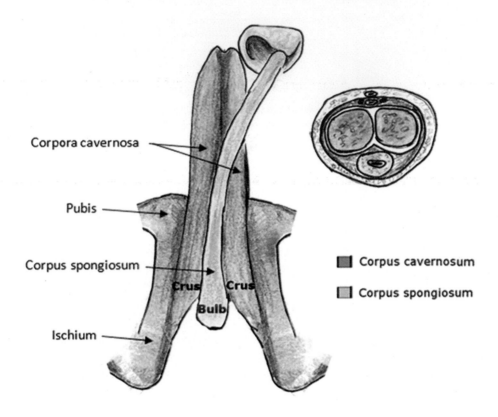

FIGURE 6.20   The corpora of the penis. (Courtesy of Gabriela Barzyk.)

The **root (radix) of the penis** consists of the following structures:

- *The bulb of the penis:* continues as the corpus spongiosum and is traversed by the spongy or penile urethra, which pierces the posterior surface of the bulb and is the outflow tract for urine and semen via the external urethral meatus. The bulb is firmly attached to the perineal membrane.
- The bulbospongiosus muscles, one on each side, cover the bulb of the penis, which helps in clearing the urethra of urine and semen.
- The **right and left crura** (*singular:* crus) **of the penis** arise from the ischiopubic rami and are covered by the ischiocavernosus muscles, which are attached to the pubic arch and help in erection; the bulbospongiosus and ischiocavernosus muscles are supplied by the perineal branch of the pudendal nerve.

The **corpora cavernosa** (*singular:* corpus cavernosum) are two cylindrical masses of porous tissue which represent the extension of the crura. They become engorged with blood on erection. Distally, they are located on the dorsal aspect of the penis.

Located on the **ventral** aspect of the penis, the **corpus spongiosum** is the third erectile tissue, containing the urethra, which ends distally as the **glans penis**. The rim of the glans is called the **corona**. Inferiorly, a thin band of tissue, the frenulum, links the glans to the **prepuce** or foreskin. The prepuce is a double

Remember: "*Sponge*Bob lives *under* the sea", which helps recall that corpus *spong*iosum is *inferior* to corpus cavernosum.

The **two suspensory ligaments of the penis** support the erect penis, anchoring it to the pubic symphysis, and are continuous with the Buck's fascia (**Figure 6.21**).

Blood Supply (Figure 6.22)

The internal pudendal artery, which arises from the anterior division of the internal iliac artery, gives rise to three branches to the corpora of the penis (distal to the origin of the perineal branch). The three branches are:

1. *Bulbourethral artery:* a short artery which supplies the penile bulb and urethra, Cowper's gland, corpus spongiosum, and glans
2. *Dorsal artery of the penis:* supplies the circumflex branches to both the corpora cavernosa and corpus spongiosum, glans, and penile skin
3. *Deep artery of the penis:* supplies the cavernosal artery, runs within the corpus cavernosum on each side (*vide infra*, mechanism of erection)

Venous Drainage of the Penis

There are three venous systems, superficial, intermediate, and deep:

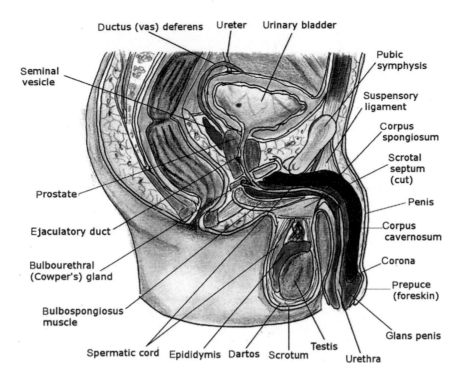

FIGURE 6.21   Midsagittal section of the male genitourinary anatomy. (Courtesy of Gabriela Baryzk.)

Superficial Venous System

The superficial veins from the penile skin drain to the **superficial dorsal vein**, which ultimately joins the superficial external pudendal vein and terminates in the long saphenous vein.

The Intermediate System

The **deep dorsal and circumflex veins, beneath the Buck's fascia**, drain the corpus spongiosum, glans, and distal two-thirds of the corpora cavernosa to the prostatic plexus.

The Deep Venous System

The deep veins (crural and cavernous) receive drainage from the proximal one-third of the penile corpora cavernosa and drain into the internal pudendal veins.

The **lymphatic drainage** of the skin of the penis, except the glans, is to the superficial inguinal lymph nodes. The glans penis drains to the deep inguinal lymph nodes. The erectile tissue and penile urethra drain to the internal iliac lymph nodes.

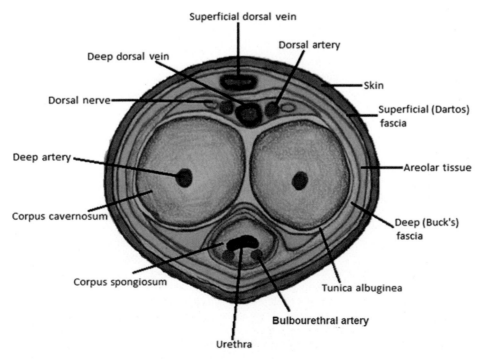

FIGURE 6.22   Axial section of the shaft of the penis showing the blood supply. (Courtesy of Neha Gadiyar.)

Nerve Supply of the Penis

The **dorsal nerve of the penis**, one arising on each side from the pudendal nerve, supplies the skin of the shaft of the penis and the glans. It travels with the dorsal artery and deep dorsal vein, in the groove between the corpora cavernosa, deep to Buck's fascia. Branches from the perineal branch of the pudendal nerve supply the ischiocavernosus and bulbospongiosus muscles.

The **sympathetic innervation** originates from the intermediolateral cell columns of T11, T12, and L1 segments of the spinal cord. Pre-ganglionic fibres synapse within the ganglia of the sympathetic chain. Post-ganglionic sympathetic fibres join the inferior hypogastric plexus (pelvic plexus) and course with the cavernous nerve. The **parasympathetic innervation** (pelvic splanchnic nerves) arises from S2, S3, and S4 (the *nervi erigentes*), which form the **cavernous nerves** that supply the three corpora.

Mechanism of Erection

Following sexual stimulation (visual, smell, tactile, and others), efferent stimuli are transmitted from the pelvic splanchnic nerves (S2–S4), reaching the spongy tissue of all three corpora, via the cavernous nerve, with nitric oxide acting as a neurotransmitter, which increases arterial blood flow (via the helicine arteries) causing vasodilation and penile engorgement. The spongy erectile tissue of the corpora cavernosa contains sinusoids separated by smooth muscle fibres.

The **ischiocavernosus muscles** surround the crura of the penis; by contracting they help to fill the corpora cavernosa with blood.

The **helicine arteries** are the terminal coiled branches of the deep (cavernous) arteries. They uncoil on parasympathetic stimulation, causing penile engorgement. The corpora cavernosa is enveloped by the tunica albuginea, an elastic tissue structure, which consists of an outer longitudinal layer surrounding them together, and an inner layer which separately surrounds each of the corpora.

The **emissary veins** from the corpora are compressed by the outer layer of the tunica albuginea, which causes the arterial blood to temporarily remain in the corpora cavernosa.

Ejaculation

The process of ejaculation is mainly under **sympathetic control** and is initiated by stimuli from the glans penis to the central nervous system (sensory fibres through the dorsal nerves of the penis). Sympathetic stimulation leads to contraction of smooth muscles in the **seminal vesicles**, **prostate**, and **epididymis** and discharge of **seminal fluid** (which is composed of **spermatozoa** and fluids from seminal vesicles, prostate, and bulbourethral glands) into the **prostatic urethra**, whilst the internal sphincter of the bladder contracts to prevent retrograde flow of semen into the bladder. The contraction of the **bulbospongiosus muscles** (supplied by the pudendal nerve) compresses the intrabulbar fossa of the urethra to aid the emission of semen (ejaculation).

CLINICAL NOTES

The **prepuce** (foreskin) is part of the penile skin covering the glans. Due to many medical, cultural, and religious reasons, males may be circumcised and have the foreskin removed. Medical reasons for this include **phimosis**, where a tight foreskin is unable to be retracted past the glans penis, which can cause discomfort. The benefits of circumcision are debated, yet it is recommended as part of a strategy to combat HIV spread, decreasing infection risk by up to 60%.

Paraphimosis is a medical emergency where the foreskin cannot be returned to its normal anatomical position, covering the glans penis. If not remedied, ischaemia can result as the blood supply of the glans is occluded.

Priapism is a continuous, painful erection which is unrelated to sexual stimulation. This is a medical emergency that, if untreated, can lead to permanent damage to the penis and erectile dysfunction. Important risk factors include haemoglobinopathies such as sickle cell anaemia and intake of medications, for example, vasoactive drugs and an overdose of sildenafil (Viagra).

Penile carcinoma is a rare type of cancer, and the majority are squamous cell carcinomas. It can occur under the foreskin in uncircumcised patients. Human papilloma virus (HPV) infection is an important risk factor.

Chancre is the ulcerative lesion which characterises the primary stage of **syphilis** and usually occurs on the glans penis.

The Urethra

The urethra is the conduit for urine and semen, extending from the bladder to the external urethral meatus. During micturition, the smooth muscle of the internal and skeletal muscle of the external urethral sphincters are relaxed.

The **internal urethral sphincter**, located inferior to the bladder, has both parasympathetic innervation from the pelvic splanchnic nerves (S2–S4) and sympathetic innervation via the hypogastric nerve (T11–L2). The **external sphincter** has somatic innervation via the pudendal nerve (S2–S4), allowing conscious constriction of the external sphincter until it is socially convenient to pass urine.

Note that in the male, the internal sphincter (also known as the sphincter vesicae) contracts during orgasm (under sympathetic stimulation) to prevent retrograde flow of semen into the bladder.

This innervation is summarised in **Figure 6.23**.

The **male urethra** can be divided into two parts, the posterior urethra and anterior urethra, as per **Figure 6.21**.

The **posterior urethra** is composed of the following:

1. **Pre-prostatic** (intramural) is about **1 cm** long, between the bladder base and prostate gland.
2. **Prostatic**, **3 to 4 cm** long, passes through the prostate gland. The urethral lumen in this segment contains the **urethral crest**, a mucosal fold in the midline posteriorly. Here, the urinary and reproductive systems meet, and the ducts of the prostate gland empty lateral to the urethral crest into the prostatic sinuses. The **seminal colliculus** (or verumontanum) is an elevation on the floor of the prostatic urethra in the middle of the urethral crest and marks the site of the **prostatic utricle** (develops from the paramesonephric ducts). The seminal (ejaculatory) ducts open on each side of the prostatic utricle. The seminal colliculus is an important operative landmark in TURP to avoid damage to the urethral sphincter.

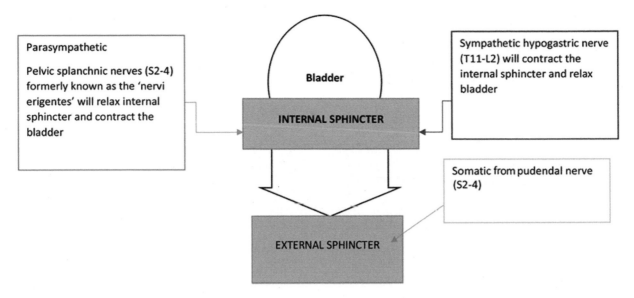

FIGURE 6.23   Mechanism of urination. (Courtesy of Faris Hussein.)

3. **Membranous**, approximately **2 to 2.5 cm** long as it passes through the deep perineal pouch. The striated external urethral sphincter surrounds the membranous urethra and inserts into the perineal body; it is reinforced by the pubococcygeus muscle (part of levator ani). This section of the urethra is the least dilatable and most fixed, and so is most liable to injury via catheterisation. A displaced pelvic fracture (with disruption of the pelvic ring) may also injure the membranous urethra (see earlier).

The **anterior urethra**, about 15 cm long, is encased in the corpus spongiosum and is in two parts:

- The **bulbar urethra** lies within the superficial perineal pouch, surrounded by the bulbospongiosus muscles, and is the widest part of the urethra. The bulbourethral glands open into the bulbar urethra. The dilated portion within the bulb of the penis is known as the intrabulbar fossa.
- The **penile, or pendulous, part** has an enlargement near the distal end called the **navicular fossa**, further distal to which is the external urethral orifice, which is the narrowest part of the urethra. The **external urethral meatus**, at the distal end of the glans, is a vertical slit, having the effect of "rifling" the urethra so urine is propelled as a straight stream on exit. There are numerous mucous glands within the submucosa of the urethra, particularly in the anterior part.

Learning Point

The perineal membrane is the anatomical landmark that divides the urethra into anterior and posterior parts.

CLINICAL NOTES

UTIs can be upper, such as **pyelonephritis**, or lower, such as **cystitis, urethritis, and prostatitis**.

Inflammation of the urethra (urethritis) can be caused by gonococcal and non-gonococcal infections. Sexually transmitted infections (STIs), such as **gonorrhoea** and **chlamydia**, are of increasing concern, due to antimicrobial resistance (AMR). Symptoms of STIs include urethral discharge and a burning sensation on urination. If untreated, urethritis may lead to urethral stricture (narrowing) formation and infertility.

Common causes of **posterior urethral rupture** include trauma (pelvic fractures) or **iatrogenic**, such as urinary catheterisation and endoscopic TURP or TURBT. **Iatrogenic injuries are the most common cause of urethral injuries worldwide**.

Extravasation of urine into the scrotum, and sometimes upwards on the anterior abdominal wall, along the attachment of Scarpa's fascia, can follow rupture of membranous or bulbar urethra.

For those who are interested in historical considerations, the death of King William I (The Conqueror) in 1087 gives an example of understanding the effects of urethral trauma (Mundy & Andrich, 2011).

Anterior urethral rupture usually follows crushing injuries such as road traffic accidents, straddle injuries, direct kicks to the perineum (bulbar urethral injury), and self-inflicted injuries.

The least dilatable part of the urethra is the membranous part and therefore is most liable to injury during catheterisation. **Thus, the anatomy of the urethra must be taken into consideration when catheterising a male patient.**

Hypospadias is a common congenital anomaly, where the external meatus opens on the ventral aspect of the penis. In hypospadias, circumcision is contraindicated, since a flap can be constructed from the foreskin later, as part of surgical treatment, depending on the type of hypospadias. Similarly, **epispadias** is a urethral birth defect whereby the urethra opens on the dorsal side of the penis. This is rarer, with a rate of 1/30,000 compared to the more common hypospadias that occurs in of 1/300 births.

The Scrotum (Figure 6.24)

The scrotum contains the **testes, epididymides**, and part of the **spermatic cord**. Embryologically, it develops from the labioscrotal swellings on each side of the embryonic genital tubercle, which fuse later to form the scrotum.

The scrotum is critical for the temperature regulation necessary for spermatogenesis. It is composed of two compartments separated by a relatively avascular septum. A **midline raphe** extends from the external urethral meatus down the ventral aspect of the penis and along the scrotal skin to the anus, signifying the line of fusion of the genital tubercles during development. Urologists access either or both scrotal compartments via a longitudinal skin incision through the septum, for example, when treating bilateral hydrocele or testicular torsion.

The skin of the scrotum is pigmented and devoid of fat but has numerous hair follicles and sweat and sebaceous glands (and so is a common site for the development of sebaceous cysts).

Deep to the skin lie the **dartos fascia** and **dartos muscle**. The dartos is an involuntary smooth muscle supplied by **sympathetic fibres** of the genital branch of the **genitofemoral nerve**. This muscle controls corrugation of the scrotum, altering its surface area. Thus, in hot weather the dartos relaxes, increasing scrotal surface area for heat loss, while in cold weather, the contracted dartos will decrease scrotal surface and retain heat.

Note that the function of the dartos is entirely different from that of the **cremasteric muscle** (involved in the cremasteric reflex). Do not confuse the two! (*Vide infra*)

Continuous with **Scarpa's fascia** of the abdominal wall is the superficial fascia of the perineum (**Colles' fascia**). This fascia covers the bulb of the penis (see **Figure 6.18**) and is attached to the ischiopubic rami on either side and to the perineal membrane posteriorly. This fascia is continuous with the dartos layer of muscle and fascia.

The **external spermatic fascia** is derived from the aponeurosis of the external oblique muscle. Deep to that is the **cremasteric fascia and muscle**, derived from the internal oblique and responsible for the cremasteric reflex.

The cremasteric reflex, by touching the skin of the medial thigh area, may result in the retraction of the testes to the top of the scrotum, or even to the distal inguinal canal, as the cremaster muscle contracts. The **femoral branch** of the **genitofemoral nerve** provides sensory innervation to the skin of the medial thigh, and the **genital branch** of the same nerve is motor to the cremaster muscle and sensory to the skin of the scrotum. The cremaster reflex can lead to diagnostic confusion, particularly in young boys, who can be misdiagnosed with **cryptorchidism** (undescended testis).

Deep to the cremasteric fascia is the **internal spermatic fascia**, formed by an extension of the transversalis fascia of the anterior abdominal wall at the deep inguinal ring.

Surrounding each testis is the **tunica vaginalis**, which is a remnant of the **processus vaginalis** of the parietal peritoneum. The tunica vaginalis has parietal and visceral layers with a potential space between them (see information on hydroceles below).

During testicular descent, the peritoneum bulges through the anterior abdominal wall as the processus vaginalis. The part of the processus vaginalis continuous with the abdominal peritoneum closes after testicular descent, with the remnant (distal) part forming the tunica vaginalis into which the testis invaginates (see **Figure 6.24**). With descent into the scrotum, the testes are enveloped by the successive tissue layers of the anterior abdominal wall, forming the spermatic fascial layers. All layers of the anterior abdominal wall contribute to the enveloping layers of the testis. A useful mnemonic is given in **Table 6.5** to help you remember the order of the tissue layers of the scrotum.

What Are the Layers of the Scrotum? (Figure 6.24, Table 6.5)

Blood supply to the scrotum is from the superficial and deep external pudendal arteries (branches of the femoral artery). Additional blood supply is from the perineal branch of the internal pudendal artery and the cremasteric artery, a branch of the inferior epigastric artery (to the cremasteric muscle and spermatic cord coverings).

Venous drainage follows the previously named arteries.

Lymphatic drainage of the scrotum is to the ipsilateral superficial inguinal lymph nodes.

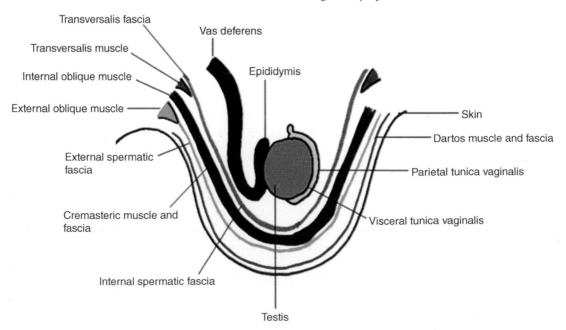

FIGURE 6.24 Midsagittal scrotum section. (Courtesy of Aditya Mavinkurve.)

TABLE 6.5: Layers of the scrotum

Layers of the Scrotum	
Skin	Some
Dartos muscle and fascia	Dangerous
External spermatic fascia, from the external oblique	Englishman
Cremasteric muscle and fascia, from the internal oblique	Called
Internal spermatic fascia, from the transversalis fascia	It
Tunica vaginalis, from the processus vaginalis of the parietal peritoneum	The
Testes	Testes

Sensory Innervation of the Scrotum

The anterior third of the scrotum is supplied by the ilioinguinal nerve (L1) via its anterior scrotal branch. The anterior scrotum also receives innervation from the genital branch of the genito-femoral nerve (L1, L2).

The posterior two-thirds are supplied by the posterior scrotal branches of the perineal branch of the pudendal nerve (S2–S4, see earlier).

The posterior femoral cutaneous nerve of the thigh (S1–S3) also contributes to supply the posterior two-thirds of the scrotum.

Testes

The testes are the male gonads and the site of spermatogenesis. As endocrine organs, the testes produce androgens, such as testosterone, from Leydig cells. During development, the testes are high up, retroperitoneally on the posterior abdominal wall. The exact mechanism of testicular descent remains largely unknown, but it has been attributed to many factors, including the influence of gonadotropin released from the placenta and testosterone produced by the fetal testes, the development of the gubernaculum, and the increase in intra-abdominal pressure.

The testes start their descent by week 12 of gestation, with the **gubernaculum**, a fibrous cord that attaches to the inferior pole of the testis, gradually shortening and pulling the testes down. At 28 weeks, the testes migrate through the inguinal canal, arriving in the scrotum by approximately 32 weeks' gestation (96% of cases) (Nemec et al., 2011). Failure of descent can occur at any stage. Thus, the testes should be within the scrotum, by birth, with the lumen of the processus vaginalis having been obliterated. Persistence of the processus vaginalis predisposes individuals to the development of indirect inguinal hernias, with or without hydrocele (**Figure 6.25**).

The Coverings of the Testis

- The **tunica vasculosa** is a network of blood vessels which forms the innermost layer of the testicular coverings.
- The **tunica albuginea** (*Latin*: "white coat") is fibrous in nature, with thick, white criss-crossing fibres. It tightly encases the anterior and lateral sides of the testis and sends partitions between the seminiferous tubules. Posteriorly, the tunica albuginea is thicker and projects as a fibrous septum called the **mediastinum testis**. The mediastinum testis is considered portal to the testis, where blood vessels, lymphatics, and genital ducts enter or leave.
- The **tunica vaginalis** has a parietal and visceral layer.

Radiating from the **mediastinum testis** are numerous **septa**, which divide the testis into 200 to 300 lobules, each of which contains one to four highly convoluted **seminiferous tubules**, in which the spermatozoa are produced. The total number of the tubules may reach 900. The production of spermatozoa (spermatogenesis) involves **spermatogonia** forming primary, and then secondary, **spermatocytes** which then form **spermatids** (haploid), which metamorphose into **spermatozoa**.

The seminiferous tubules are classed as straight or convoluted by their shape, and spermatogenesis occurs in the convoluted tubules. They become less convoluted distally (tubuli recti) and open into the mediastinum testis.

The **rete testis** is a formed by the anastomosing tubuli recti and is found in the mediastinum testis.

The rete testis is connected to the head of the **epididymis** by approximately 12 efferent ductules.

In the early embryonic life both the paramesonephric and Wolffian ducts (mesonephric ducts) are present and develop on the mesonephros. The paramesonephric ducts regress under the effect of the testis-derived androgens. The Wolffian duct gives rise to the epididymis, vas deferens, and seminal vesicles.

The epididymis is situated on the posterolateral side of the testis and is a highly coiled tube (total length of about 6 to 7 m) which acts as a conduit for the sperm cells to the vas deferens. It has head (caput), body (corpus), and tail (cauda) segments (see **Figure 6.25**). The tail is continuous with the ductus (vas) deferens. The epididymis receives arterial blood from the testicular artery, and its venous drainage is the same as for the testis. The remnants of the paramesonephric duct form the "**appendix epididymis**" and because, in most cases, it has a stalk, it is liable to twist and clinically resembles testicular torsion.

The appendix testis (hydatid of Morgagni) is a vestigial remnant of the proximal portion of the paramesonephric duct and is attached to the upper pole of the testis. Again, its twisting can mimic testicular torsion (part of the differential diagnosis of acute scrotum).

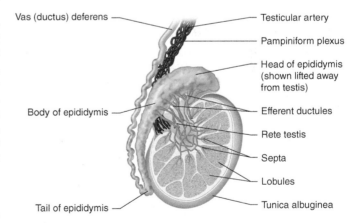

FIGURE 6.25 Midsagittal section of the testis. (Courtesy of Gabriela Barzyk.)

Testicular Blood Supply

The testes develop high up on the posterior abdominal wall and migrate downwards, bringing their blood supply with them; hence, the testicular arteries arise from the abdominal aorta at L1–L2, inferior to the origin of the renal arteries. This is the major testicular arterial supply, which is supplemented by another two arteries (the artery to the vas deferens, from the superior vesical artery, and the cremasteric artery, from the inferior epigastric artery).

The venous drainage starts as venules from the testis which form the pampiniform plexus (from *pampinus*, *Latin*: "tendril") around the artery. The left testicular vein drains into the left renal vein, whilst the right testicular vein drains into the inferior vena cava.

Learning Point

Penile and scrotal skin lymphatics drain to the inguinal lymph nodes. The testicular lymphatics drain to the para-aortic lymph nodes, following the arterial supply. This is important in cases of malignancy of the testes if lymph node clearance is planned.

CLINICAL NOTES

- **Undescended testis** (**cryptorchidism**, from the Greek *kryptos* for hidden and *orchis* for testis) is when one or both testes fail to descend into the scrotum, usually by the age of 6 months. The majority of undescended testes occur at the inguinal canal. The consequences of this condition include infertility and increased risk of testicular cancer, often associated with indirect inguinal hernia and psychological impact. It is the most common male genital anomaly and requires early surgery (usually within the first year) to bring the testis/testes down into the scrotum (orchidopexy) to avoid irreversible damage to spermatogenesis.
- **Varicocele** is an abnormal dilation of the pampiniform plexus. Clinical signs include a scrotum that feels like a "bag of worms" in addition to testicular discomfort or pain. The majority of varicoceles are left-sided, possibly due to the sharply angled junction of the left testicular and renal veins.
- **Hydrocele** is an accumulation of serous fluid, between the parietal and visceral layers of the tunica vaginalis, such that the testis is surrounded by fluid. The transillumination test (a light shone through the scrotum) is positive for a hydrocele and is the characteristic clinical sign. On palpation, it is possible to "get above" the swelling, in contrast to an inguino-scrotal hernia. Scrotal ultrasound examination is an important preoperative diagnostic tool to exclude the presence of testicular pathologies such as malignancy, which, rarely, could be the underlying cause of hydrocele.
- In **testicular torsion**, the testis twists around its pedicle (the spermatic cord), which can occlude the blood supply. Unless treated within the "golden" 6 hours, this can lead to testicular ischaemia and gangrene. There are two main types of torsion, but the most common is **intravaginal** (twisting of the testis within the tunica vaginalis). The "bell clapper" testis is a congenital anomaly where the tunica vaginalis attaches high on the spermatic cord, allowing testicular twisting. The **extravaginal** type is where torsion occurs outside the tunica vaginalis. The main symptom is sudden acute testicular pain. Testicular torsion is a surgical emergency, and when clinical suspicion arises, an expert urological opinion must be sought to avoid misdiagnosis and irreversible testicular infarction. General practitioners and clinicians in A&E should think twice before they put forth a diagnosis of epididymo-orchitis in adolescent and young men (see later).
- The majority of **testicular tumours** are malignant and can metastasise to the para-aortic lymph nodes. This is the most common malignancy in United Kingdom in men between the ages of 20 and 34 (BMJ Best Practice, 2020). Types of testicular cancers include most commonly germ cell cancers, such as seminomas, accounting for 45% of testicular cancers. The rest are non-seminomas, such as teratoma and choriocarcinoma. Because testicular cancer can spread to the para-aortic lymph nodes, an abdominal and pelvis CT is performed, in addition to an ultrasound scan of the scrotum, and checking of the tumour markers (serum alpha fetoprotein and beta-human chorionic gonadotrophin). Biopsy is usually not indicated due to the fear of cancer cells seeding.
- **Orchidectomy** is the operation of surgical removal of the testis. When indicated for testicular cancer, it is performed through the inguinal canal to avoid cancer dissemination if performed through a scrotal approach.
- **Epididymo-orchitis** (inflammation of the testis and epididymis) usually presents with scrotal pain and swelling. The testis and epididymis are tender on palpation. This condition can be caused by STIs, UTIs, and the mumps virus. **Ruling out testicular torsion is vital, as both conditions present with scrotal pain and swelling**.

QUIZ QUESTION

Q. *What is meant by acute scrotum? What is the differential diagnosis for a 10-year-old boy who presents with severe, acute left-sided scrotal pain and swelling?*

The Inguinal Canal

This is an intermuscular slit approximately 4 cm in length in adults, extending from the **deep** to **superficial inguinal rings** in the medial lower portion of the anterior abdominal wall, parallel to the inguinal ligament (**Figures 6.26** and **6.27**):

- The **deep ring** is an opening in the transversalis fascia. It is found 1.5 cm superior to the inguinal ligament, at the midpoint between the ASIS and the pubic tubercle (i.e., the midpoint of the inguinal ligament), **lateral to the inferior epigastric vessels** (see **Figure 6.26**).
- The **superficial ring** is an inverted V-shaped opening in the **external oblique aponeurosis**. It marks the end of the inguinal canal and lies **superior and lateral to the pubic tubercle**. It has lateral and medial crura.

The inguinal canal is bounded:

- *Anteriorly:* the lower part of the **aponeurosis of the external oblique** and **internal oblique muscle**
- *Posteriorly:* the **conjoint tendon** medially and **transversalis fascia** laterally, in addition to the extension of the rolled-up part of the inguinal ligament

- *Superiorly:* roof is the arching fibres of the **conjoint tendon** with fibres from the **internal oblique** and **transversus abdominis**
- *Inferiorly:* floor is gutter-like and formed by the "rolling up" of the **inguinal ligament**

Note that the description of the inguinal canal doesn't apply to neonates and very young children, as the external ring overlies the internal ring. This is of surgical importance when operating to repair their hernias, in the form of excision of the proximal part of the peritoneal sac (patent processus vaginalis), classically known as herniotomy.

The spermatic cord (in males) and the round ligament of the uterus (in females) pass through the inguinal canal, in addition to the ilioinguinal nerve, which penetrates the posterior wall of the canal.

The **spermatic cord** is a bundle of structures passing from and to the testis through the inguinal canal (**Table 6.6**).

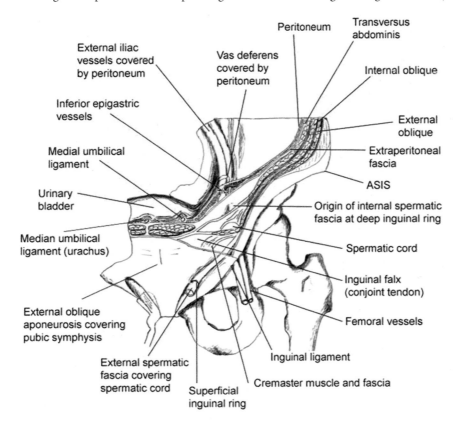

FIGURE 6.26 Left inguinal canal and related anatomy. (Courtesy of Alina Humdani.)

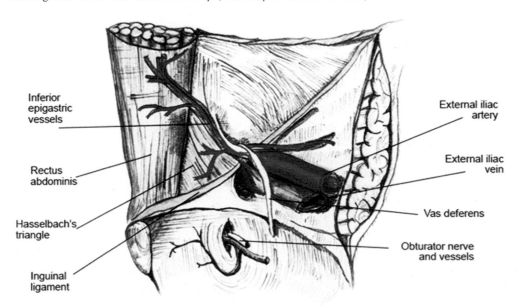

FIGURE 6.27 Posterior view of the right side of the anterior abdominal wall. (Courtesy of Calum Harrington-Vogt.)

TABLE 6.6: Contents of the spermatic cord

Three coverings (sleeves):	*Three arteries:*
• External spermatic fascia (prolongation from the external oblique aponeurosis at the superficial ring) • Cremasteric fascia and muscle (from the internal oblique muscle) • Internal spermatic fascia (prolongation from the transversalis fascia)	• Testicular artery from the abdominal aorta • Cremasteric artery from the inferior epigastric artery • Artery to the vas deferens from either the superior or inferior vesical arteries
Three nerves:	*Three tubes:*
• Sympathetic testicular nerves • Genital branch of the genitofemoral nerve (L1–L2) • Ilioinguinal nerve (L1) (travels in the inguinal canal but not through the deep ring)	• Vas deferens • Remnant of the processus vaginalis • Lymphatics to para-aortic lymph nodes

---

Learning Points

- **Inguinal ligament = Between the ASIS and pubic tubercle**
- **Midinguinal point = Halfway between the ASIS and pubic symphysis (not to be confused with the mid-point of the inguinal ligament!)**

Direct and Indirect Inguinal Hernias

An **inguinal hernia** is a protrusion of part of the contents of the abdominal cavity, commonly the bowel, within a sac of peritoneum, through the inguinal canal. It constitutes the most common type of abdominal wall hernia.

There are some clinical terms when we speak about hernias in general:

- **Sac** of the hernia is the protruding or outpouching part of the peritoneum
- **Contents** of the hernia (small or large bowel, omentum, bladder, rarely the ovary, can descend within the hernial sac)
- **Neck** of the hernia, whether it is wide or tight, which will determine the liability to incarceration and strangulation
- **Reducible or irreducible** hernia (in examinations do not attempt to reduce the hernia, and always ask the patient to reduce it while lying down)
- *Incarcerated hernia* (**Figure 6.28**): the contents are not easily returned to the abdominal cavity and may progress to strangulation

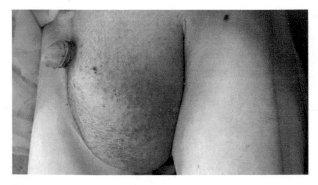

FIGURE 6.28 Incarcerated left inguinoscrotal hernia. (Courtesy of Ali M. Hasan.)

- *Strangulated hernia* (**Figure 6.29**): with cut-off blood supply and possibility of developing gangrene of the contents (commonly the small bowel) if not treated as a matter of urgency

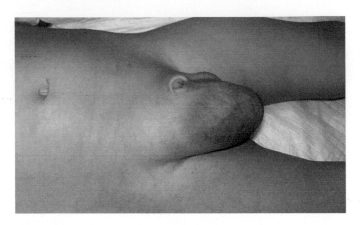

FIGURE 6.29 Strangulated right inguinal hernia (usually of indirect type) containing non-viable small bowel loops. (Courtesy of Mohammed H. Aldabbagh.)

There are two major types of inguinal hernias:

- **Direct inguinal hernia** is the protrusion of the peritoneal hernial sac, which occurs **medial** to the inferior epigastric vessels, through Hesselbach's triangle.
- **Indirect hernia**, in contrast, is a protrusion which occurs **lateral** to the inferior epigastric vessels, via the deep inguinal ring. The peritoneal sac is usually the pre-existing processus vaginalis (see discussion on testicular descent).
- In comparison to indirect hernias, direct hernias are less liable to complications such as incarceration and strangulation, due to their wide neck.
- Indirect inguinal hernias are more likely to pass into the scrotum to form an inguinoscrotal hernia.
- An inguinal hernia usually presents as a lump in the groin and needs differentiating from a femoral hernia (*vide infra*) and other causes of groin swellings.
- The patient is examined in the standing position, with full exposure of both groins, and then asked to cough. A visible swelling suggests the presence of hernia with a palpable cough impulse.
- The **occlusion test** is one of the clinical tests used to differentiate between the two main types of inguinal hernias. The test involves asking a patient to lie on the examination couch and reducing the hernia. The next step is applying digital pressure on the deep ring and asking the patient to cough. If the hernial content is controlled (remaining within the peritoneal cavity), the patient is likely to have an indirect hernia. However, if it remains protruding, the patient is said to be suffering from the direct type.
- **Examination of the scrotum is mandatory to rule out the presence of undescended testes and other causes of scrotal swellings.**

Surgical repair of inguinal hernias can be via an open or laparoscopic approach, depending on the expertise and available facilities. For adults with inguinal hernias, tension-free mesh repair is indicated to strengthen the weak posterior wall of the inguinal canal.

Differential diagnosis of a groin lump includes:

- Inguinal hernia (direct and indirect)
- Femoral hernia
- Inguinal lymphadenopathy
- Undescended testis
- Saphena varix (dilation of the terminal part of the long saphenous vein, before it joins the femoral vein)
- Femoral artery aneurysm (see **Section 7**, Lower Limb)
- Psoas abscess (TB of the lumbar vertebrae with cold abscess formation along the psoas major muscle, which presents as a lump in the groin)

QUIZ QUESTION

Q. *What is the differential diagnosis of scrotal swelling in the above patient (Figure 6.28)?*

Learning Points

- **Strangulated groin hernias are among the most common causes of bowel obstruction.**
- **Inguinal hernia is the most common type of hernia in males of all age groups.**
- **Groin hernia repair is amongst the most common general surgical procedures worldwide.**
- **Laparoscopic (keyhole) surgery is increasingly performed to treat groin hernias, especially in the elective setting.**
- **Femoral hernias occur *below and lateral* to the pubic tubercle, whilst inguinal hernias occur *above and medial* to the pubic tubercle (see Section 7, Lower Limb) and are liable to strangulation in view of the non-yielding space, especially on its medial side, where it is bounded by the sharp edge of the lacunar ligament**

Male Internal Genitalia

- Vas deferens (proximal to the deep inguinal ring)
- Seminal vesicles
- Prostate gland
- Bulbourethral glands (Cowper's glands)
- Urethra

The Vas Deferens

This is a fibromuscular duct which transports spermatozoa from the epididymis to the ejaculatory duct and is palpable in the scrotum. The vas (or ductus) deferens is 30 to 45 cm in length and **arises from the tail region of the epididymis**. It is situated on the posteromedial aspect of the testis and travels, as part of the spermatic cord, from the testis to the pelvic cavity, via the inguinal canal, entering the pelvis at the deep inguinal ring. The vas has a very narrow lumen.

The vas deferens then passes medially around the lateral side of the inferior epigastric artery, crossing the external iliac vessels, and enters the pelvic cavity. At the posterior aspect of the bladder, the vas deferens courses inferomedially **above the ureter** (important to identify during open and endoscopic surgery), joining with **the duct of the seminal vesicle**, to form the **ejaculatory duct**.

A **vasectomy** is one of the methods used for male contraception and can be performed under local anaesthetic. On each side, the vas deferens is identified by palpating the upper part of the scrotum, and a segment of the vas is excised and sent for histopathological examination to prove the correct structure has been removed (this is a medicolegal requirement). The two ends of the vas are then cauterised or ligated.

The Seminal Vesicles

These are paired sac-like structures, situated on the inferoposterior aspect (base) of the bladder, which function by producing approximately 70% of the ejaculate volume. Embryologically, they are outgrowths of the ductus deferens. The seminal vesicles produce a neutral-to-alkaline fluid to neutralise the acidic environment of the vagina, so that the spermatozoa can survive there, **but the seminal vesicles are not a store for the sperm**. The secreted fluid is rich in fructose and prostaglandins.

On both the left and right, the duct of the seminal vesicle joins the vas deferens to form the ejaculatory duct. The two ejaculatory ducts open into the prostatic urethra on each side of the seminal colliculus. Sympathetic innervation is responsible for contraction of the seminal vesicles during ejaculation. Clinically, inflamed seminal vesicles can be palpated by DRE.

The Prostate Gland

This is an unpaired, fibromuscular, glandular organ, which is located **inferior to the bladder**, has a capsule, and is in the shape of an inverted cone, the apex of which is surrounded by the **urogenital diaphragm** (the prostate gland sits on the pelvic floor; see earlier discussion on the pubococcygeus muscle). The prostate develops from the urogenital sinus. It measures about 4 cm in width at its base, 3 cm in height, and 2 cm in depth. The **base of the prostate is related to the bladder neck**.

It develops rapidly during puberty in the male. The prostate has an anterior, posterior, and two inferolateral surfaces. The **prostate is traversed by the prostatic urethra** which emerges immediately above and anterior to its apex to continue as the membranous urethra.

The prostate is related anteriorly to the lower border of the pubic symphysis and pubic arch and connected to it by the **puboprostatic ligaments**. The space posterior to the pubic symphysis and anterior to the urinary bladder is called the retropubic space (pre-vesical space or cave of Retzius). Posteriorly, it is related to the ampulla of the rectum, and it can be felt on DRE or PR examination (see information on Denonvillier's fascia earlier).

The main function of the prostate is the generation of prostatic fluid, which is produced by the branching ducts surrounded by the stroma. It contributes approximately 20% of the ejaculate, by volume, and it also produces many of the constituents of semen.

Blood supply of the prostate gland: the arterial supply is from the inferior vesical and middle rectal arteries (branches of the internal iliac artery). The **venous return** is via the prostatic venous plexus, which drains to the internal iliac vein and also receives the deep dorsal vein of the penis. The prostatic venous plexus also communicates with the venous plexus of the vertebral column, which is of clinical significance in the potential metastasis of cancer of the prostate (see **Section 5, Abdomen**).

Nerve supply is from the **inferior hypogastric plexus**. The sympathetic supply innervates the muscle, and the parasympathetic innervates the gland (see the discussion on mechanisms of erection and ejaculation earlier).

Lymphatic drainage follows the arterial blood supply to the internal iliac lymph nodes.

In current terminology, the prostate is divided into **zones**, each accounting for different-sized segments of the prostate: the **peripheral**, **transitional**, and **central zones**.

The **peripheral zone** is the largest zone of the prostate gland, comprising some 70% of the prostatic tissue and containing most of the glandular tissue of the prostate. It **is the most common site for the development of prostate cancer**. Approximately 75% of prostate cancers originate in the peripheral zone.

The **central zone** is a small area of prostatic tissue that surrounds the ejaculatory ducts. The central zone accounts for about 25% of the prostatic tissue, yet only 5% of prostate cancers.

The **transitional zone** is the area which surrounds the pre-prostatic urethra and is most commonly the site of benign prostatic hyperplasia (BPH). Despite accounting for only 5% of prostatic tissue, approximately 20% of prostate cancers originate from the transitional zone.

Benign Prostatic Hyperplasia

While the prostate gland weighs about 8 gm in youth, it enlarges with progressive age due to excessive proliferation of the epithelial cells of the prostate's **transitional zone**.

BPH is a non-cancerous disease, but the enlarged prostate can obstruct urine flow in the urethra. This can present with symptoms of lower urinary tract symptoms (LUTS): frequent micturition, dysuria, urge incontinence, hesitancy, poor stream, post-micturition dribbling, difficulty initiating urination, and nocturia. It can also lead to acute urine retention, which is a medical emergency, and which usually requires the insertion of a bladder catheter.

Clinically, an enlarged prostate gland can be palpated PR. Prostate cancers feel hard and lumpy on palpation anteriorly via the rectum. In BPH the prostate feels enlarged but is smooth.

Prostate cancer is one of the most common cancers in men, with frequent metastasis, via the prostatic venous plexus and lymphatics of the pelvis, typically to the spine and lungs. Note that the TNM (Tumour, Nodes, and Metastases) and "cancer staging" systems are used for assessing cancer progression.

A prostate-specific antigen (PSA) test measures the protein produced by cells of the prostate. Any abnormal rise may be a sign of prostate cancer, BPH, or prostatitis. Due to the many causes of raised PSA, the test is not used for screening or diagnosis of prostate cancer – an ultrasound-guided transrectal biopsy is used instead. The reliability of the PSA test is doubtful, as there can be false-positives and false-negatives; both are a source of inaccuracy and anxiety for patients.

Inflammation of the prostate (prostatitis) can be of acute onset (acute prostatitis), most commonly due to infection by *Escherichia coli* or an STD (usually from direct spread of urethritis), or of the chronic type (usually non-bacterial).

Bulbourethral (Cowper's) Glands

These are paired pea-sized glands which develop during the 12th week of gestation and are located inferior to the prostate, posterolateral to the membranous urethra in the deep perineal space, above the perineal membrane. Each gland connects to the bulbar urethra via a duct that crosses the perineal membrane to reach the superficial perineal space. The bulbourethral glands are the male equivalent of the greater vestibular (Bartholin's) glands in the female.

Cowper's glands make up about 5% to 10% of the ejaculate volume, lubricating the spongy urethra and neutralising urine acidity. The blood supply to Cowper's glands is from the bulbourethral arteries, with equivalent venous drainage. Lymphatic drainage is to the internal and external iliac lymph nodes. Cowper's glands may become inflamed in cases of infection; symptoms include fever and severe perineal pain.

Female Reproductive Organs

The **female reproductive tract is subdivided into the upper and lower genital tracts**. The lower genital tract includes the cervix, vagina, and vulva. The upper genital tract consists of the uterus, uterine tubes, and ovaries.

Embryology

Developmentally, the genital tract arises from the **paramesonephric (Mullerian) ducts** of the mesodermal germ layer and is closely related to the development of the urinary tract. This means that an anomaly in one system can be associated with an anomaly in another. The para-mesonephric ducts fuse to form the uterine tubes, uterus, cervix, and upper third of the vagina. The lower two-thirds of the vagina develop from the urogenital sinus.

The pelvic cavity in the female:

- Projects **posteriorly** from the abdominal cavity towards the buttocks.
- Has a **pelvic inlet** that is bounded by the **pelvic brim** and is oval in shape (transverse diameter is greater than the AP diameter).
- The pelvic brim delineates the **true** (lesser) from the **false** (greater) pelvis.
- The **pelvic outlet** is diamond-shaped and bounded by the symphysis pubis, inferior pubic rami, ischial rami, ischial tuberosities, sacrotuberous ligaments, and coccyx.
- True pelvis contains pelvic organs (genital, urinary, and intestinal tracts) and is assessed clinically by per vaginam (PV)/PR examination.
- The pelvic floor in the female is traversed by the urethra, vagina, and rectum.
- The pelvic diaphragm supports the pelvic viscera and directs the fetal head anteriorly.

The Female Lower Genital Tract

The **external female genitalia (vulva)** consists of the mons pubis, labia majora, labia minora, and vestibule and incorporates the structures shown in **Figure 6.30**.

Blood supply: superficial and deep external pudendal artery (branches of the femoral artery) and the perineal artery (a branch of the internal pudendal artery). The venous drainage is to the corresponding veins (external pudendal veins), which join the long saphenous vein.

Nerve supply: the anterior one-third of the labium majus is supplied by the ilioinguinal nerve (from the lumbar plexus), whilst the posterior two-thirds are supplied by branches of the pudendal nerve (S3) and the perineal branch of the posterior cutaneous nerve of the thigh (S2). The mons pubis is innervated by the genital branch of the genitofemoral nerve (L1–L2 from the lumbar plexus).

Lymphatic drainage: lymph from the skin of the vulva drains into the superficial inguinal and then to deep inguinal lymph nodes (medial to the femoral vein). Lymphatic vessels from the clitoris drain directly into the deep inguinal lymph nodes.

Labia Minora (*Singular:* **labium minus**)
Fat-free, hairless skin folds that contain some erectile tissue. They pass anteriorly to form the frenulum and prepuce of the clitoris. Posteriorly, they unite to form the frenulum of the labia minora (fourchette). The skin is non-keratinised squamous epithelium, with no sweat glands or sebaceous glands.

Vestibule
This is the space between the labia minora and contains the opening of the urethra, the introitus of the vagina surrounded by the hymen, and the openings of the vestibular glands (lesser and greater).

Clitoris
This consists of erectile tissue which has a midline glans, covered by a foreskin (or prepuce), a body, and two crura extending along the ischiopubic rami and covered by the ischiocavernosus muscles. It is innervated by the dorsal branch of the perineal nerve

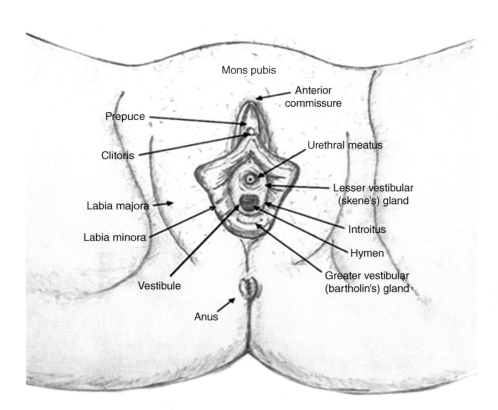

FIGURE 6.30 Diagram of the female external genitalia. (Courtesy of Naomi Bartholomew.)

Mons Pubis
The mons pubis refers to the anterior fatty eminence overlying the pubic symphysis. It is lined by keratinised, squamous epithelium with hair follicles and sebaceous and apocrine glands.

Labia Majora (*Singular:* **labium majus**)
Two longitudinal skin folds that extend from the mons pubis to the perineum, covered with hair on their lateral surface, and smooth and highly vascularised on the medial side. The two folds meet anteriorly at the anterior commissure. Posteriorly they do not join, and the area of skin between them is called the **posterior commissure**, which marks the posterior limit of the vulva.

(S2). The bulb of the clitoris is divided into two parts because of the intervening vagina.

Urethral Meatus
Also known as the external urethral orifice, through which urine exits the body. It is located approximately 2.5 cm behind the clitoris and in front of the vaginal orifice, in the vulval vestibule (important to remember whilst catheterising the bladder). The meatus is lined by non-keratinised, squamous epithelium, with a stroma that is highly vascularised, like the corpora cavernosa of the penis.

Bartholin's (Greater Vestibular) Glands
These are paired, pea-sized, mucus-secreting glands lying posterior to the bulb of the vestibule and posterolateral to the opening

of the vagina, superficial to the hymen. They produce secretions during arousal. It is possible for the Bartholin's glands to become blocked (resulting in a Bartholin's cyst, which can form an abscess). Bartholin's gland carcinoma is rare and only occurs in 1% of vulval cancers.

Skene's (Lesser Vestibular) Glands

Also known as the paraurethral glands. These are located on the anterior wall of the vagina, around the lower end of the urethra. They drain into the urethra, near the urethral opening, and may be near or a part of the so-called G-spot. They are surrounded with tissue (including part of the clitoris) that extends inside the vagina and swells with blood during sexual arousal. They are the female equivalent of the prostate gland.

Hymen

This is a membranous fold of skin that lines the vaginal opening. It has no known biological function; however, during a female's first experience of sexual intercourse, the hymen is torn, and only fragments of the hymen remain along the margins of the vaginal opening. The hymen may be imperforate, which leads to accumulation of the products of menstruation in the vagina and the uterus (haematocolpos). In some communities there is too much emphasis on the integrity of the hymen as a proof of virginity, which sadly has caused unfortunate loss of female lives in the name of "honour killing".

Physiological changes that occur during sexual arousal:

- Vaginal lubrication by increased secretions from the Bartholin's and Skene's glands, in addition to transudation from the engorged blood vessels related to the inner vaginal layer
- Enlargement of the external genitalia, involving the swelling of the clitoris and the labia
- Increased darkening or redness of the skin in these areas
- Increased heart rate and blood pressure, with flushing across the chest and upper body
- Increased blood flow to the nipples, vulva, clitoris, and vaginal walls

The **neurological control** of this is from:

- Afferent stimuli from the labia minora and clitoris via the ilioinguinal nerves (L1) and the dorsal nerves of the clitoris (from the pudendal nerve).
- Central pre-ganglionic stimuli descend the spinal cord to the sympathetic outflow (T1–L1) and then reach the sympathetic ganglia, where they synapse and give rise to postganglionic fibres which stimulate the smooth muscle of the vagina leading to their contraction.
- The external muscles (bulbospongiosus and ischiocavernosus) contract in response to stimulation from efferent fibres in the pudendal nerve.

Female genital mutilation, as defined by the World Health Organization (WHO), comprises all procedures that involve partial or total removal of the external female genitalia or other injury to the female genital organs for non-medical reasons. Unfortunately, it is still practised in many countries, mainly in Africa, the Middle East, and Asia, and is a violation of human rights of girls and women.

Vagina

This is a fibromuscular tube, which is expandable to allow passage of the fetus and for the passage of the menstrual flow. It is lined by stratified, non-keratinised squamous epithelium that extends to the uterine cervix. The upper half passes inferiorly, through the pelvic floor, and the lower half is within the perineum and opens into the vestibule, enclosed by the labia minora. The lower end is surrounded by the remnants of the hymen (vaginal orifice) forming the introitus. Note that the posterior wall is longer than the anterior (about 9 to 7.5 cm for the anterior wall). The rectouterine pouch separates the upper vagina from the rectum. Below the pouch, the vagina is related to the ampulla of the rectum, separated by the Denonvillier's fascia, in its middle part. The perineal body separates the anal canal from the lower vagina.

Anteriorly the vagina is related to the base of the bladder and urethra.

Blood Supply

The vaginal artery can arise from different origins, but commonly arises from the internal iliac artery and anastomoses with the vaginal branches of the uterine artery, forming the azygos arteries of the vagina.

Vaginal veins drain into the internal iliac veins.

Lymphatic Drainage

External and internal iliac lymph nodes (upper portion) and superficial inguinal lymph nodes (lower portion).

Nerve supply

- *Autonomic:* inferior fibres of uterovaginal plexus, derived from inferior hypogastric plexus
- *Somatic:* deep branch of the perineal nerve, a branch of the pudendal nerve

The vagina contains no glands, and so is lubricated by cervical mucus and secretions of the Bartholin's and Skene's glands. The plane of the vaginal canal is 60 degrees to the horizontal in the standing position (the same as the angle of the pelvic inlet).

The upper vagina is supported by the action of the pelvic diaphragm and the fibromuscular connective tissue (endopelvic fascia).

CLINICAL NOTES

During **pelvic organ prolapse** there is weakness of the supporting ligaments, fascia, and pelvic floor muscles. It can lead to descent of the anterior vaginal wall (cystocoele), posterior vaginal wall (rectocoele), or descent of the upper portion of the vagina into the vaginal canal after a hysterectomy (vault prolapse).

A **caudal block** will not completely anaesthetise the vulva because of the dual nerve supply. The anterior portion is supplied by the ilioinguinal (L1) and genital branch of the genitofemoral nerve (L1–L2) from the lumbar plexus, with the posterior part being supplied by the pudendal nerve (S2–S4) and the posterior femoral cutaneous nerve of the thigh, from the sacral plexus. The upper part of the vagina and the intravaginal portion of the cervix can be examined visually by inserting a vaginal speculum.

QUIZ QUESTION

Q. *What structures can be palpated on a PV exam?*

Upper Genital Tract

Three tracts pass through the female pelvis, namely the urinary, reproductive, and gastrointestinal (GI) tracts. The genital tract forms a "**genital septum**" between the GI and urinary tracts, created during development by the fusion of the two **paramesonephric (Mullerian) ducts**.

Posterior to the genital septum is the **rectouterine pouch** (of Douglas), between the anterior rectum and the posterior wall of the uterus, whilst anterior to the genital septum is the **vesicouterine pouch**, which is between the anterior surface of the uterus and the bladder.

CLINICAL NOTES

The peritoneal cavity is not completely closed in females, as it is open at the ostia of the uterine tubes. This means that organisms can spread to the peritoneal cavity, causing pelvic inflammatory disease (PID).

The close association between the rectouterine pouch (which is the lowest point of the peritoneal cavity in females in the standing position) and the posterior wall of the vagina allows for **culdocentesis**, a procedure where peritoneal fluids (e.g., blood or pus) can be aspirated from the pouch of Douglas in female patients. It involves the introduction of a needle through the posterior fornix of the vagina.

During pregnancy, the cervix has the consistency of the lips, whereas normally, it has the consistency of the nose.

The uterus has the following parts:

- *Fundus:* the part above the orifices of the uterine/fallopian tubes.
- *Corpus uteri (body):* the part below the entrance of the uterine tubes. At its superior lateral border, the body of the uterus narrows into an angle or **cornu** (Latin, "horn") on either side. The narrow portion, situated between the corpus and cervix, is known as the **isthmus** and lies at the level of the uterine artery and the **internal os** of the cervix.
- *Cervix uteri:* the narrow neck-like passage, which is generally 2 to 3 cm long and protrudes into the upper end of the vagina, creating a sulcus around the cervix and the **vaginal fornices** (*Singular:* fornix), anterior, posterior, and two laterals. The endocervical canal extends from the external os to the internal os and is lined with mucus-secreting columnar epithelium.

The cervix can be divided into **supravaginal** and **intravaginal** portions. The intravaginal portion is surrounded by the vaginal fornices and covered with non-keratinising squamous epithelium.

During pregnancy, the cervix serves to retain and protect the developing conceptus. At the early stage of pregnancy, the cervix shortens as a result of an increase in the volume of the lower amniotic cavity. At later stages, the cervix undergoes remodelling, where it softens and dilates.

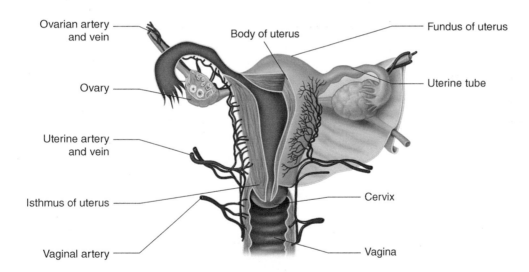

FIGURE 6.31 Diagram of the vagina, uterus, uterine tubes, uterine arteries, and ovaries. (Courtesy of Julian Bartholomew.)

Uterus

This is a hollow, pear-shaped, intraperitoneal, muscular organ, approximately 7 to 8 cm long that incubates the developing fetus for 38 weeks once an oocyte has been fertilised. The uterine wall has three components: **endometrium** (mucosal), **myometrium** (smooth muscle), and **parametrium** (mesothelial layer) (**Figure 6.31**).

The uterus allows implantation of the fertilised zygote, once it has reached the blastocyst stage, to provide an environment for the development of the fetus.

Relations:

- Base of bladder lies anterior to the cervix.
- Posterior fornix is deepest and is anterior to the rectouterine pouch.
- Nerve supply is via the pelvic splanchnic nerves (S2–S4).

Normally, the uterus and the cervix are described as **anteverted** (cervix is tilted anteriorly towards the bladder) and **anteflexed** (fundus of the uterus is directed forward). **Retroversion** means the cervix tilts posteriorly towards the spine. **Retroflexed** is when the uterine fundus is directed posteriorly, towards the rectum. Anteriorly, the bladder lies over the isthmus and the cervix.

Important relations of the uterus:

- *Anterior:* uterovesical pouch
- *Posterior:* rectouterine pouch (of Douglas)
- *Lateral:* broad ligaments
- Supravaginal cervix sits directly on top of the bladder

The ureter is an important structure related to the lateral fornix and may be palpable on clinical examination. One of the traditional questions in surgical fellowship exams was "where can you feel a stone in the lower ureter?"

At 10 to 12 weeks, the pregnant uterus becomes palpable, per abdomen, and at 20 weeks the uterus reaches the level of the umbilicus.

Blood supply

- The uterine artery is a branch of the anterior division of the internal iliac artery.
- The uterine artery is positioned superolateral to the lateral fornix and gives rise to dorsal and ventral branches.
- The ureter passes under the uterine artery.
- The uterine artery divides into ascending branches (along the lateral wall of the uterus and inferior to the uterine tube), which anastomose with the ovarian artery, from the abdominal aorta, and descending branches (along the cervix and lateral wall of the vagina) to anastomose with the vaginal arteries on the anterior and posterior surfaces of the vagina (see **Figure 6.31**).

Venous drainage: venous plexus in the broad ligament finally drains into the internal iliac veins (communicates with veins of the vagina and bladder).

Lymphatic drainage: the uterus and upper two-thirds of the vagina drain through lymph vessels that accompany the blood vessels to the internal and external iliac, obturator, and aortic lymph nodes. The lower third of the vagina and the vulva drain to inguinal lymph nodes. Some lymphatics accompany the round ligament and drain to the superficial inguinal lymph nodes.

Nerve supply

- *Sympathetic:* uterovaginal plexus mainly from the anterior and middle fibres of the inferior hypogastric plexus (sympathetic outflow from T12 to L1)
- *Parasympathetic:* pelvic splanchnic nerve (S2–S4)
- *Sensory afferents:* inferior hypogastric plexus via T10–12 and L1 nerve fibres (sympathetic)

Ligaments of the Uterus

The uterus is held on its superior aspect by the broad ligament and the round ligaments. The **broad ligament is a double sheet of peritoneum** connected to the uterus and ovaries. It can be divided into three sections:

- *Mesometrium:* surrounds the uterus and is the largest subsection of the broad ligament running laterally to cover the external iliac vessels; it also encloses the proximal part of the round ligament of the uterus.
- *Mesovarium:* associated with the ovaries, it projects from the posterior surface of the broad ligament and attaches to the hilum of the ovary, enclosing its neurovascular supply. It does not cover the surface of the ovary itself.
- *Mesosalpinx:* originates superior to the mesovarium and surrounds the uterine tubes and contains the anastomosis between the uterine and the ovarian arteries.

The **round ligaments** extend from the anterosuperior surface of the uterus, below the uterine tubes, through the deep inguinal rings and through the inguinal canals and continue to the labia majora. They are continuations of the **ligaments of the ovary**, and together, they represent the female equivalent of the gubernaculum in the male.

On its middle aspect, the uterus is supported by the cardinal, pubocervical, and uterosacral ligaments. These are condensations of endopelvic fascia.

Cardinal ligaments (Mackenrodt's or transverse cervical ligaments) form the base of the broad ligament and attach the cervix to the pelvic side wall, into the fascia of the obturator internus. The cardinal ligaments are, collectively, named the parametrium.

Pubocervical ligaments pass from the posterior aspect of the pubic bones, diverging around the urethra to the lower cervix and upper vagina.

Uterosacral ligaments run from the posterior aspect of the cervix at the level of the internal os to the anterior sacrum (S2–S4 vertebrae) (**Figure 6.32**).

The ligaments that support the uterus are, predominantly, the cardinal and uterosacral ligaments, with some assistance from the round ligament. However, the uterus is primarily aided by the pelvic diaphragm, perineal body, and urogenital diaphragm.

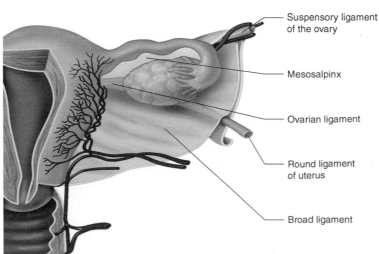

Suspensory ligament of the ovary

Mesosalpinx

Ovarian ligament

Round ligament of uterus

Broad ligament

FIGURE 6.32 Diagram of the ligaments of the uterus and ovaries. (Courtesy of Julian Bartholomew.)

CLINICAL NOTES

One or both ureters may be injured or inadvertently ligated during hysterectomy, especially during an emergency procedure. Also, the ureter/ureters can become obstructed in malignant tumours of the cervix, leading to hydroureter and hydronephrosis.

Uterine abnormalities result from the abnormal fusion of the paramesonephric duct(s) during embryogenesis. Problems may include repeated miscarriage, preterm delivery, abnormal lie of the fetus, infertility, or menstrual problems, depending on the severity of the malformation (**Figure 6.33**). Examples:

- *Uterus arcuatus:* the internal surface of the single endometrial cavity shows a shallow groove.
- *Septate uterus:* there are two uterine cavities divided by a longitudinal septum, but they look normal on the outside; the most common uterine anomaly.
- *Bicornuate uterus:* the uterus is divided into two horns.
- *Uterus unicornuate:* one rudimentary horn and only half of the uterus develop from a single Mullerian duct.
- *Uterus didelphys:* this is a type of anomaly in which the two halves of the uterus develop completely separately, with a double vagina, due to complete failure of fusion of the paramesonephric ducts.
- *Atresia* of cervix/vagina (atresia is failure of canalisation) showing as a transverse vaginal septum.
- *Agenesis of the uterus:* the uterus fails to develop.

CLINICAL NOTES

The term adnexa refers to the structures adjacent to the uterus, i.e., ovaries and fallopian tubes.

Lymphatic drainage is surgically relevant in the treatment of malignant tumours of the uterus.

Hysterectomy is the surgical removal of the uterus, coming from the Greek, *hystera*, for "womb" and *ektome*, "to cut out".

Menstrual disorders, such as menorrhagia (excessive bleeding), dysmenorrhoea (painful bleeding), and oligomenorrhoea (infrequent bleeding), are common.

Uterine prolapse occurs when the ligaments stretch or become weak so that the uterus descends into the vagina:

- *Grade 1:* uterus may descend slightly and remain above the introitus (vaginal opening)
- *Grade 2:* descent such that the cervix/lower portion of the uterus reaches the introitus
- *Grade 3:* cervix or even the entire uterus descends beyond the introitus

Uterine fibroids are benign tumours of the myometrium and are the most common tumours of the female reproductive tract (found in approximately one-third of women).

Endometriosis is when endometrial tissue is found outside the uterine cavity. Symptoms include painful periods (dysmenorrhea), pain during intercourse (dyspareunia), and excessive bleeding. Endometriosis in the myometrium is known as adenomyosis (endometriosis interna).

QUIZ QUESTION

Q. *Can uterine cancer spread to the superficial inguinal lymph nodes?*

Uterine Tubes (Fallopian Tubes/Oviducts)

These are muscular tubes developed from the paramesonephric duct or Mullerian duct that lie on the upper border of the broad ligament and extend laterally from the uterus (**Figure 6.34**).

At about 10 cm long, they are divided into four sections, medial to lateral:

- *Intramural part (shortest part):* within the myometrium.
- *Isthmus (narrowest part):* about 2 to 3 cm in length.
- *Ampulla:* about 5 cm in length, where fertilisation takes place. The widest part of the tube and the most common site for ectopic gestation and gonococcal salpingitis.
- *Infundibulum:* the funnel-shaped or trumpet-like part, with fimbriae (finger-like projections to direct the released ovum towards the infundibulum).

Blood supply: from both uterine and ovarian arteries with free anastomosis between the two:
Venous drainage: uterine and ovarian veins
Lymphatic drainage: iliac, sacral, and para-aortic lymph nodes

Ova from the ovaries are transported to the uterus through the uterine tubes during the latter half of the menstrual cycle. This happens through the contraction of smooth muscle and the wafting action of the ciliated cells on the inner layer, the mucosa. The

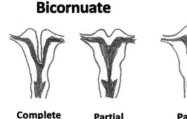

Normal   **Didelphus**   **Arcuate**

Unicornuate

Communicating   Non-communicating   No cavity   No horn

Bicornuate   **Septate**

Complete   Partial   Partial   Complete

FIGURE 6.33 Diagram showing congenital abnormalities of the female genital tract. (Courtesy of Hatidzhe Masteva.)

smooth muscle layer is sensitive to sex steroids, so peristalsis is greatest in the presence of a high amount of oestrogen.

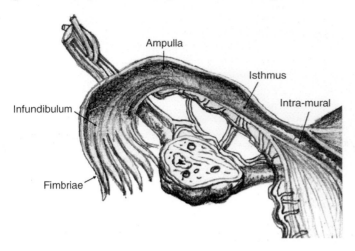

FIGURE 6.34 Parts of the uterine tube. (Courtesy of Julian Bartholomew.)

CLINICAL NOTES

The patency of the tubes/uterine cavity can be checked by a procedure called **hysterosalpingography (HSG)** by taking images after injecting a radio-opaque dye through the external cervical os.

Ectopic gestation occurs when the embryo implants outside the uterine cavity, usually in the ampulla. This is a medical emergency, as the uterine tube can rupture causing internal bleeding and hypovolaemic shock.

Pelvic Inflammatory Disease (PID) is infection of the uterus, uterine tubes, and sometimes the ovaries and pelvic peritoneum. This is mostly due to STIs (mainly *Neisseria gonococcus* and *Chlamydia trachomatis*) and mostly affects young women. Clinically manifested as bilateral lower abdominal pain, dyspareunia (painful coitus), and vaginal discharge. Its sequelae include tubal damage, higher risk of ectopic pregnancy, and chronic pelvic pain.

Salpingitis is inflammation of the uterine tubes (usually due to bacterial infection) and is a common cause of infertility in females due to the damage it causes to the tubes.

Hydrosalpinx/pyosalpinx/haematosalpinx refers to a uterine tube, which is dilated with fluid, pus, or blood, respectively, due to distal blockage.

"Chandelier sign" or "cervical excitation" is extreme tenderness on pelvic examination of the cervix, uterus, and ovaries such that women will "reach for the chandelier" to seek relief from the discomfort.

Tubal ligation is one of the methods of contraception which can be performed as an open procedure or laparoscopically (keyhole surgery).

Recent evidence suggests that many tumours thought to be ovarian in origin were in fact tubal in origin.

Ovaries

The ovaries are paired, oval organs attached to the posterior surface of the broad ligament by the mesovarium and measuring about $4 \times 2 \times 1$ cm, though they atrophy with age. Histologically,

the ovary is divided into the outer **cortex** and the inner **medulla**. The cortex contains **ovarian follicles**. The cortex has about 1 million oocytes at birth, but releases around 500 ova during life. The medulla consists of connective tissue with the neuro-vascular supply of the ovary. The cortex is lined by the germinal epithelium, which consists of cuboidal cells. The ovaries are not covered by peritoneum, but by the **germinal epithelium**.

The **ovarian fossa** is the depression on the lateral pelvic wall in which the ovary sits, below the external iliac vessels.

The ovaries develop from the **genital ridge** (mesodermal in origin) and descend from high up on the posterior abdominal wall to the level of the pelvic brim. Their function is to produce female **gametes (ova)** for fertilisation and to produce oestrogen and progesterone (sex steroids). The ovaries are closely related to the lateral pelvic wall, and the obturator nerve (L2–L4, a branch of the lumbar plexus) descends from the pelvic brim towards the obturator foramen to supply the adductor compartment of the thigh and both the knee and hip joints. Consequently, ovarian pathology, and even ovulation, can cause referred pain in the medial aspect of thigh and these joints.

Ovarian ligaments:

- *Suspensory ligament (infundibulo-pelvic ligament):* a double fold of peritoneum which contains the neurovascular supply (ovarian artery, vein, lymphatics, and sympathetic nerves) and extends from the lateral pelvic wall to the ovary; it must be divided during removal of the ovary (**oophorectomy**).
- *Ovarian ligament:* attaches the medial pole of the ovary to the fundus of the uterus, inferior to the origin of the uterine tube (posteriorly) and continues as the round ligament of the uterus (anteriorly).
- *Mesovarium:* see above.

Note that the ovaries are not directly attached to the uterine tubes.

Blood supply: ovarian arteries arise from the abdominal aorta, inferior to the renal artery, at the level of L2, to cross the pelvic brim and pass into the suspensory ligament and then enter the ovarian hilum; they also give rise to branches to the uterine tube, ureter, and round ligament of the uterus.

Venous drainage: at the ovarian hilum a pampiniform plexus forms the ovarian vein on each side. The left drains into the left renal vein; the right drains directly into the inferior vena cava (compare with the venous drainage of the testes).

Lymphatic drainage: to para-aortic nodes (compare with the lymphatic drainage of the testes).

Nerve supply: sympathetic fibres from T10 via the aortic plexus.

CLINICAL NOTES

There may be remnants of the **mesonephric (Wolffian) ducts**, which may appear as epo-ophorons and paro-ophorons, which are vestigial structures within the broad ligament. Although rare, these may develop into cysts and need surgical excision. Persistence of the lower cord of the mesonephric duct may present as a cyst in the lateral wall of the vagina (Gartner's duct cyst).

Ovarian cancer: most (80%) are epithelial in origin (the most common is serous carcinoma), whilst the remainder are stromal (10%) and germ cell (10%). Epithelial tumours originate in the cells covering the ovaries and can present as abdominal swelling.

According to the statistics from Cancer Research UK, there are around 7500 new ovarian cancer cases in the UK every year (2016–2018 statistics). Note that ovarian cancers have a poor prognosis due to late diagnosis. CT scan of the pelvis and abdomen is considered the best imaging modality to assess the spread of ovarian cancer.

Ovarian cysts: fluid-filled masses derived from graafian follicles in the ovary, which occur commonly. Most are benign (such as follicular and luteal cysts), but they might be malignant, especially with advancing age. Larger cysts may cause bleeding within the cyst and pain (**Figure 6.35**). Cyst complications include rupture, haemorrhage, and torsion and come under the differential diagnosis of acute abdomen.

Polycystic ovaries: the most common endocrine disorder affecting women of reproductive age. It is caused by increased androgen production by the ovaries. Symptoms include hormone dysfunction and infertility.

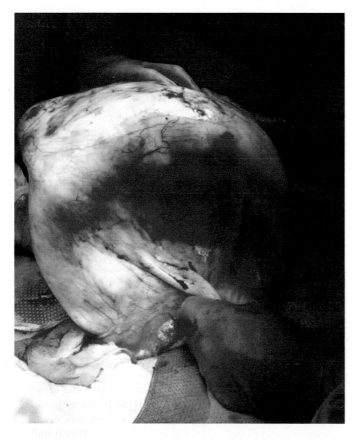

FIGURE 6.35 Large ovarian cyst draining 4 litres from it. (Courtesy of Paul Carter.)

Revision Questions

The Pelvic Girdle

Q1. What structure delineates the true (lesser) pelvis from the false (greater) pelvis?
   a. Iliac crest
   b. Ischial spines
   c. Ischial tuberosity
   d. Pelvic brim
   e. sacral promontory

Q2. Which of the following muscles DOES NOT attach to the external lip of the iliac crest?
   a. External oblique
   b. Internal oblique
   c. Latissimus dorsi
   d. Tensor fasciae latae
   e. Transverse abdominis

Q3. Which artery is a branch of the posterior division of the internal iliac artery?
   a. Inferior gluteal artery
   b. Middle rectal artery
   c. Obturator artery
   d. Superior gluteal artery
   e. Umbilical artery

Q4. What is the widest dimension of the pelvic *inlet* in a female?
   a. Anterior-posterior diameter
   b. Conjugate diameter
   c. Interspinous diameter
   d. Transverse diameter

Q5. Which pelvis type is most suitable for childbirth?
   a. Android
   b. Anthropoid
   c. Gynaecoid
   d. Platypelloid

Q6. Why is it very rare to develop diverticula in the rectum?
   a. The taenia coli in the rectum protect against them
   b. The rectum has a complete longitudinal muscle layer
   c. The rectum has a complete circular muscle layer
   d. The rectum is too short to develop them

Q7. What is the embryological origin of the epithelial lining of the upper anal canal (above the dentate line)?
   a. Ectodermal
   b. Endodermal
   c. Endodermal and mesodermal
   d. Mesodermal
   e. Mesodermal and ectodermal

Answers

A1. d
A2. e
A3. d
A4. d
A5. c
A6. b
A7. b

Male Genital Organs

Q1. Developmentally, which structure gives rise to the vas deferens?
   a. Gubernaculum
   b. Mesonephric duct
   c. Paramesonephric duct
   d. Processus vaginalis
   e. Urachus

Q2. What is the male equivalent of the labia majora?
   a. Bulbourethral gland
   b. Corpus cavernosum
   c. Corpus spongiosum
   d. Glans penis
   e. Scrotum

Q3. Which structure is closely related to the ischial spine?
   a. Ilioinguinal nerve
   b. Obturator externus muscle
   c. Obturator nerve
   d. Pudendal nerve
   e. Sacrotuberous ligament

Q4. The posterior two-thirds of the scrotum are mainly supplied by which nerve?
   a. Genitofemoral nerve
   b. Ilioinguinal nerve
   c. Obturator nerve
   d. Posterior femoral cutaneous nerve
   e. Pudendal nerve

Q5. Which structure is the bulb of the penis the proximal part of?
   a. Corpus cavernosum
   b. Corpus spongiosum
   c. Glans penis
   d. Prepuce
   e. Root of the penis

Q6. From which anterior abdominal layer does the cremasteric muscle arise?
   a. External oblique
   b. Internal oblique
   c. Peritoneum
   d. Subcutaneous fascia
   e. Transversalis fascia

Q7. In which part of the prostate does benign prostate hyperplasia arise?
   a. Capsule
   b. Central zone
   c. Peripheral zone
   d. Prostatic urethra
   e. Transitional zone

Q8. What is the parasympathetic innervation to the internal urethral sphincter, and what does it do?
   a. *Nervi erigentes* (S2–S4) will constrict the internal urethral sphincter
   b. *Nervi erigentes* (S2–S4) will relax the internal urethral sphincter
   c. Pudendal nerve (S2–S4) will constrict the internal urethral sphincter
   d. Pudendal nerve (S2–S4) will relax the internal urethral sphincter
   e. Sacral splanchnic nerves relax the internal urethral sphincter

Q9. In left testicular torsion, the testicular artery is occluded. What is the origin of the left testicular artery?
   a. Aorta (directly)
   b. External iliac artery
   c. Internal iliac artery
   d. Internal pudendal artery
   e. Left renal artery

Q10. Which layer of the anterior abdominal wall does not contribute to the layers of the scrotum?
   a. External oblique
   b. Internal oblique
   c. Parietal peritoneum
   d. Transversalis fascia
   e. Transversalis muscle

Answers

A1. b
A2. e
A3. d
A4. e
A5. b
A6. b
A7. e
A8. b
A9. a
A10. e

The Female Genital Tract

Q1.

(Courtesy of Department of Anatomical Sciences, SGUL.)

Q1. What is the structure indicated by the red arrow?
   a. Cervix
   b. Fornix
   c. Ovary
   d. Uterus
   e. Vagina

Q2. What structure is closely related to the lateral fornix and can be injured during a hysterectomy?
   a. Bladder
   b. Iliac artery
   c. Rectum
   d. Ureter
   e. Urethra

Q3.

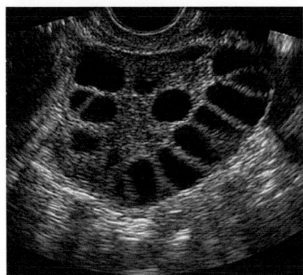

(Courtesy of Department of Anatomical Sciences, SGUL.)

Q3. What type of image is this?
   a. CT scan
   b. MRI scan
   c. PET scan
   d. Ultrasound
   e. X-ray

Q4. The image in question 3 shows an ovary. What is the pathology shown?
   a. Ectopic gestation
   b. Endometriosis
   c. Fibroid
   d. Ovarian carcinoma
   e. Polycystic ovary

Answers

A1. d
A2. d
A3. d
A4. e

Further Reading

Colorectal cancer: summary of NICE guidance. BMJ 2020;368. doi: https://doi.org/10.1136/bmj.m461.

Jin, et al. Waldeyer's fascia: anatomical location and relationship to neighboring fasciae in retrorectal space. *Surg Radiol Anat* 2011;33(10):851–854. doi: 10.1007/s00276-011-0887-6

Kao. Caudal epidural block: an updated review of anatomy and techniques. *BioMed Research International* 2017. doi: 10.1155/2017/9217145

Logsdon, et al. The role of intra-abdominal pressure in human testicular migration. *Int Braz J Urol* 2021;47(1):36–44. doi: 10.1590/S1677-5538.

Manoucheri, et al. Ureteral injury in laparoscopic gynaecologic surgery. *Rev Obstet Gynecol* 2012;5(2):106–111. doi: 10.3909/riog0182a

Mundy & Andrich. Urethral trauma, part I: introduction, history, anatomy, pathology, assessment, and emergency management. *BJU Int* 2011;108(3): 310–327.

Nemec, et al. Male sexual development *in utero*: testicular descent on prenatal magnetic resonance imaging. *J Ultrasound Obstet Gyn* 2011;38(6):688–694.

Schwertner-Tiepelmann, et al. Obstetric levator ani muscle injuries: current status. 2011. https://doi.org/10.1002/uog.11080

Sokol. The Clinical Anatomy of the Uterus, Fallopian Tubes and Ovaries. *Glob Libr Women's Med* 2011. (ISSN: 1756-2228); doi 10.3843/GLOWM.

Testicular cancer. BMJ Best Practice. July 2020. https://bestpractice.bmj.com/topics/en-gb/255

Tight foreskin (phimosis and paraphimosis). http://www.nhs.uk/conditions/phimosis/Pages/Introduction.aspx.

WHO. Female genital mutilation. 2020. https://www.who.int/news-room/fact-sheets/detail/female-genital-mutilation

WHO. A framework for voluntary medical male circumcision: effective HIV prevention and a gateway to improved adolescent boys' and men's health in eastern and southern Africa by 2021. https://apps.who.int/iris/handle/10665/246234. NHS Choices [Internet] (2015) [cited 03/08/17].

7

ANATOMY OF THE LOWER LIMB

Reviewed by Philip J. Adds and Joanna Tomlinson

Learning Objectives

- Anatomy of the gluteal region
- Osteology and arthrology of the bones and joints of the lower limb and clinical application of their injuries
- Thigh compartments and their neurovascular supply
- Muscles, neurovascular structures, and lymphatic drainage of the lower limb
- Clinical importance of lower limb ischaemia and compartment syndrome
- Common clinical conditions affecting the venous system, e.g., varicose veins and deep venous thrombosis
- Anatomy of the foot, vascular examination and diabetic foot, and common clinical problems
- Revision questions

The Gluteal Region (Figure 7.1)

- The gluteal region is a transition zone posteriorly between the trunk and the lower extremity.

- It is bounded by the iliac crests superiorly, the inferior gluteal folds inferiorly, and the lateral thigh from the iliac crest down to the greater trochanter of the femur laterally.

Muscles of the Gluteal Region

The two broad categories of gluteal muscles are:

1. **Superficial abductors and extensors of the hip** (Table 7.1 and **Figure 7.2**). These include:
   - Gluteus maximus*
   - Gluteus medius*
   - Gluteus minimus*
   - Tensor fasciae latae

(*These muscles form the main bulk of the buttock. The gluteus maximus is the thickest muscle in the body.)

2. **Deep lateral rotators of the thigh and hip**. These include:
   - Quadratus femoris
   - Piriformis
   - Gemellus superior
   - Gemellus inferior
   - Obturator internus

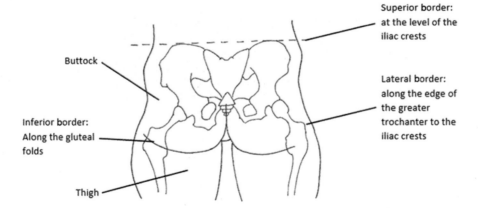

FIGURE 7.1   Boundaries of the gluteal region. (Courtesy of Calum Harrington-Vogt.)

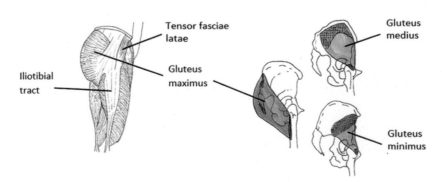

FIGURE 7.2   The main lateral muscles of the thigh and the buttock. (Courtesy of Calum Harrington-Vogt.)

DOI: 10.1201/9781003312895-8

The gluteus medius holds the pelvis steady, preventing pelvic drop. The Trendelenburg's sign is a useful indicator of nerve damage to this muscle, discussed in more detail later.

Iliotibial tract syndrome is common in young athletes (long-distance runners and cyclists) and is due to friction of the iliotibial tract against the lateral femoral epicondyle. **For information on the deep gluteal muscles, see Table 7.2.**

TABLE 7.1: The superficial abductors and extensors of the hip

Name	Origin	Insertion	Action	Innervation
Gluteus maximus: the most superficial and the largest of the gluteal muscles It is also the thickest muscle in the body	Posterior surfaces of the ilium (below the posterior gluteal line), sacrum, coccyx, and the sacrotuberous ligament	The iliotibial tract and the gluteal tuberosity on the posterior surface of the femur	Powerful extensor of the hip and assists with lateral rotation Causes the body to regain the erect position after initially stooping, when standing on one leg	Inferior gluteal nerve, arises from the ventral rami of L5–S1 and S2 of the sacral plexus
Gluteus medius: deep to the gluteus maximus, superficial to the gluteus minimus	The gluteal surface of the ilium	Greater trochanter of femur	Hip abductor, medial hip rotator (anterior fibres), lateral rotation and hip extension (posterior fibres)	Superior gluteal nerve, arises from nerve roots L4–S1 of the sacral plexus
Gluteus minimus: deep to the gluteus maximus and medius	The gluteal surface of the ilium	Greater trochanter of femur	Abducts and medially rotates the hip joint and holds the pelvis secure when walking	Superior gluteal nerve
Tensor fasciae latae: the most superficial gluteal muscle, which lies to the anterior of the iliac crest	Anterior iliac crest and the ASIS	The iliotibial tract (a fibrous reinforcement of the fascia lata)	Abduction and medial rotation of the lower limb Supports gait cycle, stabilises knee in extension	Superior gluteal nerve
The iliotibial tract or band (ITT or ITB)	Anterolateral iliac tubercle portion of the external lip of the iliac crest	Lateral condyle of the tibia (Gerdy's tubercle)	Continuation of tensor fasciae latae, part of the insertion of gluteus maximus Maintains knee stability in hyperextension Hip flexor and medial rotator	Inferior gluteal nerve (L5–S2)

TABLE 7.2: Deep gluteal muscles

Name	Origin	Insertion	Action	Innervation
Piriformis (from the Latin word for "pear-shaped"): the most superior of the deep gluteal muscles	Anterior aspect of the sacrum	Greater trochanter (via greater sciatic foramen)	Lateral rotation and abduction of the hip joint	Nerve to piriformis, arises from the posterior divisions of the ventral rami from L5, S1, and S2 of the sacral plexus
The gemelli: two thin muscles, a superior and an inferior gemellus muscle	*Superior gemellus:* ischial spine *Inferior gemellus:* ischial tuberosity	Greater trochanter of femur	Lateral rotation and abduction of the hip joint	*Superior gemellus:* nerve to obturator internus *Inferior gemellus:* nerve to quadratus femoris
Quadratus femoris: the most inferior deep gluteal muscle Small, flat, and square	Lateral aspect of the ischial tuberosity of the pelvis	Quadrate tubercle on the intertrochanteric crest of the femur	Lateral rotation of the hip joint	Nerve to quadratus femoris, which arises from ventral divisions of the roots L4–S1 of the sacral plexus
Obturator externus: makes up part of the anterior wall of the pelvic cavity and is sometimes considered part of the medial thigh compartment rather than the gluteal region	External border of the obturator foramen	Posterior femur at the trochanteric fossa	Laterally rotates and adducts the hip joint	Posterior branch of the obturator nerve (L3 and L4)
Obturator internus: makes up the lateral walls of the pelvic cavity; forms the triceps coxae with the two gemelli muscles; the levator ani muscle also originates from the tendinous arch of the obturator internus	Pubis and ischium at the obturator foramen of the pelvis through the obturator membrane	Greater trochanter of femur (via lesser sciatic foramen)	Lateral rotation and abduction of the hip joint	Nerve to obturator internus, which arises from ventral divisions of the roots L5–S1 and S2 of the sacral plexus

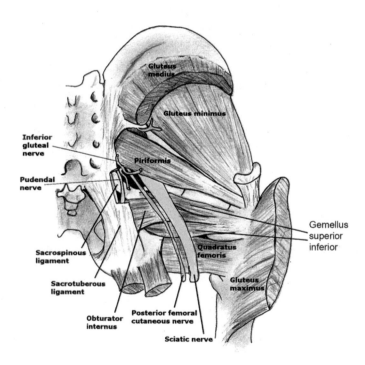

FIGURE 7.3 The main nerves of the sacral plexus and their relations with the piriformis muscle. (Courtesy of Gabriela Barzyk.)

Nerves in the Gluteal Region

These primarily arise from the sacral plexus (discussed in more detail in **Section 6**, Pelvis and Perineum) and traverse or supply the gluteal region.

Superior gluteal nerve

- *Roots:* L4–S1
- *Course:* passes through the greater sciatic foramen superior to the piriformis. Passes anterolaterally between the gluteus minimus and medius, both of which it supplies, as well as the tensor fasciae latae muscle.

Inferior gluteal nerve

- *Roots:* L5–S2
- *Course:* crosses the greater sciatic foramen inferior to the piriformis and supplies the gluteus maximus.

Pudendal nerve

- *Roots:* S2–S4
- *Course:* passes through the gluteal region. Can be seen just inferior to the piriformis before it exits the pelvis through the lesser sciatic foramen, over the sacrospinous ligament and under the sacrotuberous ligament. It travels through Alcock's canal (*vide infra*) before dividing into three branches: inferior rectal, perineal, and clitoral or penile branches.
- **Alcock's canal** (or pudendal canal) is defined as a passage formed by the separation of the obturator fascia. It contains the pudendal nerve and internal pudendal vessels. Entrapment of the pudendal nerve can occur here.
- The nerve carries sensory, autonomic, and motor signals to and from the genitals, anus, and urethra.
- For more details on the course of the pudendal nerve, see **Section 6**, Pelvis and Perineum.

The posterior femoral cutaneous nerve

- *Roots:* S1–S3
- *Course:* passes through the greater sciatic foramen inferior to the piriformis. It runs deep to the gluteus maximus in the gluteal region and runs down to the calf muscles. The nerve provides innervation to the skin of the posterior thigh and leg and the posterior part of the perineum.

The sciatic nerve

- The largest and thickest nerve in the body.
- *Roots:* L4–S3
- Divides into tibial and common peroneal nerves.
- *Course:* passes through the greater sciatic foramen and deep to the piriformis. The nerve courses inferiorly, deep to the gluteus maximus, before continuing down the middle of the posterior thigh.

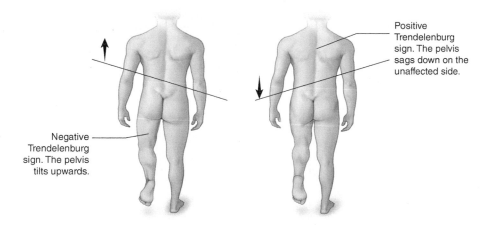

FIGURE 7.4   The image on the left shows a "normal" Trendelenburg's sign and on the right a "positive" sign. (Courtesy of Calum Harrington-Vogt.)

CLINICAL NOTES

SCIATICA

- A condition characterised by lower back pain and pain going down one or both legs.
- *Cause:* most of the cases are caused by intervertebral disc herniation, which then presses against one or more of the lumbar or sacral nerve roots (commonly L4–L5 or L5–S1). Other causes can be spinal stenosis, pelvic tumours, and compression of nerve roots by the fetus during pregnancy.

The *straight-leg-raising (SLR) test:* a positive test is when the leg is raised by a practitioner while the patient is lying on their back, pain shoots down to below the knee. Knee and ankle jerks could also be weak, depending on the nerve roots affected.

INTRAMUSCULAR INJECTIONS

The superolateral quadrant of the buttock is often used to administer intramuscular injections, as the area is relatively "nerve free", which is particularly useful as it avoids the sciatic nerve but still gives access to the very muscular gluteal region (**Figure 7.5**).

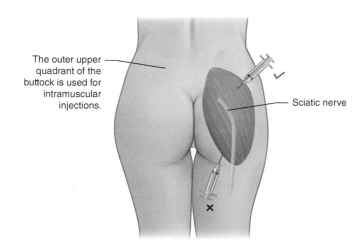

FIGURE 7.5   The safe area for intramuscular injection on the gluteal region. (Courtesy of Calum Harrington-Vogt.)

Blood Supply to the Gluteal Region

These are the superior and inferior gluteal arteries; both arise from the internal iliac artery (see **Section 6**, Pelvis and Perineum). The superior gluteal artery, the largest branch of the internal iliac artery, accompanies the superior gluteal nerve and divides into deep and superficial branches that supply the gluteal maximus and the gluteus medius and minimus, respectively. The inferior gluteal artery accompanies the inferior gluteal nerve and gives rise to a companion artery to the sciatic nerve. The gluteal veins accompany the arteries and drain into the internal iliac vein.

An anastomosis around the hip (the trochanteric anastomosis) is formed by the superior gluteal, inferior gluteal, and medial and lateral femoral circumflex arteries.

CLINICAL NOTES

SUPERIOR GLUTEAL ARTERY PERFORATOR (SGAP) FLAP

Skin and fat from the upper to middle buttock can be removed, as well as the superior gluteal artery and vein (which supply the area via perforators through the gluteus maximus). This section of skin can be used in reconstructive breast surgery as a skin donor site and is a growing field in microsurgery.

Anatomy of the Hip (Acetabulofemoral) Joint

The function of the femoral head is to articulate with the acetabulum and form what is commonly known as the hip joint.

- A multiaxial, ball and socket synovial joint.
- The socket (Latin: *acetabulum*, or "vinegar cup") is a deep depression formed by the unification of the ilium, pubis, and ischium of the pelvis, fused together by the triradiate cartilage, which keeps the three bones separate until they fuse by the age of 25 years. The acetabulum is deepened by the attached fibrocartilaginous acetabular labrum.
- Primarily functions to support the individual's weight in both static and dynamic postures.

The hip joint capsule, also known as the articular capsule, is very strong and dense . It is attached to the rim of the acetabulum superiorly, and surrounds the neck of the femur inferiorly. The attachment of the hip joint capsule is on the intertrochanteric line anteriorly and posteriorly attaches more proximal to the intertrochanteric crest.

The surface of the acetabulum differs in texture. The smoother lunate surface articulates with the head of the femur and is covered by hyaline cartilage. This is where all the weight is loaded. The deeper part, the acetabular fossa, is non-weight-bearing and is filled with fat.

There are four main ligaments of the hip joint, of which one is intracapsular.

The intracapsular ligament is the ligamentum teres (round ligament). Functionally, in our day-to-day activities, this ligament is not as important as the other three, as it is attached to the rim of the acetabulum and to a depression on the femoral head (the fovea capitis) and keeps the two fixed together, rather than affecting our ability to move. It also encloses a branch of the obturator artery, which is a part of the arterial supply of the hip joint.

The Extracapsular Ligaments of the Hip

There are three main ligaments which are continuous with the outer surface of the hip joint capsule.

Iliofemoral Ligament

This is the **strongest ligament in the body** and runs between the anterior inferior iliac spine and the intertrochanteric line of the femur and has a Y shape. Its role is to prevent hyperextension of the hip joint. It loosens on flexion of the hip, but gets twisted on standing and hip extension; this movement then draws the femur towards the ilium, so it keeps the head of the femur in the acetabulum and therefore contributes to hip stability.

Pubofemoral Ligament

The pubofemoral ligament extends between the superior pubic rami and the intertrochanteric line of the femur. It has a triangular shape. Its role is to prevent excessive abduction and extension and to resist external rotation.

Ischiofemoral Ligament

Spans between the body of the ischium and the greater trochanter of the femur. It has a spiral orientation (spirals around the neck to attach to the intertrochanteric line). Its role is to prevent excessive extension and resist internal rotation.

Blood Supply of the Femoral Head

The blood supply to the femoral head travels proximally from the distal side along the reflected part of the capsule (retinaculum), and therefore fractures of the neck of the femur can prevent blood flow to the head of the femur.

The hip joint is supplied by the medial circumflex and lateral circumflex femoral arteries, which are branches of the profunda femoris. There are numerous anatomical variations in which one or both arteries may arise from the femoral artery.

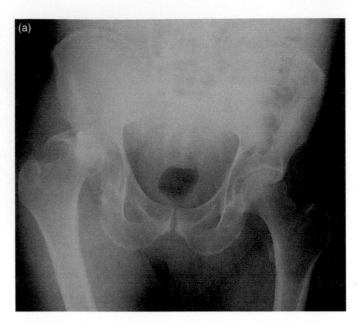

FIGURE 7.6a Right posterior hip dislocation. (Courtesy of Salam Ismael.)

CLINICAL NOTES

POSTERIOR HIP DISLOCATION

This is the most common type of hip dislocation (contrast with shoulder joint dislocation, where the majority of dislocations are anterior/inferior). It could also result in fracture of the posterior lip of the acetabulum (**Figure 7.6a**).

It usually follows severe injury to the flexed hip, e.g., where the knee is driven back in dashboard injuries. Clinically, the affected lower limb is shortened, adducted, and internally rotated.

CONGENITAL HIP DISLOCATION (CHD)

CHD, or developmental dysplasia of the hip, occurs when a child is born with an unstable hip. It is due to the malformation of the hip during early fetal development. The child may suffer from dislocation of the joint. In CHD, the cup-shaped hip socket is too shallow and the femoral head can move, as it is not held tightly in place, which can result in the femoral head lying completely outside the socket.

It can affect one or both hips; however, it is much more common in the left hip. According to National Health Service (NHS) statistics, 1 in every 1000 babies is born with developmental dysplasia of the hip. Without proper treatment, it can lead to developing a limp, chronic hip pain, and stiff joints due to osteoarthritis.

ARTHROPLASTY

This is the surgical reconstruction or replacement of a joint. The hip joint can deteriorate for many reasons, such as osteoarthritis. Total hip replacement (THR) (replacement of the femoral head and acetabulum with synthetic materials) is a choice when all other methods have been tried and tested (**Figure 7.6b**).

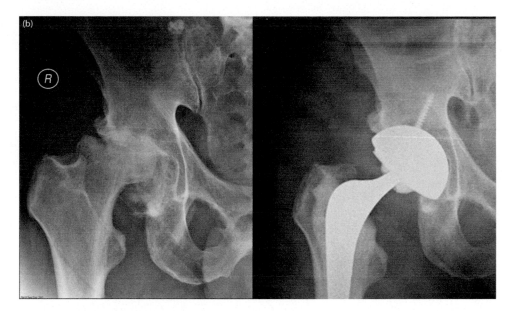

FIGURE 7.6b Total hip replacement (THR), preoperative and postoperative plain film X-rays. (Courtesy of Philip J. Adds.)

Osteology of the Femur

The femur is the longest bone in the body, measuring at about a quarter of an individual's height (**Figure 7.7**). It consists of the head, neck, shaft, and lower end (femoral condyles). The anatomy of the head of the femur has been described with anatomy of the hip joint (see earlier).

The **neck of the femur (NOF)** is cylindrical in nature and attaches to the femoral shaft at an angle of approximately 130 degrees.

Fractures in the NOF are classified as **either intracapsular (subcapital) or extracapsular** (trochanteric), and it is important to identify which fracture has taken place in the patient, as that will determine the possible consequences of the fracture, as well as potential treatment options. If the fracture has occurred above the intertrochanteric line, then it is an intracapsular fracture. If the fracture has occurred on or below this line, then it is classified as an extracapsular fracture.

Intracapsular fractures can cause a disruption to the blood supply to the head of the femur and potentially cause avascular necrosis requiring hip replacement surgery. Extracapsular fractures, although they are far more common, are less likely to cause disruption to the blood supply to the neck and head of the femur.

Fracture of the femoral neck is clinically manifested by inability of the patient to move the lower limb, which is shorter on the affected side and externally rotated.

Avascular necrosis (trauma-related avascular necrosis), also known as an osteonecrosis, is where there is interruption of blood supply to the head of the femur, which will cause necrosis and eventual collapse of the bone. It may follow hip dislocation or fracture of the NOF.

Lateral to the lower end of the neck of the femur is the **greater trochanter**, which is a projection on both anterior and posterior aspects and forms the insertion site of the muscles of the gluteal region, including the piriformis, except for the gluteus maximus, which is mainly inserted into the iliotibial tract.

On the medial side the **lesser trochanter** can be found inferior and posterior to the NOF. This is the site of attachment for the iliacus and psoas muscles (iliopsoas); both are flexors of the hip.

A bony ridge known as the **intertrochanteric line** runs anteriorly from the greater trochanter to the lesser trochanter in an inferomedial direction, and this is the site of attachment for the iliofemoral ligament. On the posterior surface of the upper femur, the intertrochanteric line continues as the pectineal line once it passes the lesser trochanter in the inferolateral direction. The **intertrochanteric crest** is found on the posterior aspect at the junction between the femoral neck and shaft.

A rounded tubercle, known as the **quadrate tubercle**, can be found on the superior half of the crest itself. This is the site of attachment for the quadratus femoris muscle.

The Linea Aspera

On the posterior aspect of the femur, the now descending pectineal line on the medial side and the gluteal tuberosity on the lateral side (where part of the gluteus maximus attaches, unlike the other gluteal muscles) meet and form a longitudinal single line of ridged bone known as the linea aspera ("rough line" in Latin), on the posterior aspect of the femoral shaft. The linea aspera gives attachment to the lateral and medial vasti muscles and adductor magnus.

The medial and lateral borders of the linea aspera diverge inferiorly to become the medial and lateral supracondylar lines, and eventually become part of the floor of the popliteal fossa. Again, it is important to observe the termination of these lines; unlike the lateral line, the medial supracondylar line stops at the adductor tubercle, and it is here where the adductor magnus attaches.

The area between the two femoral condyles is called the intercondylar fossa, which is part of the floor of the popliteal fossa and gives attachment to the anterior and posterior cruciate ligaments of the knee joint.

Blood Supply of the Femur

The femur is supplied generally by the femoral artery. This gives rise to the lateral and medial circumflex arteries (from the profunda or deep femoral artery); see above.

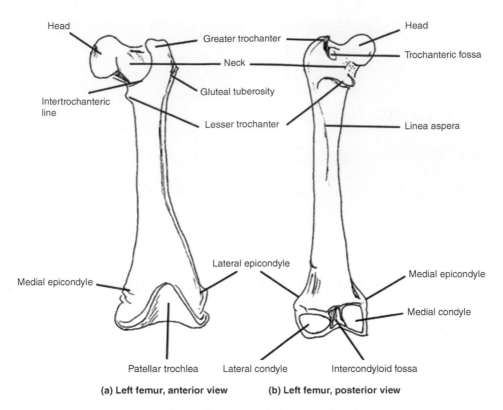

Head
Greater trochanter
Neck
Gluteal tuberosity
Intertrochanteric line
Lesser trochanter
Head
Trochanteric fossa
Linea aspera
Medial epicondyle
Lateral epicondyle
Medial epicondyle
Medial condyle
Patellar trochlea
Lateral condyle
Intercondyloid fossa

(a) Left femur, anterior view   **(b) Left femur, posterior view**

FIGURE 7.7   Anterior and posterior view of the femur. (Courtesy of Alina Humdani.)

CLINICAL NOTES

FRACTURE OF THE SHAFT OF THE FEMUR

Fractures of the shaft of this bone require very high-energy traumas such as high-speed car crashes or a pedestrian being hit by a car, gunshot wounds, etc. (**Figures 7.8** and **7.9**).

Another entity is a pathological fracture, which is where an already damaged area of a bone breaks due to other pathologies, such as metastatic tumours from other primaries (commonly from breast, lung, and prostate), infections, and osteoporosis (more commonly in elderly people who have weaker bones, falling over in a low-force incident).

In patients with fracture of the femur note that:

- **Significant blood loss can accompany femoral shaft fractures**, as the fractured bones can be very sharp and could tear a major artery such as the deep femoral artery, leading to significant blood loss.
- **The integrity of the neurovascular bundle of the lower limb should always be checked.**

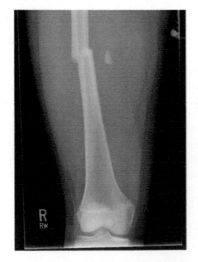

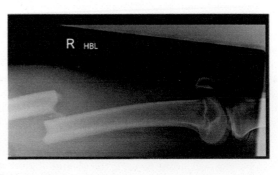

FIGURE 7.8   Anteroposterior (AP) and lateral views of a plain film radiograph of the right thigh of a 16-year-old female, who fell from a third-floor window, showing a closed transverse fracture of the midshaft of the right femur. (Courtesy of Radiology Department at St. George's Hospital NHS Trust.)

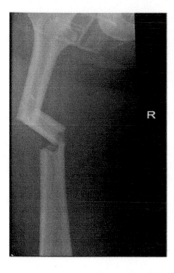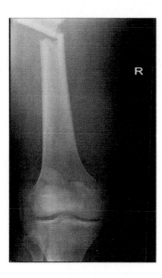

FIGURE 7.9 Plain film X-ray of the right lower limb of a 27-year-old male motorcyclist who was involved in a road traffic collision with an oncoming car. Two images have been taken: anteroposterior (AP) view of the right femur *(left image)* and an AP view of the right femur and knee joint *(right image)*. There are two closed transverse fractures in the mid third of the shaft of the right femur. (Courtesy of Radiology Department at St. George's Hospital NHS Trust.)

Femoral Triangle (Figure 7.10)

The boundaries of the femoral triangle, which contains the femoral vessels and nerve (which is located laterally) and the vein medial to the artery (important when taking venous sample in patients with difficult peripheral venous access) include the following:

- *Superior border:* the inguinal ligament
- *Lateral border:* the medial border of the sartorius
- *Medial border:* formed by the medial border of the adductor longus muscle; the rest of this muscle forms part of the floor of the triangle
- *Roof:* fascia lata (deep fascia of the thigh)
- *Floor:* pectineus, iliopsoas, and adductor longus

CLINICAL NOTES

THE FEMORAL TRIANGLE

- The femoral artery is an important clinical landmark for vascular examination and for catheterization, such as in angiogram procedures (injection of dye to delineate the arterial tree for blockages or narrowing of arteries, like the coronary arteries) and other interventional procedures, such as stenting or balloon angioplasty, and has been linked to injuries of butchers' thighs whose meat cleavers can slip and lacerate the artery.
- The femoral artery is explored within the femoral triangle in patients with acute lower limb ischaemia where emboli or thrombosis occlude the artery (embolectomy).
- Inguinal lymph node biopsy. See "Sentinel Node Biopsy".
- Exploration of the saphenofemoral junction in surgical treatment of varicose veins (ligation of the long saphenous vein at its connection to the femoral vein in addition to its tributaries at the junction).

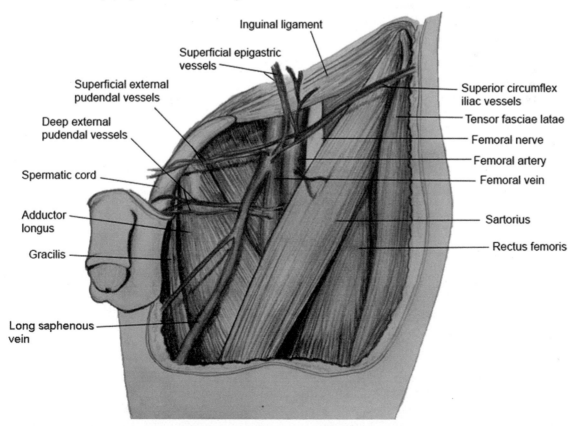

FIGURE 7.10 The femoral triangle. (Courtesy of Neha Gadiyar.)

The Femoral Canal

This is a small canal (1.5 cm in length) which passes medial to the femoral vein, at the upper end of the femoral triangle. The proximal end is called the femoral ring. It is filled with extraperitoneal connective tissue. The femoral canal is wider in females because they have a wider bony pelvis (adapted for childbirth).

Relations:

- *Anterior:* inguinal ligament
- *Posterior:* pectineal ligament, superior ramus of the pubic bone, and the pectineus muscle
- *Medial:* lacunar ligament
- *Lateral:* femoral vein

The femoral canal, femoral vein, and femoral artery are all enclosed in a fascial sheath (**femoral sheath**), which is bounded anteriorly by the transversalis fascia and posteriorly by the iliac fascia (which covers the psoas and iliacus muscles). There is a lymph node within the canal (Cloquet's node).

CLINICAL NOTE

Herniation through the femoral canal from the peritoneal cavity is called a **femoral hernia**, a protrusion of a pouch of peritoneal sac, which may contain an intra-abdominal organ, like the small bowel, through the femoral canal. This type of hernia is more common in females and can be easily missed on physical examination of the groin; it is more liable to strangulation and bowel ischaemia. However, among females, the inguinal hernia is more common.

Pes Anserinus (Latin: "Goose's Foot")

This is the arrangement of the three tendons of the sartorius, gracilis, and semitendinosus as they insert anteromedially into the proximal tibia.

Pes anserine bursitis is inflammation of the bursa underneath the common tendon and is characterised by pain and swelling on the medial aspect of the knee, commonly in athletes following overexercise.

Muscles of the Anterior Thigh (Figure 7.11)

The muscles of the anterior thigh are innervated by the femoral nerve.

The **femoral nerve** (L2–L4) is a mixed nerve and one of the branches of the posterior divisions of the lumbar plexus. It emerges underneath the inguinal ligament (lateral to the femoral artery) and supplies motor branches to the sartorius, pectineus, and quadriceps femoris. It supplies sensory branches to the anterior and medial aspects of the thigh (the intermediate and medial femoral nerves of the thigh) and continues as the saphenous nerve (see later, **Table 7.3**).

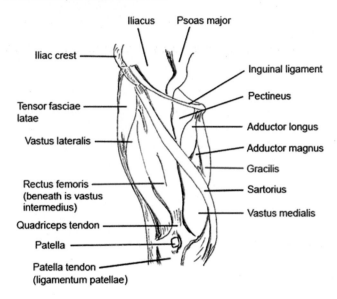

FIGURE 7.11   Musculature of the anterior compartment of the right thigh. (Courtesy of Alina Humdani.)

TABLE 7.3: Muscles of the anterior thigh*

Name	Origin	Insertion	Action
Sartorius (the longest muscle in the body)	Anterior superior iliac spine (ASIS)	Medial aspect of upper tibia (pes anserinus)	Flexion, abduction, and lateral rotation of the thigh, flexion of the knee
Rectus femoris (note that this muscle has two heads and crosses two joints)	*Straight head:* from the anterior inferior iliac spine (AIIS) *Reflected head:* along the upper part of the acetabulum at the ilium	Quadriceps tendon along with the three vasti muscles into the patella and through the patellar tendon to the tibial tuberosity	Hip flexion and knee extension
Iliacus	Iliac fossa	Lesser trochanter *Note:* before insertion, this muscle unites with the psoas major behind the inguinal ligament to form the iliopsoas	Medial rotation of thigh and hip joint flexion
Vastus lateralis (the largest of the quadriceps femoris)	Upper part of the intertrochanteric line; the greater trochanter, the outer border of the gluteal tuberosity, and outer border of the linea aspera	Lateral side of the quadriceps tendon, joining with the rectus femoris	Extends the knee. Allows the body to stand up from a squatting position
Vastus intermedius	Anterior and lateral aspects of the upper part of the femoral shaft	Quadriceps tendon into the tibial tuberosity	Extends the knee
Vastus medialis	Medial part of the intertrochanteric line and the medial lip of the linea aspera	Medial side of the quadriceps tendon into the tibial tuberosity and some fibres to the medial patellar retinaculum	Extends the knee; the lower fibres prevent lateral displacement of the patella

* Quadriceps femoris consists of rectus femoris, vastus lateralis, vastus intermedius, and vastus medialis.

Medial Compartment of the Thigh

Hip Adductors (Figure 7.12 and Table 7.4)

The medial thigh consists of muscles known together as the hip adductors:

- Gracilis
- Obturator externus
- Adductor longus
- Adductor brevis
- Adductor magnus

Some authors consider the pectineus one of the adductors. For details of the pectineus, see **Section 6**, Pelvis and Perineum.

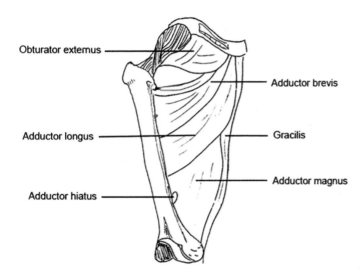

FIGURE 7.12 Musculature of the medial compartment of the thigh. (Courtesy of Alina Humdani.)

The medial thigh muscles are innervated by the obturator nerve (L2–L4); the hamstring portion of the adductor magnus is supplied by the tibial component of the sciatic nerve.

The arterial supply is the obturator artery plus profunda femoris.

The **obturator nerve** (L2–L4) enters the pelvis medial to the psoas major muscle to pass into the obturator canal and then divides into anterior and posterior divisions. It supplies sensory fibres to the medial aspect of the thigh and knee in addition to an articular branch to the knee joint (for referred pain, see **Section 6**, Pelvis and Perineum) and motor branches to the adductors (see earlier).

CLINICAL NOTES

"GROIN STRAIN"

"Groin strain" arises from strain in the adductor muscles. Usually, the most affected areas are the proximal part, where they tear near their attachments in the pelvis. Groin injuries usually occur during sports where sudden or extreme stretching leads to strain. The normal presentation in patients involves pain gradually increasing in the deep groin and proximal to the origins of the adductor muscles. The diagnosis is made clinically, but chronic pain involves utilisation of imaging.

TRANSPLANTATION

The gracilis is popularly used in reconstructive surgery, usually for muscle transfer or soft tissue coverage. The gracilis may be used to cover a damaged area in the hand or forearm. Patients with stress incontinence may have a vascularised pedicle flap transferred around the neck of the bladder, thereby strengthening it.

Another use is a free gracilis flap (through microsurgical anastomosis) to treat facial palsy. A small section is used in the face and attached to either the hypoglossal nerve or to a cross-facial nerve graft. This allows it to act as a motor muscle in the face.

OBTURATOR NERVE ENTRAPMENT SYNDROME

Obturator nerve entrapment syndrome is when the obturator nerve gets compressed. Patients consequently present with loss of sensation to the medial thigh, usually accompanied by weakness in thigh adduction. Causes include childbirth and pelvic tumours such as ovarian cysts.

Usually, obturator nerve entrapment can be diagnosed by the gold-standard electromyography or magnetic resonance imaging (MRI), which highlight the atrophy of the adductor longus and brevis muscles.

TABLE 7.4: Hip adductors

Name	Origin	Insertion	Action
Adductor longus (most anteriorly placed)	Body of pubic bone, underneath the pubic tubercle	Linea aspera of femur (broad insertion)	Adduction, flexion of the thigh
Adductor brevis (posterior to the adductor longus)	Body and inferior ramus of pubis	Linea aspera	Adduction, flexion of the thigh
Adductor magnus* Posterior to the adductor brevis	*Adductor portion:* inferior ramus of pubis, ramus of ischium *Hamstring portion:* ischial tuberosity	Adductor portion: gluteal tuberosity, inner lip of linea aspera *Hamstring portion:* adductor tubercle	Strong adductor of thigh *Adductor portion:* weak flexion and lateral rotation of the thigh *Hamstring portion:* extension and lateral rotation of the thigh
Gracilis (the most superficial of the adductor muscles)	Body and inferior ramus of pubis	Medial upper portion of tibia, inferior to medial condyle (pes anserinus)	Adduction and medial rotation of thigh, flexion of the knee joint
Obturator externus	Membrane of the obturator foramen	Posterior aspect of greater trochanter	Adduction and lateral rotation of the thigh

* The adductor magnus can be split into two parts – the adductor portion (superior) and the hamstring portion (inferior).

Posterior Thigh Compartment
(Figure 7.13 and Table 7.5)

Hamstrings

The hamstrings are a group of muscles located in the posterior compartment of the thigh. The hamstrings consist of the semimembranosus, semitendinosus, biceps femoris (consists of a long and short head), and part of the adductor magnus. Their main function is hip extension and knee flexion. The posterior compartment of the thigh is supplied by the sciatic nerve (L4, L5, S1, S2, and S3).

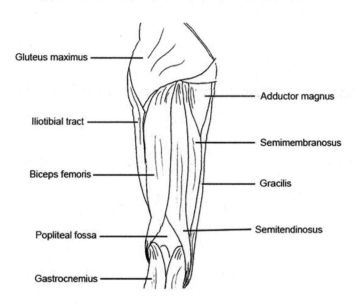

FIGURE 7.13 Musculature of the posterior compartment of the left thigh. (Courtesy of Alina Humdani.)

Vasculature of the Lower Limb

Introduction

The lower limb vasculature comprises arteries, veins, and lymphatics. In this section the lower limb vasculature is examined from the level of the inguinal ligament, beginning in the arterial system with the femoral artery. Venous vasculature is especially important, as pathologies such as deep venous thrombosis (DVT) and varicose veins commonly present in clinical settings across the population.

Arterial Supply of the Lower Limb

Femoral Artery

The continuation of the external iliac artery as it enters the thigh deep to the inguinal ligament, midway between the anterior superior iliac spine (ASIS) and the pubic symphysis. It is the main arterial supply to the lower limb and lies enclosed within the femoral sheath alongside the femoral vein and femoral canal.

The femoral artery continues deep to sartorius after giving rise to the profunda femoris (deep femoral artery). It descends along the anteromedial aspect of the thigh, passing down the adductor (subsartorial) canal to the adductor hiatus (an opening in the adductor magnus), where it becomes the popliteal artery (**Figure 7.14**).

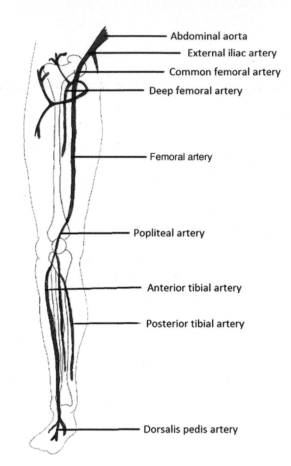

FIGURE 7.14 Arterial system of the lower limb. (Courtesy of Calum Harrington-Vogt.)

TABLE 7.5: Muscles of the posterior thigh and their innervation

Muscle	Origin	Insertion	Innervation	Function	Further Information
Semitendinosus	Upper part of the posterior surface of the ischial tuberosity	*Pes anserinus:* upper part of the medial surface of the tibia, behind the attachment of sartorius	Tibial nerve (L5–S2)	Extension of the hip and flexion of the knee	It has a very long tendon that is sometimes used for anterior cruciate ligament (ACL) reconstruction
Semimembranosus (deep to the semitendinosus)	Ischial tuberosity	Posterior aspect of the medial condyle of the tibia	Tibial nerve (L5–S2)	Extension of the hip and flexion of the knee	Superiorly becomes thin like a membrane, hence the name
Biceps femoris	*Long head:* ischial tuberosity *Short head:* lateral lip of the linea aspera and lateral supracondylar line	Head of the fibula	*Long head:* tibial nerve (L5, S1) *Short head:* common peroneal division of sciatic nerve (L5, S1)	Knee flexion, external rotation, and extension of the hip	Has a long and short head (short head acts on the knee joint only)

Six significant branches of the femoral artery include the:

- Superficial circumflex iliac
- Superficial epigastric
- Superficial and deep external pudendal
- Deep femoral (profunda femoris)
- Descending genicular

CLINICAL NOTES

ANGIOGRAPHY

The femoral artery is the most common site for angiography (**Figure 7.15**). This is a method of injecting contrast dye into the femoral artery to delineate the arterial tree, particularly the coronary arteries of the heart. During this procedure the femoral artery is cannulated using the **Seldinger's technique**, in which a catheter is guided sequentially through the external iliac artery, common iliac artery, aorta, and into the coronary arteries. Seldinger's technique is one of the most commonly used procedures and was invented by Dr Sven Ivar Seldinger (a Swedish radiologist) to access the vascular system and hollow organs (see the chest drain insertion, **Section 4A**, Thorax, for more information). The first step is getting access through insertion of a trocar and then threading a guide wire and removing the trocar. The next step is passing a wide-bore catheter or cannula over the guide wire. The guide wire is then removed. leaving the procedure done by passing different catheters and appliances through the introducer sheath.

Common examples include:
- Angiography (balloon angioplasty and stenting may be needed as well; see later). In leaking cerebral aneurysms, a coil may be inserted to stop the bleeding. Endovascular aneurysmal repair (EVAR) is another example of vascular intervention through the use of Seldinger's technique.
- Insertion of chest drains and catheters to drain collections and abscesses.
- Percutaneous endoscopic gastrostomy (PEG); see **Section 5**, Abdomen.

BALLOON ANGIOPLASTY

Balloon angioplasty is the use of an inflatable balloon to dilate occluded vessels. This procedure may also include the insertion of a stent, a mesh wire tube-like structure that continues to keep the vessel patent.

LOWER LIMB ACUTE ISCHAEMIA

Lower limb ischaemia can be caused by thrombosis (most cases), embolus, and other causes such as arterial trauma.

An embolus (*Plural:* emboli, Greek, "wedge") is any mass that travels through the bloodstream. Common emboli are blood clots (thromboembolism). In this case they commonly form in the left side of the heart (for example, due to atrial fibrillation) or within the arterial system and lodge at the common femoral artery. Acute

(Continued)

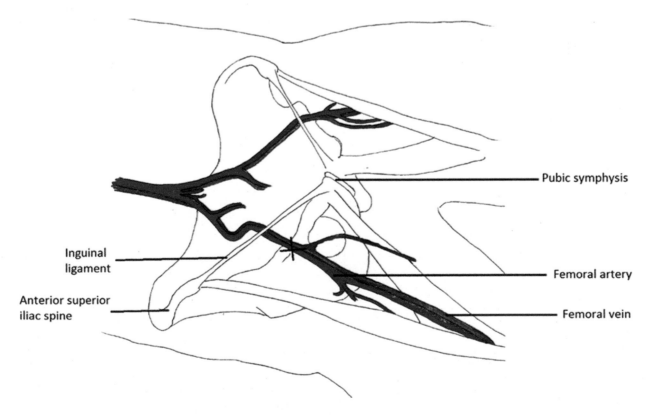

FIGURE 7.15   Location of femoral arterial puncture. (Courtesy of Calum Harrington-Vogt.)

lower limb ischaemia (ALI) is a serious condition, which can be missed, with a delay in diagnosis and treatment. On clinical suspicion of acute ischaemia, advice from the vascular surgery team is urgently needed, as the limb may still be salvageable.

It presents with the classical clinical symptoms and signs of the "**6Ps**" distal to the site of the blockage:

1. Pain
2. Pallor
3. Perishing cold (temperature of affected tissue is no longer controlled due to lack of perfusion, so normalises with external ambient temperature)
4. Paraesthesia (sensation of tingling "pins and needles")
5. Pulselessness (no peripheral pulses, i.e., popliteal, dorsalis pedis, posterior tibial)
6. Paralysis

The mere presence of the first three Ps, (sudden, severe pain; pallor; and perishing coldness) should trigger the alarm, alerting the clinician to this possibility and leading to diagnosis at this early stage, before the progression to sensory and motor deficit (the patient can usually wiggle their toes, meaning that there is time to request arterial imaging, and definitive treatment can be performed by either interventional radiology or surgery in the form of an emergency thromboembolectomy).*

FEMORAL ARTERY PSEUDOANEURYSM

The artery can become dilated (identified as an aneurysm if the dilatation of the diameter of an artery is more than 50%). Following penetrating injuries, including intra-arterial drug abuse, a pseudoaneurysm or false aneurysm may form and can be felt as an expansile swelling in the groin.

FEMORAL VENEPUNCTURE

A venous blood sample can be taken about 1 cm medial to the pulse of the femoral artery and about 1 cm inferior to the inguinal ligament. This point is useful for access to the central venous system when other veins are unavailable. A useful mnemonic to remember the relative location of the femoral vein is **NAVeL (Nerve, Artery, Vein, Lymphatics)**, which describes the femoral area from lateral to medial (lymphatics always being the most medial).

---

* Personal communication with Prof. M. I. Aldoori.

Profunda Femoris (Deep Femoral) Artery

This arises posterolaterally in the femoral triangle as the largest branch of the femoral artery, about 3.5 cm distal to the inguinal ligament. It passes posterior to the adductor longus muscle.

The profunda femoris gives rise to the following significant branches:

- Medial and lateral circumflex femoral arteries
- Descending branch of the lateral circumflex artery
- Perforating branches that supply the posterior and medial compartments of the thigh

The **subsartorial canal, or adductor (Hunter's) canal,** was named for John Hunter, a Scottish surgeon who worked at St George's Hospital, London. The femoral vessels leave the femoral triangle and enter this tendinous canal and leave at the hiatus (opening) in the adductor magnus. Its boundaries are:

- *Anteriorly:* sartorius muscle (hence the name)
- *Laterally:* vastus medialis
- *Posteromedially:* adductor longus and adductor magnus

The other contents are the saphenous nerve and the femoral nerve supply to the vastus medialis.

The **saphenous nerve** is a sensory cutaneous branch of the femoral nerve which gives rise to an articular branch to the knee joint and to the skin over the patella (the infrapatellar branch). It runs on the medial aspect of the leg alongside the long saphenous vein and supplies the medial and anterior aspects of the leg and the medial aspect of the foot down to the base of the big toe (bunion area) and is the longest nerve in the body. It might get injured during venesection of the long saphenous vein (see later), above and anterior to the medial malleolus.

Popliteal Fossa

This is a diamond-shaped area behind the knee. The boundaries of the popliteal fossa are as follows:

- *Upper lateral:* biceps femoris
- *Upper medial:* semitendinosus and semimembranosus
- *Lower lateral and medial:* the two heads of the gastrocnemius
- *Roof:* formed by the tough deep fascia and a floor which is the posterior aspect of the knee joint capsule, popliteus muscle, and posterior surface of the lower femur (**Figure 7.16**)

The popliteal fossa contains the **popliteal vein, popliteal artery, and nerves**; the sciatic and its two terminal branches; and the tibial and common peroneal (fibular), although the sciatic nerve may bifurcate more proximally.

The **sural nerve** is a cutaneous nerve that runs over the posterior aspect of the leg and is formed by roots from both the tibial and common peroneal nerves.

The **short saphenous vein** (SSV) drains into the popliteal vein. It runs superficial to the crural fascia before piercing the popliteal fascia to join the popliteal vein (important when dealing with varicose veins of the SSV).

The popliteal artery is the deepest structure (but the most anterior) and clinically not easy to palpate.

Popliteal Artery

This is the continuation of the femoral artery at the adductor hiatus, at the junction of the middle and lower thirds of the thigh.

The popliteal artery branches into two significant arteries, the anterior and posterior tibial arteries, at the inferior border of the popliteus.

It is the major contributor to the blood supply of the knee joint, by giving five genicular (related to the knee) branches

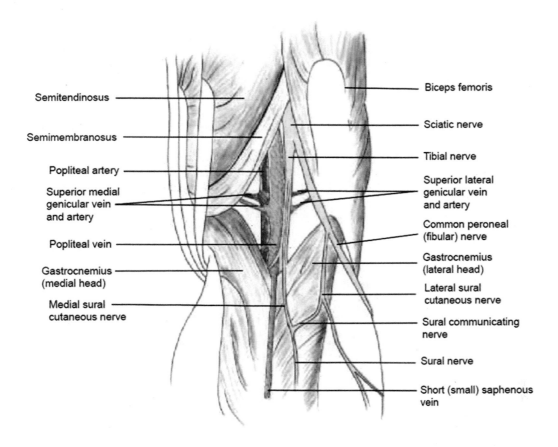

FIGURE 7.16 Structures within the popliteal fossa. (Courtesy of Xi Ming Zhu.)

(in addition to the muscular arterial branches to the hamstrings and gastrocnemii):

- Superior medial and lateral genicular
- Inferior medial and lateral genicular
- Middle genicular

The two nerves (tibial and common peroneal) are the most superficial structures. The common peroneal nerve follows the biceps femoris tendon.

CLINICAL NOTES

The **"fem-pop"** (femoro-popliteal) bypass graft is one of the most common vascular operations to improve the arterial blood supply to the leg following blockage of the femoral artery.

POPLITEAL ANEURYSM

A dilation in the popliteal artery can lead to compression of other structures in the popliteal fossa, including compression of the tibial nerve, which leads to foot/posterolateral leg paraesthesia (abnormal sensation, typically "pins and needles") and weak/absent plantar flexion. A distinction between a popliteal aneurysm and other masses can be made by applying a stethoscope to the site to detect turbulent blood flow (bruit); an aneurysm can be determined by palpable pulsation (thrill).

Learning Point

Always check both sides, as about 50% of popliteal aneurysms are bilateral.

Popliteal Block

Block of the sciatic nerve (L4–S3).

Site location is identified at a point 5 cm above the popliteal skin crease and 1 cm lateral to the line bifurcating the popliteal fossa. Usually performed under ultrasound guidance. This nerve block is performed in foot and ankle surgery.

Anterior Tibial Artery

This vessel originates posterior to the tibia at the distal aspect of the popliteus and supplies the anterior compartment of the leg and dorsal surface of the foot. Its course is between the tibia and fibula, through an oval opening at the superior aspect of the interosseous membrane. After leaving the interosseous membrane, the artery descends between the tibialis anterior and extensor digitorum longus. As it passes the anterior aspect of the ankle joint, it becomes the dorsalis pedis artery.

Posterior Tibial Artery

This artery passes deep to the gastrocnemius and soleus and supplies the posterior and lateral compartments of the leg and plantar surface of the foot. It gives rise to a large branch, the **peroneal (fibular) artery**, close to its origin from the popliteal artery, about 2.5 cm below the lower border of the popliteus, which supplies the lateral leg compartment. It then passes behind the medial malleolus (*vide infra*) and divides into the medial and lateral plantar arteries.

Dorsalis Pedis Artery

Supplies the dorsal surface of the foot as a continuation of the anterior tibial artery; arises at the anterior aspect of the ankle joint (midway between the malleoli). Runs on the dorsum of the foot to the proximal part of the first intermetatarsal space, where it divides into two branches, the **first dorsal metatarsal artery** and the **deep plantar artery,** which joins the lateral plantar artery of the posterior tibial artery, forming the plantar arch.

Pulse points in the lower limb (Figure 7.17):

- *Femoral pulse:* palpate the artery as it enters the femoral triangle. This can be found at the midinguinal point (midway between the ASIS and pubic symphysis).
- *Popliteal pulse:* this is more technically challenging to palpate. Can be found by deep palpation of the popliteal fossa; flexion of the knee can assist by relaxing surrounding fascia.

- *Dorsalis pedis pulse:* found by palpation lateral to the extensor hallucis longus tendon on the dorsum of the foot.
- *Posterior tibial pulse:* palpable behind and below the medial malleolus.

Venous Drainage of the Lower Limb

The venous drainage is by both deep and superficial veins (**Figure 7.18**).

Dorsal Venous Arch

A superficial vein that connects the short and great saphenous veins. It courses superficial to the metatarsal bones across the dorsal aspect of the foot. Lies midway between the malleoli and metatarsophalangeal joints.

Long (Great) Saphenous Vein (LSV)

The LSV is the longest vein in the body, running from the hallux to the femoral triangle. It drains the medial side of the dorsal venous arch then courses **anterior to the medial malleolus**, on the medial aspect of the leg, then posterior to the medial aspect of the patella. Ascends superficially along the medial aspect of the thigh to end in the femoral vein in the femoral triangle, after piercing the cribriform fascia (2-3 cm below the pubic tubercle). Here, it usually receives four tributary veins: the superficial epigastric, deep external pudendal, superficial external pudendal, and superficial circumflex iliac.

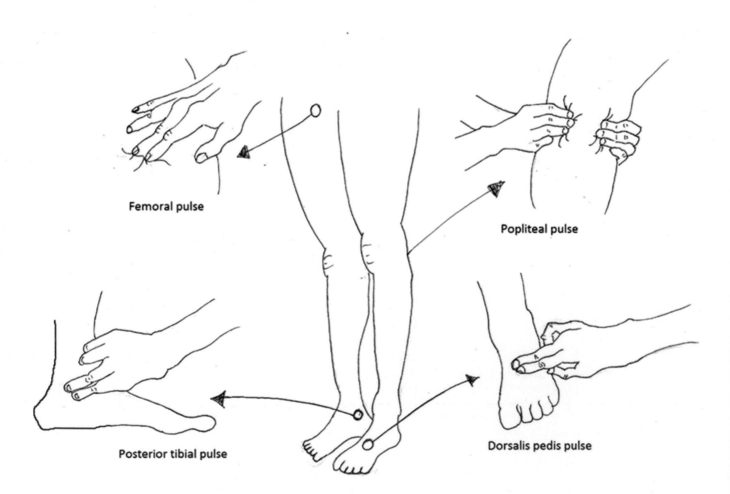

Femoral pulse

Popliteal pulse

Posterior tibial pulse

Dorsalis pedis pulse

FIGURE 7.17   Pulse points in the lower limb. (Courtesy of Calum Harrington-Vogt.)

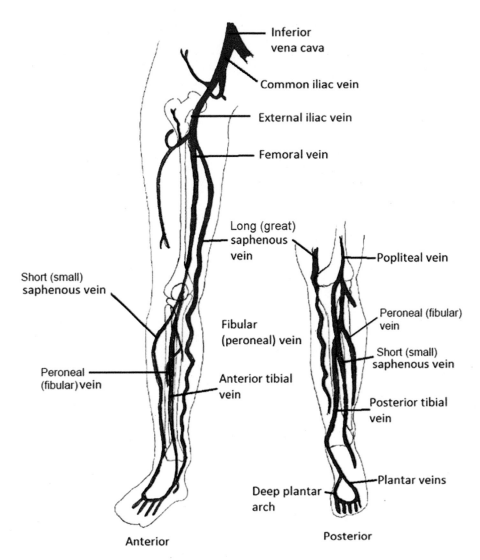

FIGURE 7.18 The venous drainage system of the lower limb. (Courtesy of Calum Harrington-Vogt.)

Short Saphenous Vein (SSV) (Figure 7.19)

Begins posterior to the lateral malleolus as it drains the lateral side of the dorsal venous arch. Ascends superficially at the midline of the posterior leg, to flow into the popliteal vein at the popliteal fossa, after piercing the deep fascia. (Saphenous: probably from the Greek *saphaina*, "to be clearly seen").

CLINICAL NOTES

CORONARY ARTERY BYPASS GRAFT (CABG)

A major operation that harvests segments of the long and/ or short saphenous veins to be used for bypass grafting in the heart, which aims to alleviate cardiac ischaemia by bypassing blockage of the coronary arteries. This is not a first-line treatment and is only considered if balloon angioplasty or stenting fails.

Note: Due to the presence of valves in these veins, these vessels must be placed in the right orientation when grafted to the heart.

Deep veins of the leg occur as venae comitantes, pairs of veins that tightly adhere to the arteries to drain deeper structures. Pulsation of the artery, and movement of the surrounding muscles, work alongside the valves to increase pressure to return the venous blood to the heart. Other veins are less intimately related and do not occur as venae comitantes.

The soleal venous plexus is formed within the soleus muscle and contributes to the calf muscle pump. It drains into the popliteal vein. DVT (*vide infra*) usually starts within this plexus and spreads proximally.

Popliteal Vein

Formed by the anterior tibial and posterior tibial venae comitantes. It lies more superficial than the popliteal artery. It becomes the femoral vein as it passes through the adductor hiatus.

The SSV drains into the popliteal vein, in addition to the genicular veins, which correspond to the five genicular arteries mentioned earlier.

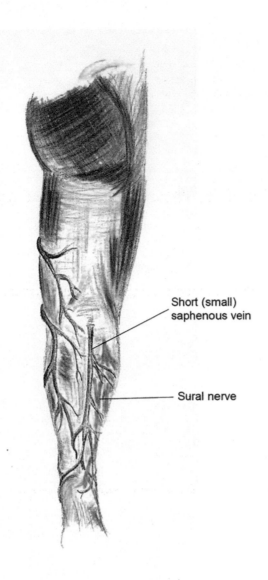

Short (small) saphenous vein

Sural nerve

FIGURE 7.19 The posterior aspect of the leg and course of the short saphenous vein. (Courtesy of Kathryn DeMarre.)

Femoral Vein

Begins at the hiatus of the adductor canal as the continuation of the popliteal vein. Runs alongside the medial side of the femoral artery in the femoral sheath. It becomes the external iliac vein as it passes deep to the inguinal ligament.

Drains significant veins such as the profunda femoris vein and LSV, at the saphenofemoral junction.

Lower Limb Lymphatics

There are both superficial and deep lymphatic vessels which drain into superficial and deep inguinal lymph nodes, respectively (**Figure 7.20**).

Deep Lymphatic Vessels

Note: *these vessels are not related to the deep inguinal lymph nodes.*

Terminate in the popliteal lymph nodes and accompany deep arteries of the lower leg only (anterior tibial artery, posterior tibial artery, peroneal artery).

Superficial Lymphatic Vessels

The superficial lymphatic vessels are more numerous and are classified into medial or lateral lymphatics (**Figure 7.21**).

Medial Superficial Lymph Vessels

Terminate in the superficial inguinal lymph nodes (lymph node positions are given relative to the saphenofemoral junction in the femoral triangle) and closely follow the course of the LSV.

Drain:

- Anteromedial lower leg (to inferior superficial inguinal nodes)
- Medial side of the gluteal region and lower abdominal wall (to superolateral superficial inguinal nodes)
- Perineum and external genitalia (to superomedial superficial inguinal nodes)

Lateral Superficial Lymph Vessels

Terminate in the popliteal lymph nodes. Closely follow the course of the SSV.

Drain:

- Superficial regions of the posterolateral aspect of the leg
- Plantar aspect of the foot

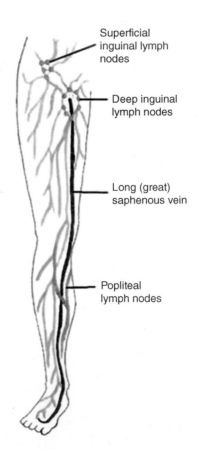

Superficial inguinal lymph nodes

Deep inguinal lymph nodes

Long (great) saphenous vein

Popliteal lymph nodes

FIGURE 7.20 Lymphatics of the lower limb. (Courtesy of Calum Harrington-Vogt.)

Inguinal Lymph Nodes

Deep Inguinal Lymph Nodes

Located deep to the cribriform fascia of the saphenofemoral junction and arranged medial to the femoral vein. These three to five nodes drain the glans penis or clitoris) and superficial inguinal lymph nodes. The deep inguinal lymph nodes drain to the external iliac lymph nodes (this is relevant to cancer metastasis).

CLINICAL NOTE

SENTINEL NODE BIOPSY

Cloquet's node is the most superomedial node of the deep inguinal lymph nodes, within the femoral canal medial to the femoral vein. It is considered to be the most often involved of the inguinal nodes in metastasis. Involvement of this node is often used to determine the extent of metastasis and whether further surgery is necessary to excise cancerous lymph nodes. Penile cancer and malignant melanoma of the skin of the lower limb are examples of the use of this lymph node to predict metastasis.

For more details on sentinel node biopsy, see **Section 4**, The Breast.

Superficial Inguinal Lymph Nodes

Located deep to the superficial fascia, within the femoral triangle. These nodes form a chain that overlies the femoral vessels and lie in a T-shape arrangement (lateral, medial and vertical) **Figure 7.21**. The roughly 10 nodes that comprise this group drain the structures of the lower limb, including the lower back up to the level of the iliac crests, anterior abdominal wall below the umbilicus, the anus below the dentate line, and the external genitalia (except the testes).

CLINICAL NOTES

Lymphadenopathy is the enlargement of lymph nodes due to different causes such as cancers and infections of the drainage area. This is because lymph nodes are a part of the immune system.

Lymphoedema of the lower limb is due to inadequate lymphatic drainage and presents as unilateral or bilateral lower limb swelling. It can be due to primary causes (congenital such as Milroy's disease) or secondary to parasitic infection by the nematode *Wuchereria bancrofti*, malignancies such as lymphomas, surgical excision of lymph nodes, and postoperative radiotherapy.

DEEP VEIN THROMBOSIS

Occurs as a result of blood clotting in the deep veins of the lower limb (mainly in the soleal venous plexus). This can be a result of inactivity (less muscle movement means less pressure exerted on veins to propel blood, leading to stasis, and thus clotting), especially after major surgical procedures; old age; certain blood disorders; and intake of certain medications (see Virchow's triad, **Section 4A**, Thorax). These factors are particularly important postoperatively, when damage to veins during surgery is likely to occur, for example, pressure on the calf while the patient is anaesthetised; this is the reason for applying thromboembolic deterrent (TED) stockings and the use of intraoperative electrical stimulation of the calf muscles and avoiding trauma to the calf muscle, in addition to the use of low-molecular-weight heparin subcutaneous injections, for example, enoxaparin (Clexane).

Pulmonary embolism (PE) can be a life-threatening condition that can complicate DVT. The clots are transported via the deep veins of the leg and pelvis to the inferior vena cava, and ultimately to the right atrium and ventricle. Massive emboli may block the main pulmonary artery and prove fatal.

Varicose veins

Varicose veins are tortuous and dilated superficial veins. The pathology of varicose veins is mainly related to leaking valves at the junctions between superficial and deep venous systems, usually occurring in the superficial veins of the leg (especially the saphenous veins). This condition is not life-threatening, primarily presenting as a cosmetic issue that can be painful in some patients. Complications of varicose veins include the development of venous ulcers (typically over the medial malleolus at the point of the highest venous pressure) and thrombophlebitis (inflammation of the veins).

Learning Point

DVT should be highly suspected and excluded (clinically and by Doppler studies) in patients with a swollen/painful leg following surgery, childbirth, and a long stay in bed for different reasons.

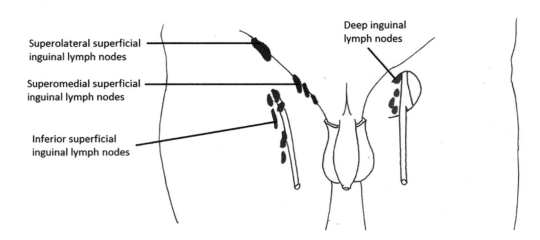

FIGURE 7.21 Inguinal lymph node clusters. (Courtesy of Calum Harrington-Vogt.)

The Knee Joint

Overview:

- The knee is a synovial joint of a modified hinge type, which is formed between the femoral condyles and the corresponding condyles of the tibia and anteriorly between the patella and the patellar surface of the femur (the latter forming the patellofemoral joint). The articular surfaces of the tibia, femur, and patella are covered by hyaline articular cartilage.
- It allows a range of motion (flexion, extension, and knee rotation) to occur in the leg, which is crucial for locomotion and allows bipedal movement.
- Extension is limited at the knee joint, but it allows a great range of flexion; this is important in the gait cycle.
- The knee joint is extended by the quadriceps femoris; flexed by hamstring muscles; and assisted by the gracilis, sartorius, and popliteus. Medial rotation is accomplished by the semitendinosus, gracilis, and sartorius, while lateral rotation is produced by the biceps femoris.
- The main stability of the knee joint depends on the muscles acting on the joint, specifically the quadriceps femoris.
- The knee joint receives innervation from the femoral, obturator, tibial, and common peroneal nerves.

The knee joint "locks" in full extension, creating a close-packed joint that requires very little energy to maintain the body in a standing position (see the discussion on the popliteus muscle later).

Osteology

The femur is categorised as a long bone; it is the longest and strongest bone in the body.

The fibula does not articulate directly with the femur; however, it articulates with the tibia and has a ligament that links it to the distal femur (the lateral collateral ligament), and thus it plays a role in stabilising the knee joint.

The patella is the smallest bone in the knee joint (see later). It plays a crucial role in bringing stability to the knee joint. The patella is a sesamoid bone that lies within the tendon of the quadriceps femoris muscle.

Capsule

A strong capsule covers the bony surfaces of the lower femur and upper tibia. Anteriorly, the capsule attaches to the edges of the quadriceps tendon, patella, and patellar tendon. The capsule receives reinforcements on the two sides, medially and laterally, from the tendons of the vastus medialis and vastus lateralis (medial and lateral retinacula, respectively) on each side of the patella. Posteriorly, it receives a reflection from the tendon of the semimembranosus (forming the oblique popliteal ligament).

The **synovial membrane** lines the inside of the joint but has an anterior pouch which extends upwards deep to the lower part of the quadriceps muscle, above the patella, forming the **suprapatellar bursa**, in addition to prepatellar and infrapatellar bursae.

The synovial cavity can also communicate with the semimembranosus bursa on the back of the knee joint (if enlarged, it is called Baker's cyst or popliteal cyst), which can present as a mass in the popliteal fossa (other masses, such as an aneurysm of the popliteal artery, must be excluded by proper clinical assessment and ultrasound imaging).

Ligaments

Like the hip joint, the knee joint has both intracapsular and extracapsular ligaments (**Figure 7.22**).

Anteriorly, the **ligamentum patellae** (patellar tendon) is the name given to the lower part of the tendon of the quadriceps muscle between the lower patella and the tibial tuberosity.

This structure is where the clinician detects the **knee jerk reflex** by eliciting contraction of the quadriceps after striking with the patella hammer (checking L2–L4 spinal segments). The knee jerk is a monosynaptic reflex between the stretch receptors in the tendon (afferent nerves), which synapse with anterior horn cells in the spinal cord, causing contraction of the quadriceps muscle.

The **popliteus** is a small muscle within the posterior knee. It arises from the lateral femoral condyle and inserts into the posterior surface of the tibia and is used for "unlocking" the knee when initiating walking. It does this by medially rotating the tibia during the closed portion of the gait cycle. Locking the knee during standing still allows the body to conserve energy. The tendon of the popliteus muscle separates the lateral collateral ligament from the lateral meniscus. Its nerve supply comes from the tibial nerve.

The Intracapsular Ligaments

Cruciate ligaments are named according to their attachment to the articular surface of the tibia. They are named from their resemblance to a cross (*crux* in Latin). The cruciate ligaments are intracapsular but outside the synovial membrane.

Anterior Cruciate Ligament (ACL)

The ACL is a diagonal ligament (runs down and medially) from the lateral femoral condyle to the anterior intercondylar eminence on the tibial plateau. With the knee flexed, it resists anterior translation of the tibia and posterior displacement of the femoral condyle. The anterior drawer test allows us to check whether damage has been inflicted to this ligament.

Posterior Cruciate Ligament (PCL)

The PCL is a diagonal (runs down and laterally) ligament running from the medial femoral condyle to the posterior part of the intercondylar eminence on the tibial plateau. It resists posterior translation of the tibia and anterior displacement of the femoral condyle when the knee is flexed, and it can be tested using the posterior drawer test. ACL injuries are more common than PCL injuries.

The Extracapsular Ligaments

Collateral Ligaments

Alongside the two cruciate ligaments are the medial and lateral collateral ligaments of the knee joint. Both exist to prevent excess varus and valgus stress on the knee.

- The **medial** (or tibial) **collateral ligament** is attached to the medial epicondyle of the femur proximally and to the medial condyle of the tibia distally and acts to prevent valgus stress on the knee joint, i.e., it prevents forces from acting medially on the joint. The medial side of the knee is responsible for bearing most of the force of weight on the knee joint and provides medial stability to the knee joint. This fibrous and broad ligament forms part of the "unhappy triad" and is more commonly injured when compared to its counterpart, due to excess valgus stress placed upon this ligament, with the knee in a slightly flexed position, causing injury.
- The **lateral** (or fibular) **collateral ligament** is a strong fibrous band, narrower than its counterpart, attached to the lateral epicondyle of the femur proximally and to the head of the fibula distally, where it splits the tendon of the biceps femoris at its insertion. It acts to prevent excess varus stress on the joint, i.e., it prevents forces acting laterally on the joint.

Menisci (Semilunar Cartilages)

The menisci are C-shaped fibrocartilage structures firmly attached to the upper surface of the tibial condyles (tibial plateau). Each meniscus is formed of a thick peripheral part and a thin concave inner part and has anterior and posterior horns. Their function is to deepen the articular surface of the tibial condyles and act as cushions between the femoral and tibial condyles.

The medial meniscus is attached to the medial collateral ligament, and its anterior horn blends with the ACL. Consequently, it is less mobile and more prone to injuries.

Osteology of the Patella

The patella (kneecap or "flat dish" in Latin) is the largest sesamoid bone in the body. It has a wide upper border and pointed lower border (patellar apex) and is located within the tendon of the quadriceps femoris. The posterior surface has articular facets that articulate with the distal femur (lateral and medial condyles). The lateral femoral condyle projects farther forward than the medial condyle, as a bony obstacle to lateral movements of the patella.

Blood Supply

The knee joint has a rich blood supply from the anterior and posterior tibial, popliteal (the five genicular arteries, see earlier), and femoral arteries and the descending branch of the lateral circumflex artery (from the femoral).

Nerve Supply of the Knee Joint

From the saphenous nerve (a branch of the femoral nerve), both tibial and common peroneal nerves, in addition to an articular branch of the obturator nerve.

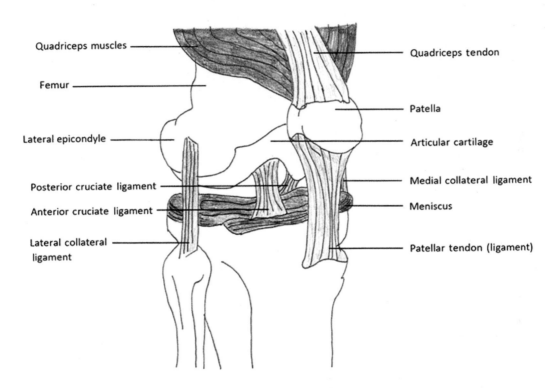

FIGURE 7.22   Structures within the knee joint. (Courtesy of Alina Humdani.)

CLINICAL NOTES

McMURRAY'S TEST

This is one of the clinical tests for meniscal injury. With the patient in the supine position, the examiner holds the heel with one hand and the knee in the other hand. It is elicited by bending the knee first, then straightening it and rotating the lower leg on both lateral and medial sides. With a palpable or audible click on these movements, the test is considered positive for a torn meniscus.

MENISCAL INJURIES

Most injuries follow sports such as football (squat and twist knee) with sudden pain in the knee and sometimes locking of the knee.

Degenerative changes in the menisci occur with aging and can follow previous knee injury.

THE UNHAPPY TRIAD

The "unhappy triad" or "O'Donoghue triad" is an injury to the ACL, medial collateral ligament, and medial meniscus. It is the among the most common injuries to the knee and can be sustained during sports such as football and rugby. It occurs as a result of excess lateral (valgus) stress to the knee. Repair often involves surgery and reconstruction of the ligaments.

ARTHROSCOPY

Arthroscopy is the surgical procedure to visualise the inside of the joint by inserting a telescope attached to a

(Continued)

camera. It is both diagnostic (for meniscal and cruciate ligament injury) and therapeutic (joint irrigation, suturing of cruciate ligament rupture, meniscectomy).

DEFORMITIES OF THE KNEE JOINT

Valgus and varus deformities can occur at the knee joint. In a valgus deformity, the distal part of the leg is deviated outward, resulting in a knock-kneed appearance. Conversely, a varus deformity occurs when the distal leg is deviated inwards, leading to a bowlegged appearance.

SWOLLEN KNEE

1. *Generalised swelling:* joint effusion (excessive fluid collection) seen in rheumatoid arthritis, osteoarthritis, septic arthritis, and haemarthrosis
2. *Localised swellings:* prepatellar bursa (anteriorly), Baker's cyst posteriorly

HAEMARTHROSIS

Collection of blood in the joint cavity. It usually follows severe trauma to the knee and can be a feature of haemophilia following a trivial trauma. It involves heavy bleeding into the joint; this can cause extreme pain and cause clots to form within the joint.

SEPTIC ARTHRITIS

Septic arthritis is defined as the deep infection of a joint, and the knee joint is the most commonly affected joint. The causative bacteria are mostly *Staphylococcus aureus* (especially in patients with previous joint implants and the immunocompromised). In young people, gonococcal arthritis is an important cause. In septic arthritis the knee joint will become inflamed (red), swollen, hot, and painful. It is a medical emergency, and prompt treatment is required to avoid septicaemia and possible death. The treatment involves an urgent referral to hospital and intravenous (IV) antibiotics along with joint aspiration.

OSTEOARTHRITIS

The knee joint is commonly affected by osteoarthritis, a type of non-inflammatory arthritis. It is generally caused by "wear and tear" and usually affects the more elderly population. However, with the increased prevalence of obesity, osteoarthritis has been affecting younger people. This condition can be extremely painful.

ABOVE- AND BELOW-KNEE AMPUTATIONS

These common operations are indicated for different reasons:

- Critical limb ischaemia, commonly due to diabetes and atherosclerosis (this the most common cause for above- or below-knee amputations)
- Severe trauma to the leg, where vascularity is irreversibly compromised
- Severe infections of the leg
- Malignant conditions of the leg

The decision between above- and below-knee amputation depends on the clinical assessment, especially making sure of enough blood supply to the skin flaps.

OSGOOD-SCHLATTER DISEASE

Osgood-Schlatter disease is inflammation of the patellar ligament at the tibial tuberosity due to repeated tension on the growth plate of the upper tibia which usually affects teenagers. It presents with a tender bump below the knee that is worse with activity and better with rest. These episodes of pain can last up to a few months. Both knees can be affected. Risk factors include excessive sports such as running and jumping. X-rays can show either a normal or fragmented attachment area.

The patella has more tendency to dislocate laterally, counteracted by the horizontally oriented fibres of the lower part of the vastus medialis.

Fractures of the patella can be of the comminuted or transverse type and impair proper knee extension.

Osteology of the Tibia

The tibia is the second longest bone in the body, found on the medial aspect of the leg. It consists of an upper end, shaft, and lower end.

The upper end of the tibia has a semi-flat articular surface on both medial and lateral tibial condyles (which is called the tibial plateau). The condyles are separated by the **intercondylar eminence**, which has anterior and posterior areas that mark the sites where the cruciate ligaments attach.

The tibial condyles articulate with the femoral condyles within the knee joint. The lateral tibial condyle below the plateau articulates with the head of the fibula (forming the superior tibiofibular joint).

The tibial plateau also forms attachment points for the medial and lateral menisci. The medial condyle forms an attachment point for the semimembranosus tendon, whereas the iliotibial tract and the popliteus tendon attach to the lateral condyle. Anteriorly, beneath the condyles is the **tibial tuberosity**, which serves as an attachment point for the patellar tendon (ligamentum patellae), a continuation of the quadriceps tendon.

Connecting the proximal and distal portions of the tibia is the **tibial shaft**, triangular in cross-section. It has an anterior, medial, and lateral (interosseus) border and three surfaces (lateral, medial, and posterior). The anterior border and the medial surface (the shin) are subcutaneous, and fractures at this site are more likely to be of the compound type (open and exposed to infection). The soleus muscle is attached to the **soleal line** posteriorly, in addition to its origin on the posterior fibular shaft. The tendons of the sartorius, gracilis, and semitendinosus attach to its upper medial surface at the *pes anserinus.* The popliteus muscle is attached posteriorly to the tibial shaft above the soleal line. The lateral surface is occupied by the muscles of the anterior compartment (see later).

The tibial shaft provides attachment points for the tibialis anterior on its lateral surface and the plantar flexors (flexor digitorum longus, tibialis posterior) and soleus posteriorly. The interosseous membrane (composed of tough, fibrous tissue) connects the lateral tibial border with the medial fibular border; some books consider it the middle tibiofibular joint.

Distally, the tibia on its medial surface forms the medial malleolus, which articulates with the talus (talocrural joint). The lateral part of the lower end (fibular notch) articulates with the fibula (lower tibiofibular joint) (**Figure 7.23**).

Osteology of the Fibula

Thinner in diameter than the tibia, the fibula is a long, non-weight-bearing bone located laterally to the tibia in the leg. The **head of the fibula** (proximal end) is oval in shape and articulates with the lateral aspect of the lateral tibial condyle and forms an attachment point for the lateral collateral ligament and the biceps femoris.

The **common peroneal nerve (a branch of the sciatic nerve) wraps around the neck of the fibula**, which is clinically significant, as the nerve may be damaged in fractures of the fibular neck or via plaster cast treatment. The common peroneal nerve also divides here into its superficial and deep branches. The **shaft of the fibula** provides attachment points for the peroneus (fibularis) longus and brevis muscles, in addition to the extensor digitorum longus and extensor hallucis longus anteriorly, and the plantar flexors tibialis posterior and flexor hallucis longus, on its posterior surface.

The **lower end of the fibula** continues as the lateral malleolus distally, which projects farther than the medial malleolus and articulates with the talus. The lateral malleolus provides attachment points for the lateral ligaments of the ankle joints, including the anterior and posterior talofibular ligaments and the calcaneofibular ligament. The tendons of the peroneus (fibularis) longus and brevis pass posterior to the lateral malleolus to their attachment points at the base of the fifth metatarsal (brevis) and medial cuneiform and first metatarsal (longus) (**Figure 7.23**).

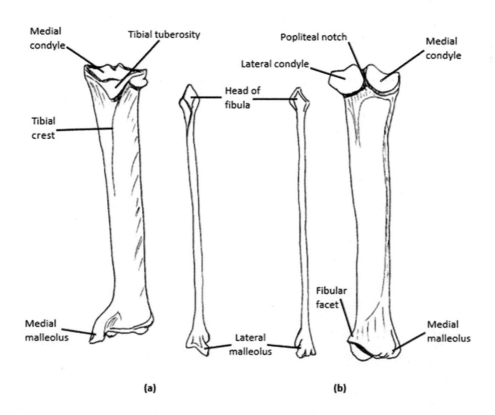

FIGURE 7.23   (a) Anterior and (b) posterior views of the left tibia and fibula. (Courtesy of Alina Humdani.)

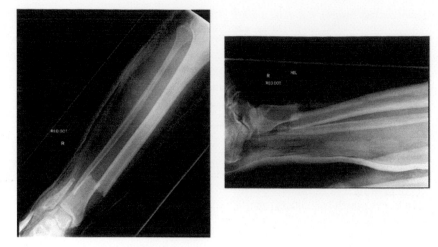

FIGURE 7.24 AP and lateral views, plain film X-ray of the right lower limb of a 21-year-old male who fell on to his right lower leg and sustained fractures of lower parts of the tibia and fibula. (Courtesy of Radiology Dept. at St. George's Hospital NHS Trust.)

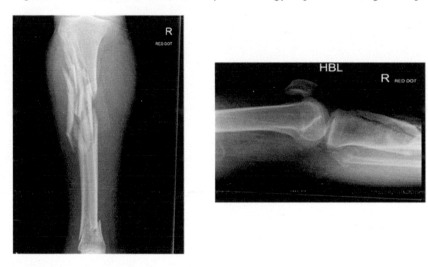

FIGURE 7.25 AP and lateral views, plain film X-ray of the right lower limb of a 36-year-old male pedestrian who was involved in a road traffic collision with an oncoming car. Closed comminuted fracture of the proximal midshaft of the right tibia and fibula. Multiple fragments can be seen of both the tibia and fibula. (Courtesy of Radiology Dept. at St. George's Hospital NHS Trust.)

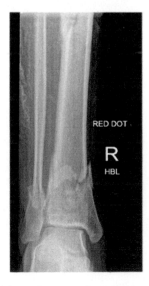
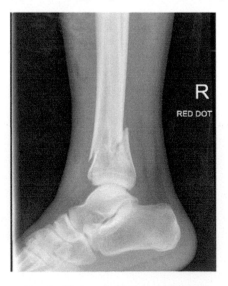

FIGURE 7.26 AP and lateral views, plain X-rays of the same patient in **Figure 4.25** showing closed transverse fracture of the distal third of the right tibia and fibula and no involvement of the talocrural joint or subtalar joints. (Courtesy of Radiology Department at St. George's Hospital NHS Trust.)

Musculature of the Leg

The muscles are divided into three distinct compartments: anterior, lateral, and posterior, which have common actions in each compartment (**Figure 7.27**).

Anterior Compartment of the Leg (Table 7.6)

All of the muscles in this compartment are innervated by the deep peroneal (fibular) nerve (L4–S1), supplied by the anterior tibial artery, and all dorsiflex the foot. Note that L4/L5 segments innervate the tibialis anterior and L5/S1 segments innervate the rest of the muscles in the anterior compartment. The deep fascia, which covers the extensor compartment, is tough and thick.

The **common peroneal (common fibular) nerve (L4, L5, S1, S2)** is the smaller of the two divisions of the sciatic nerve at the upper part of the popliteal fossa, behind the biceps femoris (of which it supplies the short head). It gives articular branches to the knee and the superior tibiofibular joint. It also contributes to the sural nerve, which supplies the posterolateral aspect of the lower leg.

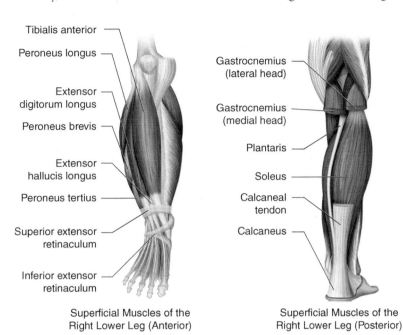

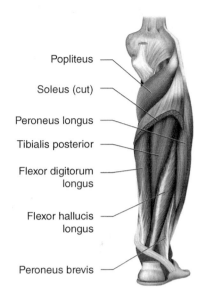

FIGURE 7.27   Muscles of the leg compartments. (Courtesy of Alina Humdani.)

TABLE 7.6: Muscles of the anterior compartment of the leg

Muscle	Attachments	Action
Tibialis anterior	Originates from the lateral surface of the lateral tibial condyle and upper part of the tibial shaft and interosseous membrane; to base of first metatarsal and to the medial cuneiform	Dorsiflexion of the ankle and inversion of the foot at the subtalar joint
Extensor digitorum longus (EDL)	Originates from the lateral condyle of the tibia and medial aspect of the fibula and interosseous membrane; converges into a tendon which splits into four and inserts into the middle and distal phalanges of the lateral four toes	Dorsiflexion of the ankle and extension of lateral four toes
Extensor hallucis longus (EHL)	Originates on the medial surface of the fibula and adjacent interosseous membrane, between the tibialis anterior and EDL; attaches to base of distal phalanx of the big toe	Dorsiflexion of the ankle, extension of the big toe
Peroneus tertius (fibularis tertius)	Originates with the EDL and attaches to the base of the fifth metatarsal	(Weak) dorsiflexion of the ankle and eversion of the foot

The **common peroneal (fibular) nerve winds around the neck of the fibula** in quite a superficial location, which makes it vulnerable to injuries like fractures and following the application of tight casts resulting in loss of eversion and dorsiflexion of the foot. Within the substance of the peroneus longus, it divides into superficial and deep peroneal nerves. The superficial peroneal supplies motor branches to the peroneus longus and brevis and sensation to the anterolateral aspect of the leg and the whole dorsum of the foot, except for the web area between the big and second toes and the lateral side of the big toe and second toe, which are supplied by the deep branch.

The deep peroneal nerve, accompanied by the anterior tibial vessels, enters the extensor compartment, deep to the extensor digitorum longus, to supply all the extensors and dorsiflexors. It enters the foot deep to the extensor retinaculum and supplies motor branches to the extensor hallucis brevis and extensor digitorum brevis.

In clinical examination of a patient with suspected common peroneal nerve injury, ask the patient to walk and check their gait for slapping gait and foot drop. Heel walking checks the dorsiflexors, while toe walking checks the tibial and superficial peroneal nerves.

The next to be checked are the tone and power of the anterior and lateral compartments, and lastly the sensation on the lateral aspect of the leg and foot and dorsum of the foot, for both light and sharp sensation compared with the uninjured side.

The Posterior Compartment of the Leg

The posterior compartment is the largest of the three compartments of the leg. Muscles in this compartment are either within the superficial or deep layer; see **Table 7.7**.

The nerve supply of the posterior compartment is the tibial nerve, one of the terminal branches of the sciatic nerve. The tibial nerve passes anterior to the superficial muscles (gastrocnemius and soleus) on the posterior surface of tibialis posterior. It then passes with the posterior tibial vessels and the tendons of the flexor digitorum longus, flexor hallucis longus, and tibialis posterior behind the medial malleolus.

The tibial nerve divides into medial and lateral plantar nerves.

The posterior tibial artery is larger than the anterior tibial and continues in the foot as the medial and lateral plantar arteries. Palpating the artery is a common question in clinical exams to assess the blood supply to the foot (see "Diabetic Foot").

TABLE 7.7: Muscles of the posterior compartment of the leg

Layer	Muscle	Attachments	Action
Superficial All muscles in this group are innervated by S1/S2 segments of the tibial nerve (the three muscles are termed the triceps surae)	Gastrocnemius (responsible for most of the bulge of the calf)	Lateral head originates from lateral femoral condyle, and the medial head arises superior to the medial femoral condyle, on the posterior surface of the femur. Both insert via the calcaneal tendon on to the posterior surface of the calcaneus	Gastrocnemius and soleus are powerful plantar flexors of the ankle joint and provide the forward propulsive force to raise the heel off the ground in walking and running. They are also flexors of the knee joint
	Plantaris	Originates from the lateral supracondylar line of the femur and oblique popliteal ligament. Has a long slender tendon which inserts on to the calcaneus, medial to the calcaneal tendon	Assists in plantarflexion of the ankle joint and (weak) flexion of the knee joint
	Soleus	Originates from soleal line of tibia, posterior aspect of fibula and the tendinous arch between tibial and fibular attachments. Inserts on to the calcaneal tendon	Plantarflexion of the ankle
Deep The superficial and deep groups are separated by the deep transverse fascia	Tibialis posterior (innervated by L4/L5)	Originates between the tibia and fibula and the posterior surface of the interosseous membrane and attaches to the plantar surface of the medial tarsal bones (navicular, medial cuneiform) and bases of second, third, and fourth metatarsals	Its main action is plantarflexion of the foot at the ankle joint and inversion of the foot at the subtalar joint. Supports medial longitudinal foot arch when walking
	Flexor digitorum longus FDL (innervated by S2/S3)	Originates from the medial surface of the tibia and attaches to the plantar surface of the bases of the distal phalanges of the lateral four toes	Flexor of the distal phalanges of the lateral four toes and plantarflexion at the ankle joint, in addition to supporting the medial and lateral longitudinal foot arches
	Flexor hallucis longus FHL (innervated by S2/S3)	From the posterior surface of the fibula. In the foot crosses medially to the base of the distal phalanx of the big toe	Plantarflexion of the distal phalanx of the big toe and the foot and supports the medial longitudinal foot arch. Note that the tendon of the FDL crosses under the tendon of FHL at the "knot of Henry"
	Popliteus (supplied by L4, L5, and S1)	Within the articular capsule from the lateral femoral condyle to the upper part of the posterior tibia. Its tendon passes between the lateral meniscus and the lateral collateral ligament of the knee joint	It has a rotatory function on the knee to slacken its ligaments (unlocking of the knee) by laterally rotating the femur on the tibia at the onset of knee flexion

CLINICAL NOTES

RUPTURE OF ACHILLES TENDON

The Achilles tendon (or tendocalcaneus) is the strongest tendon in the body. Its rupture is usually due to a direct insult or trauma, sustained during forceful plantarflexion of the foot, and usually occurs about 4 cm above its insertion into the calcaneus. The rupture can be complete or partial. Common symptoms from patients who have experienced a ruptured Achilles tendon include the patients felt like they "were shot or kicked in the ankle", as well as intense pain. The affected foot will be permanently dorsiflexed and cannot plantarflex.

ANKLE JERK REFLEX

Tapping the Achilles tendon with a rubber tendon hammer with the foot dorsiflexed results in contraction of the gastrocnemius and soleus and plantar flexion (S1 spinal segment). This is a stretch reflex and classically very slow in patients with hypothyroidism.

Negative ankle jerk can be a feature of a prolapsed intervertebral disc at the L5–S1 level.

FLEXOR RETINACULUM (TARSAL TUNNEL)

The flexor retinaculum is made up of connective tissue attaching from above the medial malleolus to the inferomedial margin of the calcaneus; this retinaculum is continuous superiorly with the deep fascia of the leg and inferiorly with the plantar aponeurosis of the foot. The flexor retinaculum forms the roof of the tarsal tunnel. The tarsal tunnel transmits the neurovascular bundle, which contains the posterior tibial artery and vein and tibial nerve and the flexor tendons. These structures run behind the medial malleolus; the tendon of the tibialis posterior is the most anterior, then that of flexor digitorum longus, the neurovascular bundle, and most posteriorly is the tendon of flexor hallucis longus (**Figure 7.28**).

TARSAL TUNNEL SYNDROME

Compression of the tibial nerve at this site is called tarsal tunnel syndrome (compare with the more common carpal tunnel syndrome in the hand).

KEY STRUCTURES NEAR THE MEDIAL MALLEOLUS

Tom Dick and A Very Nervous Harry

Key when learning how different vessels and tendons enter the foot from the lower limb, the area of the medial malleolus provides a well-documented pathway for three tendons along with an artery, vein, and nerve to enter the foot, through the tarsal tunnel, deep to the **flexor retinaculum**. To learn the precise order of the tendons and vessels, **Tom Dick and A Very Nervous Harry** is an excellent mnemonic to recall the structures.

From superior to inferior:

a. **T**om = (tendon of) **t**ibialis posterior
b. **D**ick = (tendon of) flexor **d**igitorum longus
c. and **A** = posterior tibial **a**rtery
d. **V**ery = posterior tibial **v**ein (sometimes not included in mnemonic)
e. **N**ervous = tibial **n**erve
f. **H**arry = (tendon of) flexor **h**allucis longus

Lateral Compartment of the Leg (Table 7.8)

The lateral compartment of the leg is the smallest of the three muscular compartments.

Lateral compartment muscles are supplied by the superficial peroneal nerve (L5–S1).

The tendons of the peroneus longus and brevis pass behind the lateral malleolus. **The tendon of the peroneus tertius passes anterior to the lateral malleolus**.

TABLE 7.8: Muscles of the lateral compartment of the leg

Muscle	Attachments	Action
Peroneus (fibularis) longus	Originates from the head and lateral surface of the fibula, converges into a tendon, entering the foot posterior to the lateral malleolus, attaching medially underneath the foot to base of the first metatarsal	Eversion at the subtalar joint and plantarflexion of the ankle. Also supports the lateral longitudinal and transverse arches of the foot
Peroneus (fibularis) brevis	Similar in course to the peroneus longus, but attaches from the lower two-thirds of the lateral aspect of the fibula to the lateral aspect of the base of the fifth metatarsal	Eversion of the foot

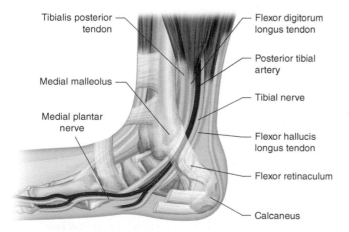

Tibialis posterior tendon
Medial malleolus
Medial plantar nerve

Flexor digitorum longus tendon
Posterior tibial artery
Tibial nerve
Flexor hallucis longus tendon
Flexor retinaculum
Calcaneus

FIGURE 7.28 Structures near the medial malleolus. (Courtesy of Alina Humdani.)

The Anatomy of the Foot

Introduction

This review will include an overview of the anatomy of the foot, including osteology, ligaments, joints of the foot, important muscles, and their attachments, as well as clinical conditions relevant to the anatomy.

Osteology of the Foot

To begin learning about the anatomy of the foot, it is important to learn first about the osteology of the foot and the functions each bone plays in forming the foot. By learning the osteology, joint and ligamentous attachments become easier to identify, as well as identifying the potential consequences of fractures or ligamentous tears or sprains in the foot. Also, key areas to learn in this section are structures deep to the medial and lateral malleoli and their organisation.

There are three sets of bones in the foot, from proximal to distal: **tarsals, metatarsals, and phalanges**. This is similar to the composition of the bones of the hand (in that the metacarpals are homologous to the metatarsals and the sequence of the phalanges in the foot are similar to the hand); the tarsals, however, vary from the carpals (**Figures 7.29** and **7.30**, **Table 7.9**).

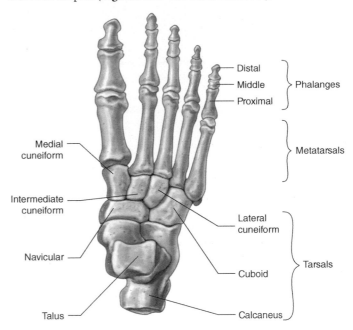

FIGURE 7.29 Osteology of the foot. (Courtesy of Gabriela Barzyk.)

The bones of the foot are arranged in longitudinal and transverse arches. When standing, the lateral margin of the foot, the ball of the foot, and the pads of the toes are the only parts of the foot that make contact with the ground.

Tarsals

There are seven bones which make up the tarsals (proximal to distal).

The articular surface of the trochlea of the talus is wider anteriorly than posteriorly. This is of significance, as the stability of the foot varies with its position: dorsiflexion is more stable than plantarflexion. The talocrural (ankle) joint is stabilised due to the wider anterior side immobilised by the articulation with the tibia. In plantarflexion, the narrower posterior part is articulating, allowing greater movement but less stability.

An important ligament which **maintains the medial foot arch**, the spring ligament or plantar calcaneonavicular ligament, passes underneath the head of the talus for its attachments to the navicular (anterior).

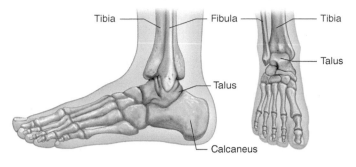

Tibia — Fibula — Tibia

Talus

Talus

Calcaneus

FIGURE 7.30 Lateral and anterior view of osteology of the foot. (Courtesy of Gabriela Barzyk.)

The Ankle Joint (Talocrural)

The ankle Joint, known as the talocrural joint, is a synovial hinge joint and is formed by the distal ends of the tibia and fibula and the proximal end of the talus. This hinge joint allows the movements of dorsiflexion (by muscles in the anterior compartment of the lower leg) and plantarflexion of the foot (posterior compartment of the lower leg. Due to the arrangement of the bony articulation, the ankle joint is considered a mortise joint (the talus fits snugly in between the lower ends of the tibia and fibula).

Ligaments within the Ankle Joint

To maintain the stability of the talocrural joint and ensure the foot arches are maintained, there are various ligaments on both the medial and lateral aspects of the ankle joint, attaching from the distal ends of the tibia or fibula to the individual tarsal bones. Important ligaments to recognise on a specimen or model are noted here, along with their points of attachment and functions.

TABLE 7.9: Bones of the foot

Bone	Location	Shape	Articulations	Important Structures
Talus	Superior to calcaneus	Trochlea of talus articulates with the distal ends of the fibula and tibia superiorly; head and neck articulate with the navicular anteriorly	Head of the talus articulates with the navicular anteriorly; body of the talus articulates with the calcaneus inferiorly Articulations with the distal ends of the tibia and fibula form the talocrural joint (ankle joint)	No muscle is attached to this bone
Calcaneus – "heel bone"	Forms the base of the foot, inferior to the talus and posterior to the cuboid The largest bone in the foot	Irregularly shaped, projects backwards to form the skeletal framework (heel) and forwards, which contains articulating surfaces	Achilles (calcaneal) tendon attaches to the posterior surface of the calcaneus Articulates with the talus superiorly and the cuboid and navicular anteriorly Also, there is an attachment for the calcaneonavicular ligament on the medial surface of the calcaneus	Stability of the foot; forms the skeletal framework of the heel. The medial surface contains a shelf-like structure called the sustentaculum tali The tendons of the peroneus longus and brevis pass on its lateral surface, separated by the peroneal tubercle
Navicular	Located on the medial side of the foot	Boat-shaped	Articulates posteriorly with the talus and anteriorly and laterally with the cuboid and cuneiform bones	Involved in the transverse tarsal (midtarsal joint), as well as an attachment point for the spring ligament Gives attachment for tibialis posterior tendon
Cuneiforms (**Medial**, intermediate, and lateral)	Three cuneiform bones, part of the intermediate/ distal tarsal bones	Wedge-shaped	Articulate posteriorly with the navicular and anteriorly with the bases of the three medial metatarsals	Provides attachment points for tibialis anterior and posterior, peroneus longus, and flexor hallucis brevis
Cuboid	Anterior to the calcaneus, lateral to the lateral cuneiform	Cube-shaped	*Points of articulation:* • Posteriorly with calcaneus • Anteriorly with bases of lateral two metatarsals • Medially with lateral cuneiform	Provides a groove for peroneus longus to pass through to reach the first metatarsal and cuneiform bones
Metatarsals	Five metatarsals, proximal to the phalanges	Each has a head distally and a base proximally joined by a shaft	Head articulates with proximal phalanx of a toe; base articulates with either cuboid or cuneiforms	Involved in the tarsometatarsal joints
Phalanges	Toes 2 to 5 have three phalanges (proximal, middle, and distal); the hallux only has proximal and distal phalanges	Each has a head distally and a base proximally joined by a shaft	Head of the distal phalanx is non-articular; base of the proximal phalanx articulates with corresponding metatarsal	Dexterity and movement

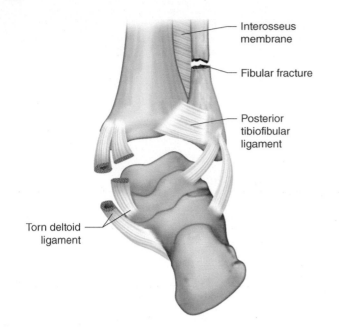

FIGURE 7.31 Ligaments of the ankle joint. (Courtesy of Gabriela Barzyk.)

Medial Aspect of the Ankle

The main ligament to be aware of is the **deltoid ligament**. This is an extremely strong ligament attaching from the medial malleolus superiorly to the navicular and talus inferiorly, which prevents excess eversion of the ankle joint. Made up of four individual ligaments, all collate to form a strong ligament and complete the same function – resisting over eversion of the ankle joint (**Figures 7.31** and **7.32**).

Lateral Aspect of the Ankle

Key ligaments to be aware of in this area are summarised in **Table 7.10**. The main function of the collective lateral ligaments is to prevent excess inversion of the ankle joint (**Figure 7.33**).

Between the Distal Ends of the Tibia and Fibula

The anterior tibiofibular ligament connects the anterior surface of the distal end of the tibia and the fibula; the posterior tibiofibular ligament connects the posterior surface of the distal end of the tibia and the fibula.

Key structures near the lateral malleolus are shown in **Figure 7.34**.

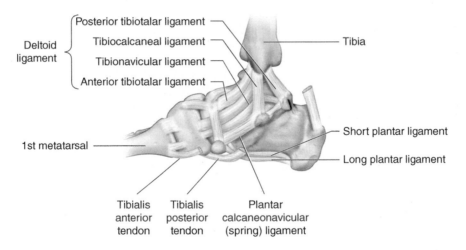

FIGURE 7.32 Ligaments, medial aspect of the ankle. (Courtesy of Alina Humdani.)

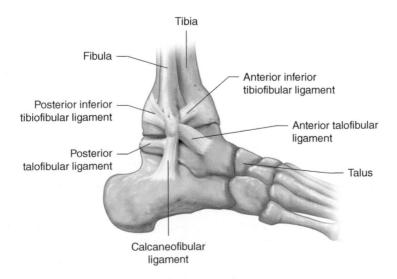

FIGURE 7.33 Ligaments of the lateral aspect of the ankle. (Courtesy of Alina Humdani.)

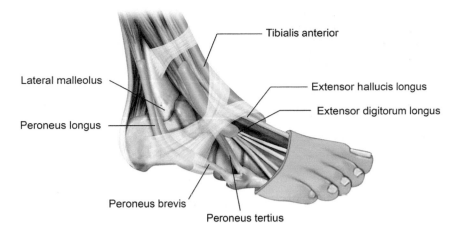

FIGURE 7.34 Key structures next to the lateral malleolus. (Courtesy of Alina Humdani.)

TABLE 7.10: Ligaments of the lateral aspect of the ankle joint

Ligament	Attachments
Anterior talofibular	From the lateral malleolus to the lateral aspect of the talus
Posterior talofibular	From the lateral malleolus to the posterior aspect of the talus
Calcaneofibular	Runs from the posteromedial side of the lateral malleolus to the lateral surface of the calcaneus

Extensor Retinacula

The extensor retinacula are made up of the superior extensor retinaculum and the inferior extensor retinaculum, both of which bind the extensor tendons to the foot during extension of the ankle (dorsiflexion) and toes.

The superior extensor retinaculum is superior to the ankle joint and attaches to the anterior borders of the tibia and the fibula.

The inferior extensor retinaculum is Y-shaped and is attached laterally to the upper surface of the calcaneus and medially to both the medial malleolus with one arm of the Y and to the medial side of the plantar aponeurosis with the other arm of the Y (**Figure 7.35**).

Arrangement of structures on the dorsal surface of the foot (lateral to medial):

- (Tendon of) peroneus tertius
- (Tendons of) extensor digitorum longus
- Dorsalis pedis artery
- (Tendon of) extensor hallucis longus
- (Tendon of) tibialis anterior

Fibular Retinacula

Also made up of superior and inferior portions, the fibular retinacula bind the peroneus brevis and longus tendons. Both parts extend from the calcaneus, with the superior portion terminating at the lateral malleolus and the inferior portion terminating at the inferior extensor retinaculum.

Nerve and blood supply of the ankle joint is from the tibial and deep and superficial peroneal nerves. The blood supply comes from the three major arteries (anterior and posterior tibial and the peroneal).

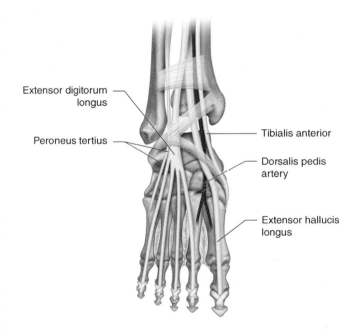

FIGURE 7.35 Anterior surface of the foot. (Courtesy of Alina Humdani). Note that the structures on the dorsal surface of the foot are encased by the extensor retinacula *(shaded)*.

CLINICAL NOTES

POTT'S FRACTURE DISLOCATION

Also known as a bimalleolar ankle fracture, this occurs after forcible foot eversion, pulling on the medial deltoid ligament and producing an avulsion fracture of the medial malleolus. An avulsion fracture indicates an injury to the bone where a ligament or tendon attaches to the bone in a specific location, and when a fracture occurs, the tendon or ligaments pulls off a piece of bone also (**Figure 7.36**).

As the talus is not held in place medially due to fracture of the bony articulation with the medial ligament, the talus moves laterally, shearing off the lateral malleolus and breaking the fibula superior to the inferior tibiofibular joint.

(Continued)

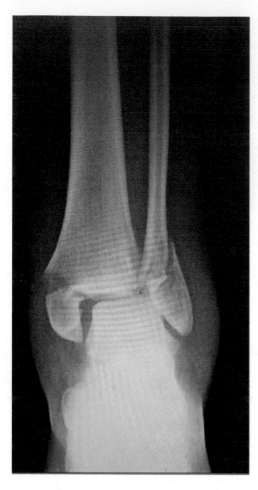

FIGURE 7.36 Fractures of the medial and lateral malleoli. (Courtesy of Salam Ismael.)

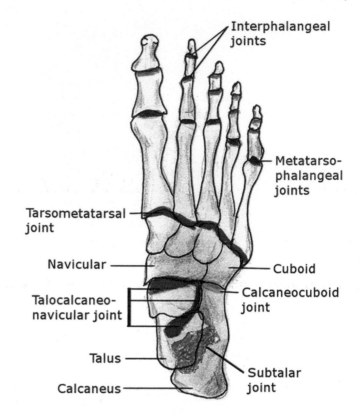

FIGURE 7.37 Joints of the foot. (Courtesy of Gabriella Barzyk.)

Note: The movements of inversion/eversion differ from movements of supination/pronation. Inversion/eversion are in a linear plane, whereas supination/pronation involves degrees of inward and outward rotation.

INVERSION AND EVERSION INJURIES

Approximately 90% of all ankle sprains are inversion injuries, which overstretch the lateral ligaments, including the anterior and posterior talofibular ligaments and the calcaneofibular ligament, generally weaker than the medial ligaments. The anterior talofibular ligament is the most common to be affected. The most common injuries occur in a plantarflexed foot which has been excessively inverted.

If a patient has an eversion injury, it is commonly caused by overstretching and tearing of the medial deltoid ligament, which is normally very strong and resists over eversion. Either inversion or eversion injuries can cause a sprained ankle if there is a partial or complete tear in its corresponding ligaments.

Joints within the Foot

The subtalar joint allows for inversion and eversion. **Other joints** which are important to identify as they are involved with the key movements of the foot are listed in **Table 7.11** and **Figure 7.37**.

CLINICAL NOTES

Boot top fracture: often sustained by skiers when they are unable to keep their balance and fall forward on top of their ski boot. The proximal tibia is bent forwards as the person falls forwards, compressive stresses and strains act on the anterior surface of the tibia due to the presence of the rigid ski boot, and the tibia and fibula become fractured at the top of the boot. The fracture is often comminuted, i.e., the bone is broken into many pieces.

Stress fracture: caused by repetitive stresses over time on an area of bone, which results in weakening of the bone and a small crack or bruising forming within the bone. These types of fractures are often seen in athletes and runners. As bones within the foot must bear the weight of the entirety of the body, stress fractures most commonly occur here, usually in the second, third, and fourth metatarsals. Moreover, non-athletes who experience a sudden change of activity or who may be using an improper technique to complete their exercises, such as doing an excessive amount of exercise too soon, may also be vulnerable to stress fractures (**Figure 7.38**) (Continues below **Table 7.11**).

TABLE 7.11: Joints of the foot

Joint Name	Type	Articulations	Movements
Subtalar (also known as the talocalcaneal joint)	Plane synovial	Two points of articulation between the talus and the calcaneus, anterior and posterior attachments	Allows for inversion and eversion of the foot. Also allows for supination and pronation of the foot
Transverse tarsal (also known as the midtarsal joint or Chopart's joint)	Joint between the midfoot and the hindfoot, comprises the talocalcaneonavicular joint and the calcaneocuboid joint	Formed by the articulation of the calcaneus with the cuboid (calcaneocuboid joint) and the articulation of the talus with the navicular (talocalcaneonavicular joint)	Joint rotates slightly to allow inversion (during plantarflexion) or eversion (during dorsiflexion)
Talocalcaneonavicular	Ball-and-socket joint	Rounded head of the talus articulates with the posterior surface of the navicular and the anterior surface of the calcaneus	Inversion and eversion of the foot. Forms the transverse tarsal joint with the calcaneocuboid joint.
Calcaneocuboid	Saddle joint	Anterior end of the calcaneus articulates with the posterior surface of the cuboidal bone	Small degree of mobility but does carry out inversion and eversion of the foot (5) Forms the transverse tarsal joint with the talocalcaneonavicular joint
Tarsometatarsal	Synovial plane joints that allow gliding (arthrodial joint)	Articulations between base of the metatarsals and the anterior surfaces of the cuneiforms and the cuboid bone	Gliding of the tarsal and metatarsal bones upon each other
Metatarsophalangeal (MTP)	*Condyloid joint:* an oval-shaped end is received into a congruent elliptical cavity	Articulations between the anterior surface of the metatarsal bones and the posterior surfaces of the proximal phalanges	Flexion, extension, abduction, and adduction of the phalanges
Interphalangeal	Hinge joint	Articulations between the head of the proximal phalanx and the end of the distal phalanx	Flexion and extension of the phalanges

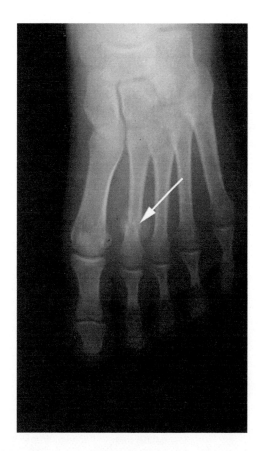

FIGURE 7.38 Stress fracture of the second metatarsal with callus formation.

Signs of alleviation of pain when resting, exacerbation of pain when using the fractured area, or tenderness at the site of the fracture may be experienced by the individual, requiring medical attention.

LISFRANC INJURY

Also known as a midfoot injury, this results from torn ligaments or fractured tarsal bones in the midfoot.

The midfoot is formed by the three cuneiform bones, cuboidal bone, and navicular bone, along with their ligaments, which are vital to maintain the arch and are also vital for walking. The Lisfranc joint describes the many individual joints between the midfoot tarsal bones and the proximal attachment of the midfoot bones to the forefoot (metatarsal) bones. Any fracture or dislocation to bone in this area or ligamentous tear will cause a Lisfranc injury (**Figure 7.39**).

Unlike stress fractures, which are commonly seen in athletes and runners, Lisfranc injuries do not require repetitive movements to cause a fracture, and instead can be caused by a twist of the foot downwards and then falling. Bruising on both surfaces of the foot, but especially the plantar surface, indicates a differential of a Lisfranc injury. Although non-surgical treatments may be recommended for individuals whose Lisfranc injury is due to a sprained ligament and nothing else, surgery is recommended for injuries involving fractures or dislocations of the bones in the midfoot or torn ligaments.

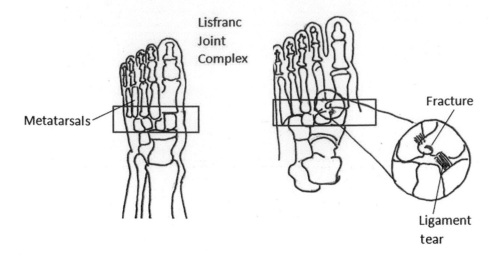

FIGURE 7.39 Lisfranc injury. (Courtesy of Alina Humdani.)

Other Anatomical Anomalies

Hammer toe: Hammer toe describes a phalanx that is permanently pushed downwards, normally as a result of pressure from the wrong size or type of footwear. The joints usually involved are the proximal interphalangeal joints from the second to the fourth toes.

Bunions: bunions are also an important finding at the base of the hallux (big toe). A bunion is a bony deformity of the joint, which may cause hallux valgus – an abnormal valgus alignment of the big toe.

Individuals with hallux valgus may notice some changes with their gait, as the hallux valgus causes a reduction in dorsiflexion when walking (**Figure 7.40**).

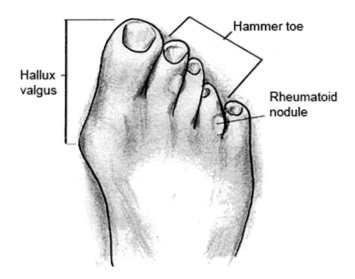

FIGURE 7.40 Abnormalities of the forefoot. (Courtesy of Gabriela Barzyk.)

Gout Affecting the Metatarsophalangeal Joints

Gout is a form of arthritis which is caused by a highly elevated level of uric acid in the blood. The uric acid then crystallises and is deposited within joints, causing them to become inflamed. A common area for gout to develop in the body is at the metatarsophalangeal joints in the foot, commonly at the first metatarsophalangeal joint, at the base of the big toe. This condition is called podagra.

Remember the five signs of inflammation: **r**edness (*rubor*), **P**ain (*dolor*), **H**eat (*calor*), **S**welling (*tumor*), and **L**oss of function (*functio laesa*).

The Spring Ligament (Figure 7.32)

Also known as the plantar calcaneonavicular ligament, it connects the navicular to the calcaneus and also supports the head of the talus. This ligament is especially important, as it helps maintain the medial arch of the foot and, by supporting the head of the talus through its attachments from the calcaneus and the navicular, bears most of the body weight.

Arches of the Foot (Figure 7.41)

To help the foot maintain its concave shape, the medial, lateral, and transverse foot arches act like a spring network to bear the weight of the body and absorb the shock produced during movement.

- The medial longitudinal foot arch is supported by the spring (calcaneonavicular ligament) and the plantar ligaments and is the higher of the two longitudinal foot arches. This arch spans over the calcaneus to the first three metatarsal bones.

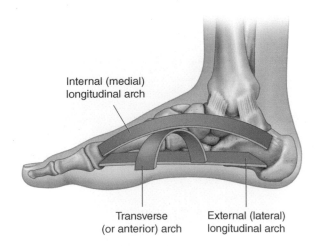

FIGURE 7.41 Arches of the foot. (Courtesy of Gabriella Barzyk.)

- The lateral longitudinal arch is slightly flatter and spans from the calcaneus to the fourth and fifth metatarsals. Similarly supported by the plantar ligaments, it is connected to the medial arch via the anterior transverse foot arch.
- The transverse foot arch lies coronally and is attached to the metatarsal bases and cuneiform bones. Supported by the plantar ligaments, it forms a connection between both longitudinal arches.

The Use of High-Heeled Shoes

Unwise, less stable, and more prone to collapse is the consequence of wearing high-heeled shoes. When a person attempts to step in high heels, the tibia moves posteriorly, pulling on the talus due to the talocrural joint. The spring ligament is attached to the talus, causing the medial foot arch (normally maintained by the spring ligament and plantar ligaments of the foot) to collapse and be less stable.

Muscles Contributing to Movements of the Foot

Movements of the foot are completed by the muscles of the lower leg (anterior, lateral, and posterior compartments), of which it is vital to recognise and identify the points of origin and insertions for each of the muscles contributing to movements of the foot, but also their innervation, blood supply, and action.

Intrinsic Muscles of the Foot

For the basic clinical sciences student, it is important to recognise that the intrinsic muscles of the foot on the plantar side are organised into four layers. Similar in composition to the intrinsic muscles of the hand, i.e., both the hand and the foot have interossei on their dorsal and ventral sides (in the case of the foot, on their dorsal and plantar sides), the toes are also equipped with lumbricals; what is important to take away is that the intrinsic muscles of the foot modify actions of the long tendons and generate fine movements of the toes.

Blood Supply and Innervation of the Foot

The foot is mainly supplied by branches of the posterior tibial artery and the dorsalis pedis artery.

The Posterior Tibial Artery

This artery enters the plantar aspect of the foot, posterior to the medial malleolus, and branches into the medial and lateral plantar arteries. The lateral plantar artery (the largest branch) turns medially and joins with the dorsalis pedis artery at the first intermetatarsal space to form the plantar arch to supply the digital branches to the toes. The medial plantar artery supplies the medial side of the big toe.

The Dorsalis Pedis Artery

Anterior to begin with, this artery passes inferiorly past the cuneiform bones, lateral to the extensor hallucis longus tendon, to join the plantar arch. It supplies the dorsum of the foot and both sides of the big toe.

Innervation of the Foot (Figure 7.42)

There are five nerves which innervate the skin of the foot:

- *Tibial nerve:* it runs through the calcaneal branches to the heel, medial plantar nerve to skin on the medial side of the sole, and medial three and half toes including their nail beds. The lateral plantar nerve supplies the skin on the lateral aspect of the sole and fifth toe and lateral aspect of the fourth toe including their nail beds (compare with the distribution of the median and the ulnar nerves in the hand).
- *Deep fibular (deep peroneal):* see above.
- *Superficial fibular (superficial peroneal):* see above.
- *Sural nerve:* it supplies the lateral aspect of the dorsum of the foot.
- *Saphenous nerve:* running with the LSV, this is a terminal branch of the femoral nerve and is sensory in function and found in subcutaneous tissue; it supplies the medial aspect of the dorsum of the foot to the base of the hallux.

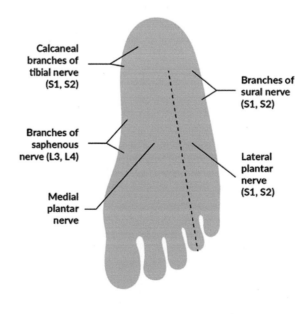

FIGURE 7.42 Sensory innervation of the foot, dorsal and plantar surfaces. (Courtesy of Ali Baker.)

An important rule to adhere to here is that the muscles of the foot are mainly innervated by the tibial nerve (via its lateral and medial plantar nerves), except for the extensor digitorum brevis, extensor hallucis brevis, and the first two dorsal interossei, which are innervated by the deep peroneal nerve.

CLINICAL NOTE

PLANTAR FASCIITIS

Plantar fasciitis is also known as a common cause in the UK of "heel pain". It is caused by the straining and inflammation of the plantar aponeurosis and can result from high-energy exercises such as running or high-impact aerobics. This may be further exacerbated by patients wearing inappropriate footwear such as worn-out shoes.

Patients present to the physician with a "stabbing or knife-like" heel pain, relieved with rest and aggravated with activity – both core symptoms for a diagnosis of plantar fasciitis. Patients may often experience post-static dyskinesia, the medical term for pain being felt upon walking the first few steps after rising from a seated or lying position.

Ankle Examination and Testing the Movements of the Foot

Four main movements of the foot are clinically tested in the musculoskeletal ankle examination, through both active, passive, and resisted movements. The following commands next to the movements are the recognised method to test for active movements of the ankle joint:

- *Dorsiflexion:* ask the patient to point their toes up to the ceiling.
- *Plantarflexion:* ask the patient to point their toes to the ground.
- *Inversion:* ask the patient to turn their feet inwards together.
- *Eversion:* ask the patient to turn their feet outwards.

After asking the patient to complete these movements on the examiner's command and unaided, the examiner will then do these movements on the patient whilst the patient remains relaxed. This is called passive movement. The examiner will then ask the patient to "stop me doing these movements" or "push against me". As the examiner is performing a movement, e.g., dorsiflexion, they will ask the patient to "push against my hand". This is to test resisted movement of the foot.

Any weakness in any of these movements will indicate which group of muscles or which area has potentially been affected and/or injured.

Assessing for the Integrity of the Achilles Tendon

As part of the ankle examination in the clinic, to test the function of muscles of the posterior compartment (plantarflexion) and the integrity of the Achilles tendon, the Simmonds-Thompson test can be performed. One of the techniques to do this test is by asking the patient to kneel one leg on the chair, with the other leg hanging down. The clinician then squeezes the back of the leg, and if the Achilles tendon is intact, the suspended foot should plantarflex. Feeling a gap within the tendon is another way to check the integrity of the calcaneal tendon.

Vascular Examination of the Foot

Palpate the dorsalis pedis artery as noted earlier. The posterior tibial artery is usually palpated halfway between the medial malleolus and the calcaneus on the medial side, where its coverings is at its thinnest.

Palpation points are clinically significant, as these locations are heavily used in the peripheral vasculature examination to assess the blood supply to the distal ends of the lower limbs, which may be commonly affected by microvascular disease, often caused by poorly controlled diabetes mellitus.

Furthermore, the ankle brachial pressure index (ABPI) can also be performed as part of the peripheral vasculature medical examination to assess for peripheral arterial disease. ABPI compares the blood pressure at the ankle to the blood pressure in the brachium (arm). If there is a narrowing of the lower limb arteries, the systolic pressure in the arteries of the foot will be reduced.

ABPI = highest foot systolic blood pressure/brachial systolic blood pressure (**Table 7.12**).

Values are acquired by measuring the blood pressure over the brachium and the ankle separately, listening for turbulent blood flow when the cuff is inflated by using Doppler ultrasound both times. When acquiring a value for the highest systolic blood pressure in the ankle, two values are taken: one for the dorsalis pedis

TABLE 7.12: Ankle brachial pressure index (ABPI)

Description	Value
Normal	≻1.0
Intermittent claudication (obstruction of the arteries, usually during exercise, causing pain)	0.5–0.95
Rest pain	0.3–0.5
Critical ischaemia	< 0.2

and another for the posterior tibial, and the highest systolic blood pressure is used.

Diabetic Foot

The umbrella term "diabetic foot" describes a pathology of the foot, such as ulceration, peripheral neuropathy, or microvascular disease, resulting from poorly controlled diabetes mellitus and its complications.

There are three main components to the development of diabetic foot:

- Neuropathy of the sensory, motor, and autonomic nerves. Sensory neuropathy leads to impaired skin sensation and susceptibility to injury. Motor neuropathy causes dysfunction of the intrinsic foot muscles and deformities. Autonomic neuropathy results in impaired sweating of the foot and crack formation.
- Angiopathy of the arteries of the foot causes reduced blood supply and delayed healing of ulcers.
- Immunosuppression (diabetic patients show more susceptibility to develop infections) (**Figure 7.43**).

Remember, diabetes mellitus is a systemic disease and can affect other organs such as the retina (diabetic retinopathy) or kidneys (diabetic nephropathy).

In addition to these factors, poor footwear makes things worse. Patients with poorly controlled diabetic foot are at risk of leg amputations.

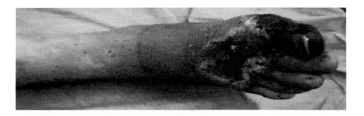

FIGURE 7.43 Advanced gangrene of the right foot due to uncontrolled diabetes mellitus. (Courtesy of Aqeel S. Mahmood.)

Revision Questions

Q1.

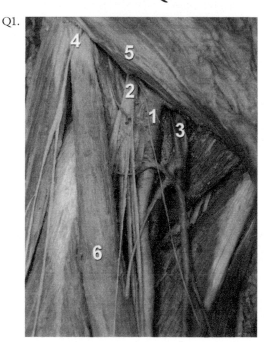

(Courtesy of Department of Anatomical Sciences, SGUL.)

Q1. Which vessel is indicated by the number 1 in the image?
a. Femoral artery
b. Femoral vein
c. Long saphenous vein
d. Popliteal artery
e. Short saphenous vein

Q2. What is the clinical significance of the indicated vessel?
a. Can be palpated for a pulse
b. Can be harvested for use in a CABG operation
c. Is a common site for development of thrombi
d. Is prone to enlarging and becoming an aneurysm
e. Is often used for taking bloods when venous access on the upper limb is impaired

Q3.

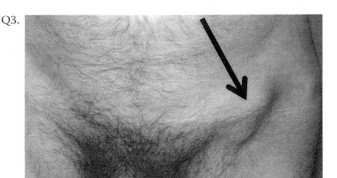

(Courtesy of Department of Anatomical Sciences, SGUL.)

Q3. Which of the following best describes the enlarged lymph node shown in the image?
a. Deep inguinal lymph node
b. External iliac lymph node
c. Internal iliac lymph node
d. Para-aortic lymph node
e. Superficial inguinal lymph node

Q4. Where does this structure drain to?
a. Deep inguinal lymph nodes
b. External iliac lymph nodes
c. Internal iliac lymph nodes
d. Para-aortic lymph nodes
e. Superficial inguinal lymph nodes

Q5.

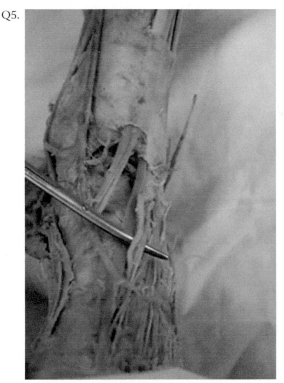

(Courtesy of Department of Anatomical Sciences, SGUL.)

Q5. Which vessel is indicated in the image?
a. Dorsalis pedis artery
b. Dorsal venous arch
c. Medial plantar artery
d. Lateral plantar artery
e. Posterior tibial artery

Q6. What is the clinical significance of the indicated vessel?
a. Most commonly affected by DVT
b. Related to incidence of arterial ulcers
c. Used to take the pulse from the lower limb
d. Used in coronary angiography
e. Used in reconstructive surgery grafting

Q7A. A 40-year-old man presented to mountaineering emergency services with a fracture sustained while skiing. The patient commented that he is a novice skier and remembered falling forwards over a rock in his path. The patient is in excruciating pain and is unable to weight-bear on his left foot.
Which sort of injury is consistent with this presentation?
a. Left malleolar fracture
b. Lisfranc injury
c. Pott's fracture
d. Stress fracture

Q7B. Which is the most common site for this injury to occur?
a. First metatarsophalangeal joint
b. Within the second and third metatarsals
c. Proximal interphalangeal joints, from the second to the fourth digit
d. Medial aspect of talus

Q8. An elderly female patient presented to A&E complaining of pain in her left calf, which is also heavy, achy, and warm. The doctor in charge of her care is concerned that she may be experiencing deep venous thrombosis and would like to send her for an ultrasound scan.
Where does the long saphenous vein drain to?
a. Femoral vein
b. Internal iliac vein
c. Popliteal vein
d. Small saphenous vein

Q9. A 20-year-old male cross-country runner sustained a fracture in his forefoot. The patient has been training for the past 4 months for this race and is in severe pain when he tries to continue running. This pain reduced after rest.
Q9A. Which sort of injury is consistent with this presentation?
a. Lisfranc injury
b. Navicular bone fracture
c. Pott's fracture
d. Stress fracture

Q9B. Which is the most common site for this injury to occur?
a. First metatarsophalangeal joint
b. Within the second and third metatarsals
c. Proximal interphalangeal joints, from the second to the fourth digit
d. Anterior surface of the distal aspect of the tibia

Q10. A group of middle-aged women were walking in Oxford Street, shopping at the nearby department stores. All were wearing stiletto high heels and were complaining of discomfort when walking and were unable to walk stably.
Which ligament has been pulled to cause the medial foot arch to collapse?
a. Calcaneofibular ligament
b. Deltoid ligament
c. Plantar calcaneonavicular (spring) ligament
d. Talocrural ligament

Q11. What are the causes of acute compartment syndrome and its earliest sign? (See text.)

Q12. What are the structures that leave the pelvis to enter the gluteal region under the piriformis muscle? (See text.)

Q13. What are the main factors which lead to the development of diabetic foot? (See text.)

Q14. What are the lower limb injuries which possibly occur following a fall from a height?

Q15. List three dashboard injuries that may happen to a front seat occupant.

Q16.

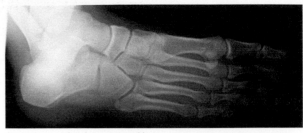

(Courtesy of Salam Ismael.)

Q16. A 21-year-old male with a history of a twisting injury of the right foot over the edge of a curb. He sustained a fifth metatarsal fracture that is minimally displaced. The risk with these fractures is non-union due to the pulling effect of the muscles attached to it. Name the two muscles attached to the fifth metatarsal that can cause non-union by their pulling action.

Answers

A1. a
A2. a
A3. e
A4. a
A5. a
A6. c
A7A. b
A7B. b
A8. a
A9A. d
A9B. b
A10. c
A11,12,13. See text
A14. Fracture of the calcaneus, tibial plateau, shaft of femur, acetabular fracture (central hip dislocation).
A15. Fracture of the patella, femoral shaft, and posterior hip dislocation.
A16. Peroneus tertius and peroneus brevis.

Further Reading

Ball T. Acute leg ischaemia. *BMJ* (2013) 346:f2681 doi: https://doi.org/10.1136/bmj.f2681
Baker QF, Aldoori MI. Chronic critical limb ischaemia and diabetic foot. Clinical Surgery: A Practical Guide (2009) pp. 242–250.
Developmental dysplasia of the hip. https://www.nhs.uk/conditions/developmental-dysplasia-of-the-hip/
Lim CS, et al. Diagnosis and management of venous leg ulcers. *BMJ* (2018) 362:k3115 doi: 10.1136/bmj.k3115
Shelbourne KD, Nitz PA. The O'Donoghue triad revisited. Combined knee injuries involving anterior cruciate and medial collateral ligament tears. *Am J Sports Med* (1991) 19(5):474–477. doi: 10.1177/036354659101900509

INDEX

Note: Locators in *italics* represent figures and **bold** indicate tables in the text.

A

AAA, *see* Abdominal aortic aneurysm
Abdomen
    anterior abdominal wall, 149–155
    blood supply, 158, 160
    colon, 182–185
    duodenum, 164–166
    gallbladder and biliary system, 173–176
    gut, 158–159
    ileum and jejunum, 176–180
    kidneys, 190–193
    large bowel/large intestine, 180–182
    liver, 170–173
    lumbar plexus, 187–189
    nerve supply, gut and pelvic organs,
        159–160
    nerve supply and lymph drainage, 161–164
    pancreas, 166–168
    peritoneum, 155–158
    posterior abdominal wall, 185–187
    retroperitoneal space, 189–190
    spleen, 168–170
Abdominal aorta, 158
Abdominal aortic aneurysm (AAA), 158
Abdominal policeman, 156
Abducens nerve (CN VI), 51
ABPI, *see* Ankle brachial pressure index
ACA, *see* Anterior cerebral artery
Accessory nerve (CN XI), 52–53
Acetabulofemoral joint, *see* Hip joint
Achalasia, 161, *162*
Achilles tendon, 259
ACL, *see* Anterior cruciate ligament
Acoustic neuroma, 45
ACS, *see* Acute compartment syndrome
ACTH, *see* Adrenocorticotropic hormone
Acute compartment syndrome (ACS), 260
Acute pancreatitis, 167, *167*
Acute poliomyelitis, 27
Acute respiratory distress syndrome (ARDS),
    127
Acute urinary retention, 207
Adamkiewicz, artery of, 24, 29
Adnexa, 229
Adolescent idiopathic scoliosis (AIS), 116
Adrenocorticotropic hormone (ACTH), 5, 190
AF, *see* Atrial fibrillation
Afferent pain fibres, 136
Age-related calcification, normal valve, 140
AIS, *see* Adolescent idiopathic scoliosis
Alar and basal plates, 15–17, 29
Alcock's canal, 213, 236
Allergic rhinitis, 47
Amygdala, 4
Anal canal; *see also* Pelvic organs
    anal cushions, 210
    anal valves, 210
    conjoint longitudinal muscle, 211
    continence, 211
    dentate, 210
    external anal sphincter, 210
    haemorrhoids, 211

    internal sphincter, 210
    lower rectum, *210*
    painful perianal conditions, 211
    pectinate, 210
    PR examination, 211
    upper and lower, 210, **210**
Angina pectoris, 136
Angiography, 245
Ankle brachial pressure index (ABPI), 268, **268**
Ankle jerk reflex, 259
Ankle joint
    deltoid ligament, 262
    examination, 268
    lateral aspect, 262, *262*, **263**
    ligaments, 261–262, *262*
    medial aspect, 262, *262*
ANS, *see* Autonomic nervous system
Ansa cervicalis, 53, 60, 61, 63, 77
Anterior abdominal wall
    anomalies, 153
    blood supply, 152
    burst abdomen, 154, *155*
    divisions, 149, *149*
    flat muscles, 151, **152**
    hernia, 153
    intertubercular plane, 149
    layers, 149
    muscles, 150
    necrotising fasciitis, 154
    pyramidalis, 150
    rectus abdominis, 150
    rectus sheath, *150*, 150–151
    skin, 149
    superficial fascia, 149
    surgical incisions, 154
    transpyloric (Addison's) plane, 149
Anterior cerebral artery (ACA), 13, 32
Anterior cord syndrome, 26
Anterior cruciate ligament (ACL), 252
Anterior superior iliac spine (ASIS), 197, 198,
    244
Antral cancer, *164*
Aorta, 122, *122*, 140
Aortic aneurysms, 123
Aponeurosis, 33
Arachnoid mater, 11
ARDS, *see* Acute respiratory distress
        syndrome
Arterial vasculature, brain
    ACA, 13
    anterior circulation, 12
    CCA, 12
    circle of Willis, 12, 13, *13*
    ICAs, 12, 13
    MCA, 13
    posterior circulation, 12
    stroke, 13
Arteria pancreatica magna, 169
Arteries, anterior forearm
    anatomical snuffbox, 95
    radial artery, 95, 96
    ulnar artery, 95
Arthroplasty, 238

Arthroscopy, 253–254
Ascending tracts
    dorsal column and spinothalamic, 22, *22*
    neuronal arrangement, **23**
    nociceptive flexion reflex, 22
Ascites, 157
ASD, *see* Atrial septal defect
ASIS, *see* Anterior superior iliac spine
Asthma, 127
Atresia, 229
Atrial fibrillation (AF), 137
Atrial septal defect (ASD), 138
Auerbach's/myenteric plexus, 162
Auriculotemporal nerve, 50
Autonomic nervous system (ANS), spinal cord
    dermatome, 20, **20**, *21*
    movements, **20**
    myotome, 20
    opposing effects, SNS and PNS, **20**
    PNS, 20
    SNS, 19–20
Avascular necrosis, 239
Axilla
    axillary artery, 105–106
    axillary lymph nodes, 106, **106**, *106*
    axillary vein, 106
    boundaries, **105**
    brachial plexus, 106, *107*
    contents, 105
    muscles, 105, **106**
    surgical importance, **107**
Axillary nerve, 83, 85, 86, *87*
Azygos system, 124, 133, 140, 196

B

Babinski's sign, 22
Bachmann's bundle, 136
Balloon angioplasty, 136, 241, 245
Barrett's oesophagus, 161
Bartholin's (greater vestibular) glands,
    225–226
Basal ganglia
    caudate nucleus, 6
    dopamine, 6
    internal capsule, 6
    lentiform nucleus, 6
    Mulligan's stain, *6*
    nucleus accumbens, 6
    striatum, 6
    subthalamic nucleus, 6
    and thalamocortical circuits, *7*
Batson's plexus, 187
BCS, *see* Breast-conserving surgery
Beck's triad, 134
Bell's palsy, 52
Benign prostatic hyperplasia (BPH), 224
Bicipital aponeurosis, 90
Bicuspid aortic valve, 140
Bilharziasis, 169, 173, 208
Bimalleolar ankle fracture, 263
BI-RADS, *see* Breast Imaging Reporting and
        Data System

Bladder
    acute urinary retention, 207
    cystitis, 207
    cystoscopy, 208, *208*
    detrusor muscle, 207
    distended, *207*
    haematuria, 208
    injuries, 208
    micturate, urge to, 207
    stone formation, 208, *209*
    suprapubic cystostomy, 207
    trigone, 208
    tumours, 207
    urothelium, 207
Blastocyst, 15
Blood supply, spinal cord
    segmental arteries, 24, *25*
    venous drainage, 25
    vertical arteries, 24
Boot top fracture, 264
BPH, *see* Benign prostatic hyperplasia
Brachial artery, 90, 91
Brachial plexus, *84*
    axillary sheath, 84
    cords, 85
    distal aspect of forearm injury, 88
    inferior to elbow injury, 88
    middle part of upper arm injury, 87
    musculocutaneous nerve injury, 87
    nerves, 85
    radial nerve injury, axilla, 87
    roots, 85
    sensory distribution, 86
    terminal branches, 85–86
Brain, anatomy of
    arterial vasculature, 12–13
    basal ganglia, 6, *7*
    brainstem, *7*, 7–8
    cerebellum, 4, *5*
    cerebrum, 1–4
    cranial nerves, 8, *9*, **10**
    CSF circulation and ventricular system, 11–12
    diencephalon, 5
    embryology, 1
    medulla oblongata, 8
    midbrain, 7–8
    pons, 8
    sagittal section, *2*
    skull base, 11
    venous vasculature, 13–14
Brainstem, 7, *7*
    interpeduncular fossa, 7
    medulla oblongata, 8
    midbrain, 7–8
    parts, 7
    pons, 8
    surface features, *7*
    tectal plate, 7
Branchial cyst, 72, *72*
Breast
    anterior view, *141*
    blood supply, 142, *142*
    boundaries, 141–142
    cancer, *143*, 143–144
    Cooper's ligaments, 142
    NAC, 142
    sagittal section, *141*
    triple assessment, 143–144, *144*

Breast-conserving surgery (BCS), 144
Breast Imaging Reporting and Data System
    (BI-RADS), 144
Broca's area, 3
Brown-Séquard syndrome, 25–26
Buck's fascia, 214, 215
Bulbourethral glands, 224
Bunions, 266
Burst abdomen, 154

C

CABG, *see* Coronary artery bypass graft
CABG surgery, *see* Coronary artery bypass
    graft
CAD, *see* Coronary artery disease
Caecum
    acute appendicitis, 182
    inflamed distended appendix, *182*
    retrocaecal appendicitis, 182
    taeniae coli, 182
    vermiform appendix, 182
Calot's triangle, 174
Camper's chiasm, 95, *95*
Camper's fascia, 149
Cannonball metastatic lung cancer, *128*
Cardiac plexus, 120
Cardiac tamponade, 133–134
Carpal tunnel syndrome, 100
Cataracts, 41
Cauda equina syndrome, 27
Cavernous sinus thrombosis, 14
CCA, *see* Common carotid artery
Central cord syndrome, 26, 27
Cerebellum
    anatomical lobes, 4
    anterior view, *5*
    arbor vitae, 4
    peduncles, 4
    vermis, the, 4
Cerebrospinal fluid (CSF)
    choroid plexus, 11
    circulation, 11–12
Cerebrum
    anatomical lobes, 1, *2*
    corpuscallosum, 2, *2*
    frontal lobe, 3
    functions, lobe, **1**
    gyri, 2
    limbic lobe, 4
    longitudinal fissure, **1**
    occipital lobe, 4, *4*
    parietal lobe, 4
    sulcus, 2
    temporal lobe, 3
Cervical excitation, 230
Cervical lymph nodes, 71
Cervical oesophagus
    anatomical relations, 75
    blood supply, 75
    dysphagia, 75, **76**
    lymphatic drainage, 75
    nerve supply, 75
Cervical rib, 115
Cervical spine injury, 59–60
Cervical sympathetic trunk, 60–61
Chancre, 216
Chassaignac's (carotid) tubercle, 60

CHD, *see* Congenital hip dislocation
Chest drains, 130
Cholecystectomy, 156
Cholecystostomy, 175
Cholelithiasis, 175
Choroid plexus, 11
Chronic obstructive pulmonary disease
    (COPD), 127
Chylothorax, 130
Cingulate sulcus, 4
Circle of Willis, 12, *13*
Clavicle (collar bone)
    conoid tubercle, 80
    roles, 80
    superior and inferior surfaces, *80*
Clitoris, 225
Coeliac plexus, 160
Collateral ligaments, knee, 252
Colles' fascia, 149
Colles' fracture, 92, *92*
Colon
    ascending, 183
    caecum, 182–183
    colostomy, 183
    CRC, 183
    descending, 183
    diverticulosis, 184, *184*
    Hirschsprung's disease, 184, *185*
    ileostomy, 183
    ischaemic colitis, 184
    sigmoid, 183
    sigmoid volvulus, 184, *185*
    stomas, 183
    transverse, 183
Colorectal cancer, 210
Colorectal carcinoma (CRC), 183
Colostomy, 183
Common carotid artery (CCA), 12, 52
    carotid body, 63, *63*
    carotid sinus, 63, *63*, 64
    endarterectomy, 63, *63*
Congenital diaphragmatic hernia, 119
Congenital hip dislocation (CHD), 238
Congenital pyloric stenosis, 164, *164*
Conjunctivitis, 41
Cooper's ligaments, 142
COPD, *see* Chronic obstructive pulmonary
    disease
Coronary angiogram, 136
Coronary artery bypass graft (CABG) surgery,
    116, 133, 136, 249
Coronary artery disease (CAD), 137
Coronary circulation
    left coronary artery, 134
    right coronary artery, 134
Coronavirus disease 2019 (COVID-19),
    127–128
Corpus cavernosum, 214
Corpus spongiosum, 214, 232
Corticobulbar tract fibres
    facial nucleus, 24
    LMNs, 23
    pseudobulbar palsy, 24
Corticospinal tract
    lateral, 23
    lesions, **24**
    LMNs, 23, 24
    medulla, 22–23

neurons, 29
UMNs, 23, 24
Costochondritis, 115
Coverings, spinal cord
bony, *18*
denticulate ligaments, 17
epidural space, 17
meningeal, 17, *19*
pia mater, 17
sub-arachnoid space, 17
Cowper's glands, 224
Cranial nerves, 8, **10**
brain, anatomy of, 8, *9*, **10**
cavity, internal view, *9*
CN III (oculomotor), 50
CN II (optic), 49
CN I (olfactory), 49
CN IV (trochlear), 50
CN IX (glossopharyngeal), 52
CN VI (abducens), 51
CN VII (facial), 51–52
CN VIII (vestibulocochlear), 52
CN V3 (mandibular), 50
CN V2 (maxillary), 50
CN V (trigeminal), 50
CN XI (accessory), 52–53
CN XII (hypoglossal), 53
CN X (vagus), 52
CV, V1 (ophthalmic), 50
function and path, **10**
recurrent laryngeal, 52
roots II to XII, *9*
Craniosynostosis, 34
CRC, *see* Colorectal carcinoma
Cricothyroidotomy, 67
Crista terminalis, 136, 137
Crohn's disease, 179, **179**
Cryptorchidism, 218, 220
CSF, *see* Cerebrospinal fluid
Cubital fossa, 90
Cubital tunnel syndrome, 97
Culdocentesis, 227
Cushing's syndrome, 190
Cystic hygroma, 72
Cystitis, 207
Cystogastrostomy, 167
Cystoscopy, 208, *208*

D

Dacryoadenitis, 41
Deafness, 45
Deep inferior epigastric perforator (DIEP) flap, 154
Deep vein thrombosis (DVT), 128, 251
Degeneration, spinal, 27
Degenerative disc disease, 187
Denonvillier's fascia, 209, 226
Denticulate ligaments, 17
Dermatome, 20, **20**, *21*
Descending tracts
corticobulbar, 23–24
corticospinal, 22, 23, *23*
Developmental dysplasia, hip, 238
Diabetic foot, 268–269, *269*
Diaphragm
abdominal surface, *118*
attachments, **117**

embryology, 116–117
ligaments, 117
motor innervation, 117
phrenic nerve, 117, 119
respiration, 119
Diaphragma sellae, 11
Diencephalon, 5, *5*
DIEP flap, *see* Deep inferior epigastric perforator
Digital rectal examination (DRE), 211
Digits
extensors, 102
pulley system of, 101–102
DIP joint, *see* Distal interphalangeal (DIP) joint
Distal interphalangeal (DIP) joint, 95
Distal radio-ulnar joint, 93–94
Diverticulosis, colon, 184, *184*
Dopamine, 5
Dorsal venous arch, lower limb, 248
Down's syndrome, 138
DRE, *see* Digital rectal examination
DU, *see* Duodenal ulceration
Duodenal ulceration (DU), 165
Duodenum
blood supply and venous drainage, 166
D1, superior part, 165
D2, descending part, 166
D3, inferior part, 166
D4, ascending part, 166
nerve supply and lymphatic drainage, 166
parts, 164, *165*
peptic ulcer, 165, *165*
Dura mater, 11, 13, 17
DVT, *see* Deep vein thrombosis
Dysphagia
causes of, **76**
definition, 75

E

Ear
anatomy, *45*
auditory ossicles, 43
auditory tube, 43
auricle/pinna, 41, *42*
blood supply, 42, 44, 45
canal, 42
cochlea, 44
external, 41–42, *42*
hearing loss, 45
infections, 44
inner, *44*, 44–45
innervation, 42, 44, 45
labyrinth, 44–45
mastoiditis, 44
middle, *43*, 43–44
muscles, middle, 43
otitis externa, 42
scala vestibuli, 44
tympanic membrane, 43
EBUS, *see* Endobronchial ultrasound bronchoscopy
Ectopic gestation, 230
Elbow
dislocation, 93
joint, 93, *93*
Embolism, 13, 32
Emphysema, 129

EMR, *see* Endoscopic mucosal resection
Endobronchial ultrasound bronchoscopy (EBUS), 123
Endocardium, 134
Endometriosis, 229
Endoscopic mucosal resection (EMR), 164
Endoscopic retrograde cholangiopancreatography (ERCP), 174, *174*, *175*
Endoscopic thoracic sympathectomy, 121
Endotracheal intubation, 67
ENS, *see* Enteric nervous system
Enteric nervous system (ENS), 160
Epicardium, 134
Epididymo-orchitis, 220
Epidural space, 17
Epidural *vs.* spinal anaesthesia, 27–28
Epigastric hernia, 153
Epiglottitis, 67
Epispadias, 217
Epistaxis, 48
ERCP, *see* Endoscopic retrograde cholangiopancreatography
External carotid artery, 64
Extracapsular ligaments, hip, 238
Eye
accommodation reflex, 39
aqueous humour chambers, 39
arterial supply, 39
cataracts, 41
ciliary ganglion, 39
conjunctivitis, 41
dacryoadenitis, 41
exophthalmos, 39, *39*
extraocular muscles, 39–40, **40**, *40*
glaucoma, 41
innervation, 38–39
intrinsic muscles, 40
lacrimal gland, 40
layers, *37*, 37–38
lymphatics, 39
occlusion, retinal artery, 39
oculomotor nerve (CN III), 38, 40
open angle glaucoma, 76
ophthalmic artery, 76
optic disc, *38*
optic nerve (CN II), 38, *38*
optic neuritis, 41
orbital blowout fracture, 41
pituitary adenoma, 41
pupillary light reflex, 38
retinal detachment, 41
retinoblastoma, 41
venous drainage, 39

F

Facial nerve (CN VII), 51–52
Fallopian tubes/oviducts, 229–230, *230*
False/pseudoaneurysm, 158
Falx cerebri, 11
Fascia, neck
ansa cervicalis, 61
cervical plexus, 61
cervical sympathetic trunk, 61
deep cervical, 60
infrahyoid muscles, 60, **61**
nerves, 61

phrenic nerve (C3–C5), 61
suprahyoid muscles, 60
vagus nerve (CN X), 61
Fasciculus cuneatus, 22
Fasciculus gracilis, 22
Fasciotomy, 260
FDP, *see* Flexor digitorum profundus
Felon, 103
Female genital mutilation, 226
Female lower genital tract, *225*
    Bartholin's (greater vestibular) glands,
        225–226
    blood supply, 225
    caudal block, 226
    clitoris, 225
    hymen, 226
    labia majora, 225
    labia minora, 225
    lymphatic drainage, 225
    mons pubis, 225
    nerve supply, 225
    paraurethral glands, 226
    pelvic organ prolapse, 226
    posterior commissure, 225
    Skene's (lesser vestibular) glands, 226
    urethral meatus, 225
    vagina, 226
    vestibule, 225
Female reproductive organs
    embryology, 224
    lower genital tract, 224–226
    upper genital tract, 227–231
Female upper genital tract
    culdocentesis, 227
    ovaries, 230–231
    rectouterine pouch, 227
    uterine tubes, 229–230
    uterus, 227–229
Femoral artery, 244
Femoral artery pseudoaneurysm, 246
Femoral nerve (L2–L4), 188, 242
Femoral venepuncture, 246
Femoro-popliteal bypass graft, 247
Femur
    aneurysms, 246
    anterior and posterior view, *240*
    blood supply, 239
    canal, 242
    femoral artery, 241
    femoral ring, 242
    fractures, shaft, 240, *240, 241*
    greater trochanter, 239
    hernia, 242
    intercondylar fossa, 239
    intertrochanteric crest, 239
    intertrochanteric line, 239
    intracapsular fractures, 239
    lesser trochanter, 239
    linea aspera, 239
    NOF, 239
    quadrate tubercle, 239
    triangle, 241, *241*
Fibula
    anterior and posterior view, *255*
    fractures, 255, *256*
    lower end, 255
    peroneal nerve, 255
    shaft of, 255

Filum terminale, 17
Flail chest, 116
Flat muscles
    conjoint tendon, 151
    external oblique, 151, *151*
    internal oblique, *151*
    lateral abdominal wall, **152**
    right transversus abdominis, *151*
Flexion-distraction fractures, 187
Flexor digitorum profundus (FDP), 95
Flexor retinaculum, 259, *259*
Follicle-stimulating hormone (FSH), 5
Foot
    anatomical anomalies, 266
    ankle joint, 261–262
    anterior surface, *263*
    arches, *266*, 266–267
    blood supply, 267
    bones, **261**
    diabetic, 268–269, *269*
    extensor retinacula, 263, *263*
    fibular retinacula, 263
    forefoot, abnormalities of, *266*
    high-heeled shoes, use of, 267
    innervation, *267*, 267–268
    intrinsic muscles, 267
    joints, 264, *264*, **265**
    muscles and movements, 267
    osteology, 260, *260*, *261*
    plantar fasciitis, 268
    tarsals, 260–261
    vascular examination, 268
Forearm and wrist
    arteries, 95–96
    bones, 91, *91*
    Colles' fracture, 92, *92*
    distal radio-ulnar joint, 93–94
    elbow joint, 93, *93*
    Galeazzi's fracture, 92
    Monteggia's fracture, 92, *93*
    muscles, anterior compartment, **94**, *94*, 94–95
    nerves, 96–97
    neurovascular structures, 95–99
    posterior compartment, 97–99
    radius, 91–92
    Smith's fracture, 92
    ulna, 92
    veins, 96
Fossa ovalis, 138
Fournier's gangrene, 154
Froment's test, 97
FSH, *see* Follicle-stimulating hormone
Funny bone, 85

G

Galeazzi's fracture, 92
Gallbladder and biliary system
    biliary obstruction, 175–176
    biliary tree, 174
    blood supply, 174
    cholelithiasis, 175
    divisions, 173
    ERCP, *174*, 174–175, *175*
    extra hepatic biliary system, 174
    gallstones, 175, *175*, *176*
    Hartmann's pouch, 173, *174*
    hepatobiliary triangle, 174

    jaundice, 176, *176*
    lymphatic drainage, 174
    Murphy's sign, 175
    nerve supply, 174
    post-hepatic (obstructive) jaundice, 175
Gangrene, *269*
Gastric cancers, 164
Gastro-oesophageal reflux disease (GORD),
    161
Gastroschisis, 153
Gastrostomy feeding, 164
Gastrulation, 15
GBS, *see* Guillain-Barré syndrome
Genitofemoral nerve, 188
GH, *see* Growth hormone
Glaucoma, 41
Glisson's capsule, 170
Glossopharyngeal nerve (CN IX), 44, 52, 54,
    55, 56, 63, 73, 78
Gluteal region
    blood supply, 237
    boundaries, *234*
    deep gluteal muscles, 235, **235**
    gluteus minimus and medius, 236
    lateral muscles, thigh and buttock, *234*
    muscles, 234–235
    nerves, 236
    superficial abductors and extensors of hip,
        234, **235**
    Trendelenburg's sign, 236, *237*
Goitre, 69
GORD, *see* Gastro-oesophageal reflux disease
Gout, 266
Gracilis, 243
Gridiron (McBurney's) incision, 154
Groin lump, 223
Groin strain, 243
Growth hormone (GH), 5
G-spot, 226
Guillain-Barré syndrome (GBS), 27
Gut
    coeliac trunk, 159
    divisions, 159
    duodenum, 158
    foregut, 159, *159*
    mesenteries, 159
    midgut, 158, 159
    nerve supply, 159–160
    omphalomesenteric duct, 159
    splanchnic nerves, 159, 160
    stomach, 158

H

Haemarthrosis, 254
Haematuria, 208
Haemoperitoneum, 157
Haemorrhage, 13, 32
Haemorrhoids, 211
Haemothorax, 130
Hammer toe, 266
Hamstrings, 244
Hand; *see also* Wrist and hand
    anatomical snuffbox, 99, *99*
    arches, 104
    arteries, 101
    bones, 101
    carpometacarpal joints, 101

digits, 101–102
felon, 103
grips, 104, *104*
infections, 103
intercarpal joints, 101
intrinsic muscles, 102–103
IP joints, 101
joints, 101
metacarpophalangeal joints, 101, *101*
nerves, 103–104
neurovasculature, 103–104
skin, 101
tenosynovitis, 103
wrist (radiocarpal) joint, 101
Hay fever, 47
Head and neck
arterial supply, 63–64
cervical oesophagus, 75–76
cranial nerves, 49–53
ear, 41–45
eye, 37–41
hyoid bone, 65
larynx, 65–67
lymphatic drainage, 71
nose, 45–49
oral cavity/mouth, 53–56
orbit, 36–37
parathyroid glands, 70
pharynx, 73–75
salivary glands, 56–58
scalp, 33
skull, bones of, *34*, 34–36
thyroid gland, 67–70
trachea, 67
venous drainage, 64
Hearing loss, 45
Heart
AF, 137
angina, 136
apex beat, 132
attack, 136
block, 137
borders, *132*
conductive system, 136, *137*
coronary arteries, *135*
coronary circulation, 134–136
coronary sinus, 134
coronary veins, *135*
cross-section, *139*
electrical conduction diagnosis,
136, *137*
great vessels, 140
internal cardiac anatomy, 137–138
mitral valve, 139
murmurs, 139–140
myocardial infarction, 136
nerve supply, 136–137
pericardium, 132–133
surfaces and borders, 132
tissue, 134
valves, *139*, 139–140
VF, 137
Helicine arteries, 216
Hepatic plexus, 172
Hepatomegaly, 172, *172*
Hernia, 153
colon, 115, *115*
femoral, 242

hiatus, 161, *161*
inguinal, 222–223
Hiatus hernia, 161, *161*
Hilum, 125, *125*
Hip adductors, 243, **243**, *243*
Hip joint
articular capsule, 237
blood supply, femoral head, 238
CHD, 238
dislocation, 238, *238*
extracapsular ligaments, 238
ligaments, 238
socket, 237
THR, 238, *239*
Hippocampus, 4
Hirschsprung's disease, 184, *185*
Horner's syndrome, 128
Houston's valves, 209
HSG, *see* Hysterosalpingography
Humerus
anatomical features, **82**
bony landmarks, 81, *82*
brachial plexus, 84–88
glenohumeral joint (shoulder joint), 83, *84*
ligaments, 81, 83
Hunter's canal, 246
Hydrocele, 220
Hydrocephalus, 12
Hydronephrosis, 229
Hydrosalpinx/pyosalpinx/haematosalpinx, 230
Hydrothorax, 130
Hydroureter, 229
Hymen, 226
Hyoid bone, 65
Hyperparathyroidism, 70
Hypogastric plexus, 160
Hypoglossal nerve (CN XII), 53
Hypoperfusion, 13, 32
Hypospadias, 217
Hypotension, 28
Hypothalamus, 5
Hysterectomy, 229
Hysterosalpingography (HSG), 230

I

IBD, *see* Inflammatory bowel disease
ICA, *see* Internal carotid artery
Ileostomy, 183
Ileum and jejunum, 176–177
Crohn's disease, 179
differences, **178**
IBD, 179, **179**
intussusception, 180, *180*
lymphatic drainage, 177
Meckel's diverticulum, 179–180, *180*
nerve supply, 177
SMA, 177, 179, *179*
small bowel obstruction, 177, 179
Iliofemoral ligament, 238
Ilioinguinal nerve, 188
Iliotibial tract syndrome, 235
Incisional hernia, 153
Inferior alveolar nerve, 50
Inferior gluteal nerve, 236
Inferior hypogastric plexus, 160
Inferior turbinate hypertrophy, 50
Inferior vena cava (IVC), 136, 158, 201

Inflammatory bowel disease (IBD), 179, **179**
Inguinal canal
deep ring, 220
hernias, 222–223
left, *221*
posterior view, right side, *221*
spermatic cord, 221, **222**
superficial ring, 220
Inguinal lymph nodes
deep, 250
superficial, 250
Innominate/coxal bone *(os coxa)*, 197–198
Intercondylar fossa, 239
Intercostal nerve block, 116
Internal cardiac anatomy
ASD, 38
atria, 137–138
ventricles, 138
Internal carotid artery (ICA), 12, 13, 14, 32, 52
Internal jugular vein (IJV), 52
Intracerebral aneurysm, 11
Intracranial bleeding, 11, **12**
Intramuscular injections, 237, *237*
Intrinsic muscles, hand
adductor pollicis, 102
dorsal interossei, 102
hypothenar eminence, 103
lumbricals, 102
palmar aponeurosis (palmar fascia), 103
palmar interossei, 102
palmaris brevis, 102
thenar eminence, 102
Intussusception, 180, *180*
Inversion and eversion injuries, 264
Ischaemic colitis, 184
Ischial spine, 199, 232
Ischioanal fossa, 213
Ischiocavernosus muscles, 216
Ischiofemoral ligament, 238
Ischium
greater sciatic notch, 199
ischial spine, 199
ischial tuberosity, 199
lesser sciatic notch, 199
parts, 198–199
Isthmus, 227
IVC, *see* Inferior vena cava

J

Jejuno-ileum, *see* Ileum and jejunum
Jobe's test, 88
Jugular venous pressure (JVP), 64
JVP, *see* Jugular venous pressure

K

Kidney
agenesis, 192
anatomical relations, 191–192
arterial blood supply, 191, *192*
developmental anomalies, *191*
embryology, 190, *190*
examination, 193
functions, 191
horseshoe, 192, *193*
infections, 192
injuries, 192

lymphatic drainage, 192
measurements, 190
mesonephros, 190
metanephros, 191
nerve supply, 192
palpation, 193
pelvic, 192
polycystic, 192, *193*
pronephros, 190
renal artery stenosis, 192
supernumerary arteries, 192
transplantation, 193
tumours, 192
urogenital ridge, 190
Killian's triangle, 74–75, *75*
Knee joint
    amputations, 254
    blood supply, 253
    capsule, 252
    deformities, 254
    extracapsular ligaments, 252, *253*
    haemarthrosis, 254
    intracapsular ligaments, 252, *253*
    ligamentum patellae, 252
    menisci (semilunar cartilages), 253
    nerve supply, 253
    osteology, 252
    patella, 253
    popliteus, 252
    swollen knee, 254
Kocher's incision, 154
Kocher's manoeuvre, 166
Kyphoscoliosis, 116, *117*
Kyphosis, 116

L

Labia majora, 225
Labia minora, 225
Lacrimal gland, 40
LAD arteries, *see* Left anterior descending
Laminectomy, 187
Lanz's incision, 154
Laparoscopic cholecystectomy, 174, 176
Large bowel/intestine
    arterial supply, colon, *181*
    colon layers, 180–181
    function, 180
    lymphatic drainage, 182
    marginal artery of Drummond, 181
    rectum, 181
    small bowel, differentiation from, 182
    taeniae coli, 181
Larry's point, 133
Laryngeal cancer, 67, *67*
Laryngeal obstruction, 67
Laryngeal papillomatosis, 67
Laryngopharynx, 74
Larynx
    anterior, posterior, and lateral views, *65*
    arytenoid cartilage, 65
    cricoid cartilage, 65
    cricothyroid membrane, 66
    epiglottis, 65
    hyoepiglottic ligament, 66
    innervation, 66
    ligaments of, 65–66
    muscles of, 66

quadrangular membrane, 66
rima glottidis, 66
superior laryngeal aperture, 66
suprahyoid muscles, 66
thyrohyoid membrane, 65
thyroid cartilage, 65
vallecula, 66
vocal cord, 66, *66*
Latissimus dorsi (LD), 116
LD, *see* Latissimus dorsi
Left anterior descending (LAD) arteries, 134
Leg, musculature of, *257*
    Achilles tendon, 259
    anterior compartment, 257, *257*
    lateral compartment, 259, **259**
    posterior compartment, 258, **258**
Leg ulcers, causes of, 260
Levator ani muscle, 199
Levator palpebrae superioris, 37, 38, 39, 77
Ligament of Treitz, 166
Linea alba, 150
Linea aspera, 239, *240*
Lingual nerve, 50
Lisfranc injury, 265, *266*
Liver
    anatomical relations, 170
    blood supply, 171
    functions, 170
    Glisson's capsule, 170
    gross anatomy, 170–171
    hepatomegaly, 172, *172*
    lobes, 170, *171*
    lymphatic drainage, 172
    metastasis, 173
    nerve supply, 172
    peritoneal recesses, 171
    porta hepatis, 170
    portal hypertension, 173
    segments, 171, *171*
    transjugular liver biopsy, 173
    transplant, 173
    visceral surface, *172*
LMNs, *see* Lower motor neurons
Long saphenous vein (LSV), 248
Lordosis, 116
LOS, *see* Lower oesophageal sphincter
Lower GI bleeding, 166
Lower limb
    anterior thigh, 242, **242**
    anterior tibial artery, 247–248
    arterial supply, *244*, 244–248
    dorsalis pedis artery, 248
    femoral artery, *244*, 244–245
    femoral vein, 250
    femur, 239–242
    fibula, 255–256
    foot, 260–269
    gluteal region, 234–237
    hip (acetabulofemoral) joint, 237–239
    ischaemia, 245–246
    knee joint, 252–254
    lymphatics, 250, *250*
    musculature, 257–260
    pes anserinus, 254
    piriformis, 236
    popliteal artery, 246–247
    popliteal block, 247

popliteal fossa, 246, *247*
popliteal vein, 249
posterior thigh, 244, **244**, *244*
posterior tibial artery, 248
profunda femoris (deep femoral)
        artery, 246
pulse points, *248*
thigh, 243–244
tibia, 254–255
vasculature, 244–251
venous drainage, 248–249
Lower motor neurons (LMNs), 23, 24
Lower oesophageal sphincter (LOS), 160, 161
Lower urinary tract symptoms (LUTS), 224
LSV, *see* Long saphenous vein
Ludwig's angina, 63
Lumbar plexus
    branches, *188*
    femoral nerve, 188
    genitofemoral nerve, 188
    ilioinguinal nerve, 188
    nerves, *188*, **189**
    obturator nerve, 188
    saphenous nerve, 188
Lumbar puncture, 27, *28*
Lumbar sympathetic trunk, 159
Lumpectomy, 144
Lungs
    apex, 124
    ARDS, 127–128, *128*
    asthma, 127
    borders, 124
    cancer, 127, 128, *128*
    COPD, 127
    innervation, 126
    lobes, 124, *124*
    lymphatic drainage, 127
    PE, 128
    pleura, 127, 129
    pleural recesses, 127
    pneumonia, 127
    pulmonary oedema, 127
    respiratory tree, 125–126
    right and left, comparison, **124**
    root and hilum, 125, *125*
    safe triangle, 130, *130*
    surfaces, 124
    trachea, *125*, 125–126
LUTS, *see* Lower urinary tract symptoms
Lymphadenopathy, 72, 251
Lymphatic drainage, 67
Lymphoedema, 251

M

Main pancreatic duct (MPD), 167
Male external genitalia
    penis, 214–216
    scrotum, 218–219
    testes, 219–220
Male genital tract
    external anatomy, 213, *213*
    inguinal canal, 220–223
Male internal genitalia
    bulbourethral (Cowper's) glands, 224
    prostate gland, 223–224
    seminal vesicles, 223
    vas deferens, 223

Malignant melanoma, 131
Mandibular nerve (CN V3), 50, 56, 77
Marginal artery of Drummond, 181
Masseter muscles, 50, 56, 77
Mastectomy, 144
Mastoiditis, 44
Maxillary nerve (CN V2), 50
Maxillary sinus, 36, *48*, 49, 77, 78
Maxillary sinusitis, 49, *49*
MCA, *see* Middle cerebral artery
McBurney's incision, 154, *154*
Mcmurray's test, 253
Meckel's diverticulum, 179–180, *180*
Medial lemniscus, 22
Medial malleolus, 246, 248, 251, 255, 258, 259,
 259, 262, *263*, 267, 268
Median nerve (C5–C8, T1), 85
Mediastinal tumours
 EBUS, 123
 mediastinitis, 123
 mediastinoscopy, 123
 neurogenic neoplasms, 123
 perforated oesophagus, 123
 retrosternal goitre, 123
Mediastinitis, 123
Mediastinoscopy, 123
Mediastinum
 anterior, 120, 121
 inferior, 120
 middle, 121
 posterior, 120, 121
 superior, 120–121
 thoracic oesophagus, 121–122
 thoracic sympathetic trunks, 120–121
Medulla oblongata/medulla, 8
Meissner's plexus, 162
Melanocyte-stimulating hormone, 5
Meningitis, 11
Meningocoele, 16–17, *17*
Meniscal injury, 253
Menisci (semilunar cartilages), 253
Menstrual disorders, 229
Mesenteries, 157
Mesonephric duct, 230, 232
Mesorectum, 209
MI, *see* Myocardial infarction
Midbrain
 cerebral aqueduct, 7
 substantia nigra, 8, *8*
 tectum, 7
 tegmentum, 8
Middle cerebral artery (MCA), 13
Midfoot injury, *see* Lisfranc injury
Mirizzi's syndrome, 175
Mitral valve, 139
Modified Allen's test, 96
Mons pubis, 225
Monteggia's fracture, 92, *93*
Montgomery's tubercles, 142
Mouth, *see* Oral cavity
MPD, *see* Main pancreatic duct
MS, *see* Multiple sclerosis
Multiple sclerosis (MS), 27
Mumps, 57
Murphy's sign, 175
Muscles of mastication, 56
Musculocutaneous nerve, 85
Myelomeningocoele, 17, *17*

Myocardial infarction (MI), 136
Myocardium, 134
Myotome, 20

N

NAC, *see* Nipple-areola complex
Nasal septum deviation, 47
Nasopharynx, 74
National Health Service (NHS), 238
NAVeL, *see* Nerve, Artery, Vein, Lymphatics
Neck; *see also* Head and neck
 atlas (C1), 58, *58*
 axis (C2), 58, *59*
 cervical degenerative diseases, 60
 cervical spine injury, 59–60
 cervical vertebrae, 58
 fascia, 60
 lump, 72–73
 lymphatic drainage, *71*, 71–72
 swellings, 71–72
 triangles, 61–63
 vertebra prominens (C7), 58, *59*
Neck of the femur (NOF), 239
Necrotising fasciitis, 154
Needle thoracostomy, 130
Nerve, Artery, Vein, Lymphatics
 (NAVeL), 246
Nerve root compression, 26–27
Nerves, forearm and wrist
 median, 96
 motor innervation, 96–97
 sensory innervation, 97
 ulnar nerve (C8–T1), 97
Nerves, named
 abducens nerve (CN VI), 51
 accessory nerve (CN XI), 52–53
 auriculotemporal nerve, 50
 axillary nerve, 83, 85, 86, *87*
 brachial plexus, 85
 genitofemoral nerve, 218
 ilioinguinal nerve, 188
 inferior alveolar nerve, 50
 inferior gluteal nerve, 236
 mandibular nerve (CN V3), 50, 56, 78
 maxillary nerve (CN V2), 50
 median nerve (C5–C8, T1), 85
 musculocutaneous nerve, 85
 obturator nerve, 188
 oculomotor nerve (CN III), 36–40, 50, 77
 olfactory nerve (CN I), 49
 ophthalmic nerve (CV, V1), 50
 optic nerve (CN II), 38, *38*, 49
 phrenic nerve, 120
  accessory, 117
  C5 part, 117
  paralysis of, 119
 posterior femoral cutaneous
  nerve, 236
 pudendal nerve, 204, *204*, 232, 236
 radial nerve, 86
 saphenous nerve, 188, 246, 267
 sciatic nerve, 202, 204, 236, 237
 splanchnic nerves, 121, 159, 160
 sural nerve, 246, 267
 sympathetic visceral nerves, 159
 tibial nerve, 267
 trigeminal nerve (CN V), 50

 trochlear nerve (CN IV), 50
 ulnar nerve (C8–T1), 85
  cubital tunnel syndrome, 97
  cutaneous branches, 97
  Froment's test, 97
  function, 97
  injury, 97
 vagus nerve (CN X), 44, 52, 120–121
 vestibulocochlear nerve (CN VIII), 45, 52
Nervi erigentes, S2–S4, 204, 209, 232
Nervus intermedius (CN VII), 45
Neurogenic neoplasms, 123
NHS, *see* National Health Service
Nipple-areola complex (NAC), 142
Nociceptive flexion reflex, 22
NOF, *see* Neck of the femur
Nose
 allergic rhinitis, 47
 blood supply, 46, 47–48
 conchae and meatuses, 46–47
 epistaxis, 48
 external part, 45
 foreign body trapped, 47, *47*
 inferior turbinate hypertrophy, 47
 innervation, 48, **48**
 Little's area, 48
 lymphatic drainage, 48
 maxillary sinusitis, 49, *49*
 muscles, 45–46, **46**
 nasal cavity and internal parts, 46, **46**
 nasal septum, *46*
 oro-antral fistula, 49
 paranasal sinuses, 48, *48*, **49**
 pituitary tumour removal, 49
 turbinate bones, *46*
 venous drainage, 47–48

O

Obturator externus muscle, 199
Obturator foramen, 199
Obturator internus muscle, 199
Obturator nerve, 188
Obturator nerve entrapment syndrome, 243
Oculomotor nerve (CN III), 36–40, 50, 77
O'Donoghue triad, 253
Oedema, *152*
Oesophageal cancer, 76
Oesophagogastroduodenoscopy (OGD), 160
Oesophagus
 cancer, 76, 161, *161*
 distal end, 160
 LOS, 160
 lymph drainage, 161
 perforated, 123
 thoracic, 121–122
OGD, *see* Oesophagogastroduodenoscopy
Olfactory nerve (CN I), 49
Olfactory sulcus, 3
Omphalocele, 153
Ophthalmic nerve (CV, V1), 50
OPSS, *see* Overwhelming post-splenectomy
 sepsis
Optic nerve (CN II), 38, *38*, 49
Optic neuritis, 41
Oral cavity
 divisions, 53
 muscles of mastication, 56

palate, 55–56
papillae, 53
tongue, 53–55
Orbit
boundaries, 36, *36*
eyelids, 37
foramina, 36–37
inferior orbital fissure, *36*, 37
optic canal, 37
superior orbital fissure, 37
Orbital blowout fracture, 41
Orbitofrontal cortex, 3
Orchidectomy, 220
Oro-antral fistula, 49
Oropharynx, 75
Osgood-Schlatter disease, 254
Osteoarthritis, 60, 254
Osteonecrosis, 239
Otitis externa, 42
Ovarian cancer, 231
Ovarian cysts, 231, *231*
Ovaries
blood supply, 230
cancer, 231
cortex, 230
cysts, 231
function, 230
germinal epithelium, 230
ligaments, 230
lymphatic drainage, 230
mesonephric duct, 230
nerve supply, 230
polycystic, 231
venous drainage, 230
Overwhelming post-splenectomy sepsis
(OPSS), 170

P

Paget's disease, 143, *143*
Painful arc syndrome, 88
Palate
cleft, 56, *56*
hard, 55
soft, 55, *55*
Palatine tonsils, 55, 71, 72, *74*, 75, 78
Pancoast syndrome, 128
Pancreas
accessory pancreatic duct, 167
acute pancreatitis, 167, *167*
blood supply and lymphatic drainage, 167
cancer, 167–168, 176
duct system, 167
nerve supply, 167
pancreaticoduodenoectomy, 168
pancreatic pseudocyst, 167
parts, *166*, 166–167
Whipple's procedure, 168
Pancreaticoduodenoectomy, 168
Parahippocampal gyrus, 4
Paramesonephric (Mullerian) ducts, 227
Paraphimosis, 216
Parasympathetic nervous system (PNS), 20, 21
Parathyroid glands, 70
Paraumbilical hernia, 153, *153*
Paraurethral glands, 226
Parotid gland, 56–57
Patent ductus arteriosus (PDA), 140

Patent foramen ovale, 138
PCL, *see* Posterior cruciate ligament
PD, *see* Peritoneal dialysis
PDA, *see* Patent ductus arteriosus
PE, *see* Pulmonary embolism
Pectineus muscle, 198
Pectoral girdle
clavicle, 80, *80*
scapula, 81, *81*
Pectus carinatum, 115
Pectus excavatum, 115
PEG, *see* Percutaneous endoscopic gastrostomy
Pelvic floor/diaphragm
iliococcygeus, 205
ischiococcygeus, 205
levator ani, 205
male, *205*
nerve supply, 205
pubococcygeus, 205
puborectalis, 205
Pelvic inflammatory disease (PID), 227
Pelvic organs
anal canal, 210–211
bladder, *207*, 207–208
embryology, 205
rectum, 209–210
ureter, 205–206, *206*, *207*
Pelvis, *197*
ala, the, 197
arcuate line, 198
arterial blood supply, 200, *201*
brim, 197
components, 197
female, 201–202
female reproductive organs, 224–231
floor, 205, *205*
fracture, 200
functions, 197
inguinal canal, 220–223
innervation, 202–204
innominate/coxal bone, 197–198
ischium, 198–199
lateral pelvic wall, 199
lymphatics, 201
male genital tract and inguinal canal, 213,
213
male internal genitalia, 223–224
organs, 205–211
outlet, 197
penis, 214–216
perineum, 212–213
pubic bone, 198
pudendal nerve block, 204, *204*
sacral plexus, 202–204
sacrum, *199*, 199–200
sciatic nerve, 202, 204
scrotum, 218–219
sympathetic innervation, pelvic part of, 204
testes, 219–220
types, 202
upper genital tract, 227–231
urethra, 216–217
venous return, 201
Penile carcinoma, 216
Penis
blood supply, 214, *215*
bulb, 214
bulbospongiosus muscles, 214

chancre, 216
corpora, *214*
corpora cavernosa, 214
crura, 214
ejaculation, 216
erection mechanism, 216
glans, 214
lymphatic drainage, 215
nerve supply, 216
paraphimosis, 216
penile carcinoma, 216
phimosis, 216
prepuce (foreskin), 216
priapism, 216
root (radix), 214
shaft of, 214
suspensory ligaments, 214
syphilis, 216
venous drainage, 214–215
Percutaneous endoscopic gastrostomy (PEG),
164
Percutaneous image-guided liver biopsy, 172
Perforated oesophagus, 123
Pericardial effusion, 133
Pericardial rub, 133
Pericarditis, 133
Pericardium
blood supply, 133
cardiac tamponade, 133–134
innervation, 133
internal serous layer, 132
Larry's point, 133
layers, 132, *133*
pericardial effusion, 133
pericardial sinuses, 133, *133*
pericarditis, 133
Perineum
anterior urogenital triangle, 212
boundaries, 212
divisions, 212
female, 212, *212*
male, 212–213
perineal body, 212
posterior (anal) triangle, 212
Periosteum (pericranium), 33
Peritoneal dialysis (PD), 157
Peritoneal ligaments
bare area, the, 158
coronary (crown- like) ligament, 158
falciform ligament, 157
ligamentum venosum, 158
round ligament, 157
Peritoneum
ascites, 157
epiploic foramen, 156
greater omentum, 156
haemoperitoneum, 157
intraperitoneal organs, 155
lesser omentum, 156
mesentery, 156, 157
mesoappendix, 157
omentum, 156
PD, 157
peritoneal attachment, 156, *156*
peritoneal cavity, 155, 156
peritoneal ligaments, 157–158
peritonitis, 157
retroperitoneal organs, 155–156

sigmoid mesocolon, 157
transverse mesocolon, 157
umbilical folds, 158
visceral and parietal layers, 155
Peritonitis, 157
Per rectum (PR) examination, 211
Pes anserine bursitis, 242
Pharynx
blood supply, 75
circular muscles, 73
inferior constrictor muscle, 73
inner and outer muscles, 73, 74
Killian's triangle, 74–75, 75
laryngopharynx, 75
layers, 73
longitudinal muscles, 73
middle constrictor muscle, 73
nasopharynx, 74
oropharynx, 74
palatopharyngeus, 74
parts, 74–75, 75
pharyngeal cancer, 74
salpingopharyngeus, 73
stylopharyngeus, 73
superior constrictor muscle, 73
Phimosis, 216
Phrenic nerve, 120
accessory, 117
C5 part, 117
paralysis of, 119
Pia mater, 11, 29
PICA, see Posterior inferior cerebellar artery
PID, see Pelvic inflammatory disease
Pineal gland, 5
PIP joint, see Proximal interphalangeal
Piriformis, 236
Pituitary adenoma, 41
Pituitary gland, 5
Plantar calcaneonavicular ligament, 266
Plantar fasciitis, 268
Pleomorphic adenoma, 57
Pleura
cervical, 129
layers, 127
nerve supply, 127
recesses, 127
Pleural effusion, 130, 131
Plummer-Vinson syndrome, 76
Pneumonia, 127
Pneumothorax, 129, 129
PNS, see Parasympathetic nervous system
Poland syndrome, 107
Polycystic ovaries, 231, 233
Pons, 8
Popliteal aneurysm, 247
Popliteal artery, 246–247
Popliteal block, 247
Popliteal fossa, 246, 247
Popliteal vein, 249
Portal hypertension, 160, 173
Posterior abdominal wall
anatomical planes, 187
flexion-distraction fractures, 187
intervertebral disc, 185, 186
laminectomy, 187
ligamenta flava, 185, 186
lumbar vertebrae, 185, 186
psoas abscess, 187

psoas major, 187
quadratus lumborum, 187
spondylosis, 187
Posterior commissure, 225
Posterior cord syndrome, 26
Posterior cricoarytenoid muscle, 65, 67, 78
Posterior cruciate ligament (PCL), 252
Posterior femoral cutaneous nerve, 236
Posterior superior iliac spine (PSIS), 197, 198
Posterior inferior cerebellar artery (PICA), 24
Post-hepatic (obstructive) jaundice, 175
Pott's fracture dislocation, 263
Precentral gyrus, 3
Presacral fascia, 209
PR examination, see Per rectum
Priapism, 216
Pringle's manoeuvre, 156
Prostate cancer, 224
Prostate gland, 223
Prostate-specific antigen (PSA) test, 224
Proximal interphalangeal (PIP) joint, 95
PSA test, see Prostate-specific antigen
Pseudoaneurysm, 246
Pseudobulbar palsy, 24
PSIS, see Posterior superior iliac spine
Psoas abscess, 187
Psoas major, 187
Pubic symphysis, 244
Pubofemoral ligament, 238
Pudendal nerve, 204, 204, 232, 236
Pulmonary embolism (PE), 128, 251
Pulmonary oedema, 127
Pulmonary plexus, 121
Purkinje fibres, 136
Pyloric stenosis, 164
Pyothorax, 130
Pyramidalis, 150

Q

Quadrangular space, 86, 87
Quadrate tubercle, 239
Quadratus lumborum, 187

R

Radial nerve, 86
Radial pulse, 96
Radius
articulations, 91–92
neck of, 91
radial styloid process, 91
shaft, 91
surfaces, 91
Rectal ampulla, 209
Rectosigmoid junction, 209
Rectum
blood supply, 209
colorectal cancer, 210
Denonvillier's fascia, 209
Houston's valves, 209
longitudinal muscle layer, 209
lymphatic drainage, 210
mesorectum, 209
nerve supply, 209
presacral fascia, 209
rectal ampulla, 209
rectosigmoid junction, 209

related fascial layers, 209–210
venous drainage, 209
Waldeyer's fascia, 209
Rectus abdominis, 150
Rectus sheath, 150, 150–151
Rectus sheath haematoma, 154
Recurrent laryngeal nerve (RLN), 52, 69, 70, 120
Recurrent papillomatosis, 67
Reflexes
Babinski's sign, 22
deep tendon, **21**
muscle spindles, 21
plantar, 22
Renal artery stenosis, 192
Respiratory tree, 125–126
Retinal artery occlusion, 39
Retinal detachment, 41
Retinoblastoma, 41
Retroperitoneal space
blood supply, 190
contents, 189
lumbar region, cross-section of, 189
suprarenal glands, 190
Retropubic space, 223
Retrosternal goitre, 68, 69, 123
Rheumatic heart disease, 140
Ribs
atypical, 112
cervical, 115
false, 110
floating, 110
fracture, 115
head of, 110
neck of, 110
subclavian vessels and brachial plexus,
111, 111
true, 110, 111
tubercle, 110, 111
RIF, see Right iliac fossa
Right dominance, 134
Right iliac fossa (RIF), 156
RLN, see Recurrent laryngeal nerve

S

Sacral plexus
branches, 202, **203**
inferior hypogastric plexus, 203
lumbosacral trunk, 202
nervi erigentes, 204
sciatic nerve, 202
superior hypogastric plexus, 203
Salivary glands
parotid gland, 56–57
sublingual, 57
submandibular, 57
Salpingitis, 230
Saphenous nerve, 188, 246, 267
Scalp
arterial supply, 33
innervation, 33
layers, 33
venous drainage, 33
Scapular anastomosis, 81
Scapula (shoulder blade), 81, 81
Scarpa's fascia, 149, 218
Sciatica, 237
Sciatic nerve, 202, 204, 236, 237

Scoliosis, 116
Scrotum, *218*, 232
　　cremasteric reflex, 218
　　cryptorchidism, 218
　　dartos fascia, 218
　　dartos muscle, 218
　　external spermatic fascia, 218
　　layers, 218, **219**
　　midline raphe, 218
　　Scarpa's fascia, 218
　　sensory innervation, 219
　　tunica vaginalis, 218
Seldinger's technique, 130, 245
Seminal vesicles, 223
Sentinel lymph node biopsy, 144, *144*
Sentinel node biopsy, 251
Septicaemia, 175
Septic arthritis, 254
Sexually transmitted infections
　　　(STIs), 217
SGAP flap, *see* Superior gluteal artery
　　　perforator
Short saphenous vein (SSV), 246, 249,
　　　250
Shoulder
　　deltoid muscle, 88, **88**
　　rotator cuff muscle, 88, **88**
Sigmoid mesocolon, 157
Sigmoid volvulus, 184, *185*
Skene's (lesser vestibular) glands, 226
Skull
　　base, 11, 34
　　bones of, *34*, 34–36
　　cranial fossae, **35**, *35*
　　fontanelles, 34
　　foramina, **36**
　　fossae, 34, *35*
　　fractures, *35*, 35–36
　　neurocranium, 34
　　pterion, 34
　　sutures, 34
SLR test, *see* Straight-leg-raising
Small bowel obstruction, 177, 179,
　　　179
Smith's fracture, 92
SNS, *see* Sympathetic nervous system
Solar plexus, 160
Somatostatin, 5
Sonic hedgehog protein, 15
Spermatozoa, 219
Sphenoethmoidal recess, 8
Sphenoid sinus, 5, *48*, 49, 78
Spigelian hernia, 153, *153*
Spina bifida occulta, 16, *17*
Spinal anaesthesia, 27–28, *28*
Spinal cord, anatomy of, *18*
　　alar and basal plates, 15–17
　　ascending tracts, 22, *22*, **23**
　　autonomic nervous system, 19–21
　　blood supply, 24–25
　　bony covering, *18*
　　coverings, 17, *18*, *19*
　　cross-section, 19, *19*
　　damage, traumatic causes of, 25–26
　　descending tracts, 22–24
　　development, 15–17
　　epidural *vs.* spinal anaesthesia, 27–28
　　gastrulation, 15

germ layers, 15, **15**
injuries, epidemiology of, 26
injury/defect, compressive causes
　　　of, 26–27
injury/defect, non-traumatic causes
　　　of, 27
ischaemia, 25
L1/L2 vertebra, 17
lumbar puncture, 27
neural tube, 15, *16*
pathology, 25–27
reflexes, 21–22
segments, 17
Spinal stenosis, 27
Spinal tap, 27
Spinothalamic tract, 22, 29
Splanchnic nerves, 121, 159, 160
Spleen
　　arteria pancreatica magna, 169
　　blood supply and drainage, 169
　　diaphragmatic and visceral surface, 168,
　　　168
　　gastrosplenic ligament, 169
　　lienorenal ligament, 169
　　nerve supply and lymph drainage,
　　　169
　　OPSS, 170
　　peritoneal ligament, 169
　　splenectomy, 169–170
　　splenic notch, 168
　　splenomegaly, 169
　　splenorraphy, 170
　　surface anatomy, 168
Splenectomy, 169–170
Splenomegaly, 169
Splenorraphy, 170
Spondylolisthesis, 187
Spondylosis, 60, 187
Spring ligament, 266
SSS, *see* Superior sagittal sinus
SSV, *see* Short saphenous vein
Stellate ganglion, 121
Sternotomy, 116
Sternum
　　bony anatomy, *110*
　　manubriosternal joint, 109, 110
　　suprasternal/jugular notch, 109
　　xiphisternal, 109, 110
Stertor, 67
STIs, *see* Sexually transmitted infections
Stomach
　　anatomical relations, 162
　　arterial blood supply and venous drainage,
　　　163, *163*
　　cardia, 162
　　functions, 162
　　fundus, 162
　　gastric cancers, 164
　　gastric wall layers, 162
　　gastrostomy feeding, 164
　　greater curvature, 162
　　layers, *163*
　　lesser curvature, 162
　　lymph drainage, 164
　　nerve supply, 164
　　pyloric region, 162
　　pyloric stenosis, 164
　　rugae, 162

Stomas, 183
Straight-leg-raising (SLR) test, 237
Stress fracture, 264, *265*
Stria of Gennari, 4, *4*
Stria terminalis, 4
Stridor, 67, 70
Stroke, causes, 13, 32
Subacute infective endocarditis, 140
Subarachnoid space, 11
Subclavian
　　artery, 64
　　vein, 64
Submandibular salivary glands, 57
Sulcus limitans, 15
Superficial forearm flexor muscles, **94**
Superior gluteal artery perforator (SGAP) flap,
　　　237
Superior hypogastric plexus, 160
Superior sagittal sinus (SSS), 13
Superior vena cava (SVC), 140
Supracondylar fracture, 91, *91*
Suprapubic cystostomy, 207
Suprarenal glands, 190
Sural nerve, 246, 267
SVC, *see* Superior vena cava
Sylvian fissure, 3
Sympathetic nervous system (SNS), 19–20,
　　　29
Sympathetic visceral nerves, 159
Syphilis, 216
Syringomyelia, 27
Systemic sclerosis, 76, *76*

T

Talocrural joint, *see* Ankle joint
Tarsal tunnel syndrome, 259
TEE, *see* Transoesophageal echocardiography
Tenosynovitis, 103
Tension pneumothorax, 129, *130*
Tentorium cerebelli, 11
Testes
　　appendix, 219
　　blood supply, 219–220
　　coverings, 219
　　epididymis, 219
　　epididymo-orchitis, 220
　　gubernaculum, 219
　　hydrocele, 220
　　mediastinum, 219
　　midsagittal section, *219*
　　orchidectomy, 220
　　rete, 219
　　torsion, 220
　　tumours, 220
　　undescended, 220
　　varicocele, 220
Testicular torsion, 220
Tetralogy of Fallot, 138, *138*
Thalamus, 5
Thigh
　　medial compartment, 243, *243*
　　muscles, anterior, 242, **242**
　　posterior compartment, 244, **244**, *244*
Thoracic cavity
　　mediastinal tumours, 123
　　mediastinum, 119–122
　　right and left pleural cavities, 119

Thoracic duct, 121
Thoracic oesophagus, 121
Thoracic outlet syndrome, 115
Thoracic wall
    accessory muscles, respiration, 112
    auscultation, 115
    azygos venous system, 113, *114*
    components, 109
    costochondritis, 115
    diaphragm, 116–119
    endothoracic fascia, 113
    flail chest, 116
    functions, 109, *110*
    hemiazygos vein, 114
    Innervation, chest wall, 114
    intercostal muscles, 112, **112**, *113*
    intercostal nerve block, 116
    lymphatic drainage, 114
    muscles, 116, **117**, *118*
    musculature, 112–113
    pectus carinatum, 116
    pectus excavatum, 115
    ribs, 110–112
    skeleton and joints, 109
    sternotomy, 116
    sternum, 109–110, 116
    superior thoracic aperture, 109
    thoracic spine, 116
    thoracotomy, 116
    vasculature and innervation, 113–114
    venous drainage, posterior intercostal
        veins, **113**
    vertebrae, 112, *112*
Thoracotomy, 116
THR, *see* Total hip replacement
Thrombosis, 13, 32
Thymus gland, 121
Thyroid gland
    arterial supply, 68, *68*
    cancer, 68
    embryology, 67–68
    goitre, 68, *68*, *69*
    laryngoscopy, 70
    retrosternal goitre, 68, *69*
    surface anatomy, 68
    surgery, 69
    thyroglossal cyst, 70, *70*
    thyrotoxicosis, 69
    venous drainage, 68
Thyroid-stimulating hormone (TSH), 5
Tibia
    anterior and posterior views, *255*
    condyles, 254
    fractures, 255, *256*
    intercondylar eminence, 254
    plateau, 254
    soleus muscle, 254
    tibial shaft, 254
    tibial tuberosity, 254
Tibial nerve, 267
Tietze's syndrome, 115
TIPSS, *see* Transjugular intrahepatic
        portosystemic shunt
Tongue
    blood supply, 54
    divisions, 53
    examination, 54
    extrinsic muscles, 53, **54**, *54*

hypoglossal nerve paralysis, 55
    intrinsic muscles, 53, *54*
    lymphatic drainage, 54
    papillae, 53
    sensory supply, 54
    sublingual absorption, drugs, 54
    ulcers, 55
Total hip replacement (THR), 238, *239*
Trachea, 67
    bifurcation, *125*, *126*
    breathing, control of, 126
    bronchial arteries, 126
    bronchial veins, 126
    bronchopulmonary segments, 126
    bronchoscopy, *126*
    tracheobronchial tree, *126*
Tracheostomy, 67, 70
TRAM flap, *see* Transverse rectus abdominis
        myocutaneous
Transjugular intrahepatic portosystemic shunt
        (TIPSS), 173
Transjugular liver biopsy, 173
Transoesophageal echocardiography (TEE),
        139, 140
Transverse mesocolon, 157
Transverse myelitis, 27
Transverse rectus abdominis myocutaneous
        (TRAM) flap, 154
Trapezius muscles, 53, 60, **61**, 62, 77, 80, 81,
        109, **117**
Traumatic diaphragmatic hernia, 115
Trendelenburg's sign, 235, 236, *237*
Triangles, neck
    anterior, 62–63
    posterior, 61–62, *62*
    scalene muscles, 62, **62**
Trigeminal nerve (CN V), 50
Trigeminal neuralgia, 50
Trochlear nerve (CN IV), 50
Trophectoderm, 15
Tubal ligation, 230

U

UC, *see* Ulcerative colitis
Ulcerative colitis (UC), 179, **179**
Ulna, 92
Ulnar nerve (C8–T1), 85
    cubital tunnel syndrome, 97
    cutaneous branches, 97
    Froment's test, 97
    function, 97
    injury, 97
Umbilical folds, 158, 195
Umbilical hernias, 153
Umbilicus, 150
UMNs, *see* Upper motor neurons
Undescended testis, 220
Unhappy triad, 253
Upper arm
    arterial supply, 90
    brachial artery, 90, 91
    muscles, 89, **89**, *89–90*
    posterior compartment, 89, *90*
Upper GI bleeding, 166
Upper limb
    arterial supply and venous drainage,
        arm, 90

axilla, 105–107
    bicipital aponeurosis, 90–91
    brachial plexus, 84–88
    cubital fossa, 90
    forearm and wrist, 91–99
    hand, functional anatomy of, 104–105
    humerus, 81–84
    neurovasculature, hand, 103–104
    pectoral girdle, 80–81
    shoulder, 88
    upper arm, 89–90
    wrist and hand, 99–103
Upper motor neurons (UMNs), 23, 24
Urachus, 158
Ureter, 205–206, *206*, *207*
Urethra
    anterior, 217
    external urethral sphincter, 216
    hypospadias, 217
    inflammation, 217
    innervation, 216
    internal urethral sphincter, 216
    male, *215*, 216
    posterior, 216–217
    urethral rupture, 217
Urethral meatus, 225
Urethritis, 217
Urogenital triangle, 212
Uterine fibroids, 229
Uterine prolapse, 229
Uterine tubes, 229–230, *230*
Uterus, *227*, 232
    blood supply, 228
    cervix uteri, 227
    congenital abnormalities, *229*
    corpus uteri, 227
    endometrium, 227
    fundus, 227
    ligaments of, 228, *228*
    myometrium, 227
    nerve supply, 228
    parametrium, 227
    relations, 228
    retroflexed, 227–228
    retroversion, 227
    ureter, 228

V

Vagina, 226
Vagus nerve (CN X), 44, 52, 120–121
Valvular disease, 140
Varicocele, 220
Varicose veins, 251
Vasculature, brain
    arterial, 12–13
    venous, 13–14
Vas deferens, 223, 232
Vasectomy, 223
Venous vasculature, brain
    cavernous sinus thrombosis, 14
    drainage, *14*
    ICA, 14
    SSS, 13
Ventral hernias, 153
Ventricular fibrillation (VF), 137
Ventricular septal defect (VSD), 138

Ventricular system, 11–12
Vestibule, 225
Vestibulocochlear nerve (CN VIII),
        45, 52
VF, *see* Ventricular fibrillation
Viral encephalitis, 52, *52*
Virchow's triad, 137
Vocal cord nodules (singer's nodules), 67
Volvulus, sigmoid colon, 184, *185*
VSD, *see* Ventricular septal defect

W

Waldeyer's fascia, 209
Waldeyer's ring, 71
Wartenberg's syndrome, 88
Wernicke's area, 3
Whipple's procedure, 168
Wolffian ducts, 230
Wrist and hand
        anatomical snuffbox, 99, *99*
        bones, 99

carpal tunnel, 100
and digits, 101–102
scaphoid, 99, *99*

Z

Zenker's diverticulum, 74
Zona fasciculata, 190
Zona glomerulosa, 190
Zona reticularis, 190